Seventh Edition

Nursing Diagnosis Handbook
with NIC Interventions
and NOC Outcomes

Judith M. Wilkinson, PhD, ARNP, RNC

Prentice Hall Health
Upper Saddle River, NJ 07458

Publisher: Julie Alexander
Editor-in-Chief: Cheryl Mehalik
Acquisitions Editor: Nancy Anselment
Editorial Assistant: Beth Ann Romph
Marketing Manager: Kristin Walton
Marketing Coordinator: Cindy Frederick
Director of Production and Manufacturing: Bruce Johnson
Senior Production Manager: Ilene Sanford
Managing Editor: Wendy Earl
Production Editor: Sharon Montooth
Text Design and Composition: Brad Greene
Cover Coordinator: Maria Guglielmo
Cover Designer: Wanda España/Wee Design Group
Printer and Binder: Banta Company, Menasha, Wisconsin

Previously published by Addison-Wesley Nursing,
a Division of the Benjamin/Cummings Publishing Company, Inc.
Menlo Park, California 94025

Care has been taken to confirm the accuracy of information presented
in this book. The authors, editors, and publisher, however, cannot
accept any responsibility for errors or omissions or for consequences
from application of the information in this book and make no warranty,
express or implied, with respect to its contents.

Permission from North American Nursing Diagnosis Association (1999).
NANDA Nursing Diagnoses: Definitions and Classifications 1999-2000. PA:
NANDA. [copyright 1999 by the North American Diagnosis Association]

Prentice-Hall International (UK) Limited, London
Prentice-Hall of Australia Pty. Limited, Sydney
Prentice-Hall Canada Inc., Toronto
Prentice-Hall Hispanoamericana, S.A., Mexico
Prentice-Hall of India Private Limited, New Delhi
Prentice-Hall of Japan, Inc., Tokyo
Prentice-Hall Asia Pte. Ltd., Singapore
Editora Prentice-Hall do Brasil, Ltda., Rio de Janeiro

Acknowledgements

I would like to thank the following colleagues for their contributions to this text, particularly to the "Clinical Conditions Guide to Nursing Diagnoses and Collaborative Problems."

Kathy Carver, RN, MSN
Professor of Nursing
Johnson County Community College
Overland Park, KS
"Pediatric Conditions"

Carol Green-Nigro, PhD, RN
Professor of Nursing
Johnson County Community College
Overland Park, KS
"Medical and Surgical Conditions"

Sylvia J. McMorris, RN, EdS
Professor of Nursing
Johnson County Community College
Overland Park, KS
"Psychiatric Conditions"

Table of Contents

Preface   *vi*
   New Features   *vi*
   Other Features   *vii*
   Audience   *viii*

Introduction   *ix*
Background   *ix*
Nursing Process in Relation to Nursing Diagnosis   *x*
Standards of Care in Relation to Nursing Diagnosis   *x*
Case Management and Critical Paths   *x*
   Case Management   *xi*
   Critical Paths and Managed Care   *xi*

Components of Nursing Diagnosis Care Plans   *xiii*
Plans of Care   *xiii*
   Nursing Diagnosis   *xiii*
   Definition   *xiii*
   Defining Characteristics   *xiii*
   Related Factors   *xv*
   Risk Factors   *xv*
   Suggestions for Use   *xv*
   Suggested Alternative Diagnoses   *xv*
   NOC Suggested Outcomes   *xvi*
   Goal Statements/Evaluation Criteria   *xvi*
   NIC Priority Interventions   *xvii*
   Nursing Activities   *xvii*
Clinical Conditions Guide to Nursing Diagnoses
   and Collaborative Problems   *xviii*

How to Create a Nursing Diagnosis Care Plan   *xxi*
Assessment   *xxi*
Diagnosis   *xxi*
NOC Suggested Outcomes   *xxii*
Goal Statements/Evaluation Criteria   *xxii*
Nursing Interventions and Activities   *xxii*
Creating a Critical Path   *xxiii*

Plans of Care in Alphabetical Order *1–524*

Each plan of care contains the following information:
Taxonomy number
Definition
Defining Characteristics
Related Factors
Risk Factors
Suggestions for Use
Suggested Alternative Diagnoses
NOC Suggested Outcomes
Goals/Evaluation Criteria (Examples of NOC and Other)
NIC Priority Interventions
Nursing Activities (NIC and Other)

Clinical Conditions Guide to Nursing Diagnoses   *525*

Medical Conditions   *526*
Surgical Conditions   *555*
Psychiatric Conditions   *567*
Antepartum and Postpartum Conditions   *578*
Newborn Conditions   *586*
Pediatric Conditions   *596*

Bibliography   *611*

Appendix A 1999–2000 NANDA-Approved Nursing Diagnoses   *626*
Appendix B NANDA-Approved Nurses Diagnoses (1999–2000)   *630*
Appendix C Diagnosis Qualifiers (NANDA)   *634*
Appendix D Multidisciplinary (Collaborative) Problems
   Associated with Diseases and Other Physiologic Disorders   *635*
Appendix E Multidisciplinary (Collaborative) Problems
   Associated with Tests and Treatments   *645*
Appendix F Multidisciplinary (Collaborative) Problems
   Associated with Surgical Treatments   *646*

Index   *649*

Preface

The *Nursing Diagnosis Handbook with NIC Interventions and NOC Outcomes*, 7th edition, is designed to help nurses and students develop individualized patient care plans. The new edition has been expanded to include all nursing diagnoses approved by the North American Nursing Diagnosis Association (NANDA) for 1999-2000, as well as linkages to current "NOC" and "NIC" research-based outcomes and interventions. Special features contribute to the book's usefulness and make it an indispensable tool for planning patient care.

New Features

NOC "Suggested Outcomes"

To facilitate use of a unified nursing language and computerized patient records, each nursing diagnosis lists the "suggested outcomes" based on the research of the Iowa Outcomes Project (Nursing Outcomes Classification, 1997). These suggested outcomes are nurse-sensitive—that is, they may be influenced by the nursing care given for a particular NANDA diagnosis. This text also demonstrates ways to use NOC outcomes, outcome indicators, and measuring scales to state patient goals.

Updated NIC Priority Interventions

NIC interventions have been updated to reflect the continuing work of the Iowa Interventions Project. As in the previous edition, the interventions given and defined for each nursing diagnosis are those designated by the Nursing Interventions Classification (1996) as the treatments of choice for that diagnosis. NIC interventions were developed and linked to the NANDA categories by a research team using a multimethod process that included the judgments of experts in nursing practice and research.

Inclusion of NIC Nursing Activities

In an effort to further promote use of standardized language, some of the "Nursing Activities" for each nursing diagnosis are written in NIC language. This helps to illustrate how the NIC activities, as well as the broader NIC interventions, can be used in care planning.

Expanded Family, Community, and Collaborative Content

More family- and community-oriented goals have also been included in the "Goals/Evaluation Criteria Examples" section.

More collaborative, family, and community nursing interventions and activities have also been included.

Collaborative Problems

In the "Clinical Conditions Guide to Nursing Diagnoses and Collaborative Problems," each disease or medical condition now includes the associated multidisciplinary (collaborative) problems. Appendices D, E, and F contain the most comprehensive listing of multidisciplinary problems available, organized for (1) diseases/pathophysiology, (2) tests and treatments, and (3) surgical treatments.

Other Features

Organized for Easy Use

The book is divided into two main parts: (1) Complete plans of care for each NANDA nursing diagnosis; and (2) a list of medical, surgical, psychiatric, perinatal, and pediatric conditions, each accompanied by nursing diagnoses and collaborative problems commonly associated with those conditions. This organization allows the nurse to begin the care planning process with either a medical condition or a nursing diagnosis.

Suggestions for Using NANDA Diagnoses

Author suggestions help to clarify the nursing diagnosis labels and to advise how they can best be used.

Organization of Defining Characteristics

These cues have been alphabetized and categorized as "subjective" or "objective." NANDA no longer designates "major," "minor," and "critical" defining characteristics.

Easy to Individualize

Each plan of care is comprehensive and allows nurses to select specific content according to the patient's condition and situation. Each nursing diagnosis includes related factors or risk factors that make it easy to individualize the care plan to the specific patient situation. Creative nurses will tailor standardized outcomes, interventions, and related/risk factors to meet the needs of each individual patient.

Assessment, Teaching, and Collaborative Nursing Activities

Nursing activities are grouped under the headings: Assessments, Patient/Family Teaching, Collaborative Activities, and

Other. This makes it easier to locate a particular activity and helps assure that the nurse considers each type of activity.

Critical Paths

An up-to-date discussion of nursing diagnosis and critical paths is featured, along with an example of a format for a multidisciplinary care plan (critical path).

Care Planning Checklist

A checklist (see back cover flap) is provided to assist the practitioner in evaluating the finished care plan for completeness and suitability for the client.

<u>Audience</u>

This pocket guide is intended to facilitate care planning for nursing students, staff nurses in a variety of settings, clinical nurse specialists, and staff development instructors.

Introduction

Background

In 1973 the American Nurses Association (ANA) mandated the use of nursing diagnosis. That same year, clinicians, educators, researchers, and theorists from every area of nursing practice came together to offer labels for conditions they had observed in practice. From that beginning, the North American Nursing Diagnosis Association (NANDA) was established as the formal body for the promotion, review, and endorsement of the current list of nursing diagnoses used by practicing nurses. The NANDA membership convenes every two years. The current list of 150 diagnoses (see inside front and back covers) will undoubtedly expand as nurses explore the breadth and depth of nursing practice.

As the list of nursing diagnoses expanded, NANDA developed a classification system, or taxonomy (1992, Taxonomy I, Revised, p. 1) for organizing the diagnostic labels. The current taxonomy is found in Appendix B. Work continues to address a number of issues (for example, there is some overlapping among the diagnostic labels). A completely new taxonomy (Taxonomy II) is being developed. It will probably be completed and accepted for use shortly after the year 2000.

NANDA has been working with the ANA and other organizations to include the NANDA labels in other classification systems, for example the World Health Organization International Classification of Diseases (ICD). NANDA diagnosis-related articles are presently indexed in the Cumulative Index of Nursing and Allied Health and in the National Library of Medicine Medical Metathesaurus for a Unified Medical Language.

The growing use of computerized patient records demands a standardized language for describing patient problems. Nursing diagnosis fulfills that need and helps define the scope of nursing practice by describing conditions the nurse can independently treat. Nursing diagnosis highlights critical thinking and decision making, and provides a consistent and universally understood terminology among nurses working in various settings, including hospitals, ambulatory care clinics, extended care facilities, occupational health facilities, and private practice.

Nursing Process in Relation to Nursing Diagnosis

The nursing process provides a structure for nursing practice—a framework in which nurses use knowledge and skills to express human caring. The nursing process is used continuously when planning and giving nursing care. The nurse considers the patient as the central figure in the plan of care and confirms the appropriateness of all aspects of nursing care by observing the patient's responses.

Assessment (also called data collection) is the initial step in the critical thinking and decision making that lead to a nursing diagnosis. The nurse uses the definition and defining characteristics of the nursing diagnosis to validate the diagnosis. Once the nursing diagnosis and the related factors or risk factors are determined, the plan of care is created. The nurse selects the relevant patient outcomes, including the patient's perceptions and suggestions for the outcomes, if possible. The nurse next works with the patient to determine which activities will help achieve the stated outcomes. Finally, after implementing the nursing activities, the nurse evaluates the care plan and the patient's progress. Is the nursing diagnosis still appropriate? Has the patient achieved the desired goals? Are the documentation interval and the target date still appropriate and realistic? Are certain interventions no longer needed? The individualized plan of care is revised as needed.

Standards of Care in Relation to Nursing Diagnosis

Nursing diagnosis care planning and standards of care are interrelated. Standards of care are developed for groups of patients about whom generalized predictions can be made. These standards direct a set of common nursing interventions for specific patient groups (e.g., for all patients having a total hip replacement). Where there are written standards of care, nursing diagnosis care planning is not used to communicate routine nursing actions. Nursing diagnosis care planning is used for those exceptional patient problems that are not addressed in the standards of care.

Case Management and Critical Paths

Escalating health care costs and the demand for health care reform have brought about a restructuring of traditional practice patterns. Two multidisciplinary clinical systems that have emerged are case management and managed care.

Case Management

Case management is a system in which health care professionals coordinate care for high-risk, complex patient populations. These are the unusual, uncommon cases seen in an agency—patients whose condition changes frequently and unpredictably, and whose needs cannot be addressed by a standardized plan or critical path. The case manager, often an advanced practice nurse, focuses on roles and relationships and provides a well coordinated care experience for patients and families in all settings in which the patient receives care.

Critical Paths and Managed Care

Managed care is used to standardize practice for the common, most prevalent case types in an agency. For example, case types in a cardiac care unit might be "myocardial infarction" and "cardiac catheterization." Managed care uses a tool called a critical path as a guide for achieving predictable client outcomes within a specified time frame. The critical path is a multidisciplinary plan of care that outlines crucial activities to be performed by nurses, physicians, and other health team members at designated times in order to achieve the desired patient outcomes (see the figure on p. xxiv).

In managed care systems, the standardized critical path replaces the traditional nursing care plan for many clients. Some agencies have incorporated nursing diagnoses directly into the critical paths. Others use nursing diagnoses to name variances and develop an individualized plan for achieving revised outcomes. A variance occurs when desired outcomes are not achieved at the specified times.

Nursing Diagnosis Incorporated into Critical Path As an example, when incorporating a nursing diagnosis into a critical path for a newly diagnosed insulin-dependent diabetic, the following nursing diagnosis would be a part of the preprinted multidisciplinary care plan:

> *Ineffective management of therapeutic regimen* related to limited information and limited practice of skill, as evidenced by verbalization of limited knowledge, inaccurate follow-through of instruction, and inaccurate performance on tests.

Client goals might be that by day 3, the client will recognize signs and symptoms of hypo/hyperglycemia, and by day 5, be able to self-inject the required dose of insulin.

Nursing Diagnosis Used to Name Variance In this system, the critical path for a newly diagnosed insulin-dependent diabetic would not include a nursing diagnosis, but rather would list "teaching needs" for each day. On day 5, if the patient is unable to meet the outcome of self-injection, this variance would be identified and analyzed. At that point the nursing diagnosis of *Ineffective management of therapeutic regimen*...would be used to individualize the nursing care for this patient's variance from the critical path.

Even in organizations using managed care, the nursing process is used to plan and deliver patient care via a multidisciplinary care plan, and nursing diagnoses are valuable in individualizing critical paths to meet unique, individual patient needs. It is vital that today's nurse be well versed in using nursing diagnoses in order to effectively identify and address nursing care issues within the multidisciplinary team.

Components of Nursing Diagnosis Care Plans

This book is organized into two parts: "Plans of Care" and "Clinical Conditions Guide to Nursing Diagnoses and Collaborative Problems." Information regarding these two parts, with some examples of how to use them, follows.

Plans of Care

Each plan of care includes a nursing diagnosis label, the label definition, defining characteristics, related factors or risk factors, suggestions for use, suggested alternative diagnoses, NOC outcomes, client goals, NIC priority interventions, and nursing activities. See the figure on page xiv.

The nursing diagnosis care plans are organized alphabetically to make the labels easy to locate. The diagnoses are worded in order to set forth the key concept in the first word of the label. For example, *Ineffective denial* is easier to find in an index when it is written as *Denial, ineffective*.

Nursing Diagnosis

The nursing diagnosis is a concise label that describes patient conditions observed in practice. These conditions may be actual or potential problems. Using NANDA terminology, potential problems are labeled *Risk for*. Appendix C contains a list of definitions of the "qualifier" words that are used in many of the diagnostic labels (eg, acute, altered, impaired). Add other qualifying words as needed to make diagnoses precise and descriptive.

Definition

The definition for each nursing diagnosis helps the nurse verify a particular nursing diagnosis. Unless otherwise specified, the definitions in this text were taken from the NANDA taxonomy.

Defining Characteristics

Defining characteristics are cues that describe patient behavior, either observed by the nurse (objective) or verbalized by the patient/family (subjective). After assessing the patient, nurses organize the defining characteristics into meaningful patterns that alert them to the possibility of a patient problem. Usually, the presence of two or three defining characteristics verifies a nursing diagnosis.

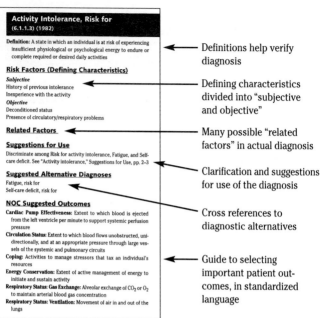

Activity Intolerance, Risk for
(6.1.1.3) (1982)

Definition: A state in which an individual is at risk of experiencing insufficient physiological or psychological energy to endure or complete required or desired daily activities.

← Definitions help verify diagnosis

Risk Factors (Defining Characteristics)

Subjective
History of previous intolerance
Inexperience with the activity
Objective
Deconditioned status
Presence of circulatory/respiratory problems

← Defining characteristics divided into "subjective and objective"

Related Factors

← Many possible "related factors" in actual diagnosis

Suggestions for Use

Discriminate among Risk for activity intolerance, Fatigue, and Self-care deficit. See "Activity intolerance," Suggestions for Use, pp. 2–3

Suggested Alternative Diagnoses

Fatigue, risk for
Self-care deficit, risk for

← Clarification and suggestions for use of the diagnosis

← Cross references to diagnostic alternatives

NOC Suggested Outcomes

Cardiac Pump Effectiveness: Extent to which blood is ejected from the left ventricle per minute to support systemic perfusion pressure
Circulation Status: Extent to which blood flows unobstructed, unidirectionally, and at an appropriate pressure through large vessels of the systemic and pulmonary circuits
Coping: Activities to manage stressors that tax an individual's resources
Energy Conservation: Extent of active management of energy to initiate and sustain activity
Respiratory Status: Gas Exchange: Alveolar exchange of CO_2 or O_2 to maintain arterial blood gas concentration
Respiratory Status: Ventilation: Movement of air in and out of the lungs

← Guide to selecting important patient outcomes, in standardized language

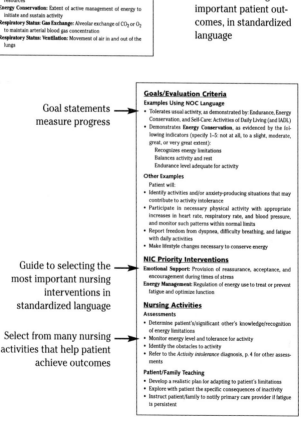

Goal statements measure progress →

Goals/Evaluation Criteria
Examples Using NOC Language
• Tolerates usual activity, as demonstrated by: Endurance, Energy Conservation, and Self-Care: Activities of Daily Living (and IADL)
• Demonstrates **Energy Conservation**, as evidenced by the following indicators (specify 1–5: not at all, to a slight, moderate, great, or very great extent):
 Recognizes energy limitations
 Balances activity and rest
 Endurance level adequate for activity

Other Examples
Patient will:
• Identify activities and/or anxiety-producing situations that may contribute to activity intolerance
• Participate in necessary physical activity with appropriate increases in heart rate, respiratory rate, and blood pressure, and monitor such patterns within normal limits
• Report freedom from dyspnea, difficulty breathing, and fatigue with daily activities
• Make lifestyle changes necessary to conserve energy

NIC Priority Interventions
Emotional Support: Provision of reassurance, acceptance, and encouragement during times of stress
Energy Management: Regulation of energy use to treat or prevent fatigue and optimize function

Guide to selecting the most important nursing interventions in standardized language →

Nursing Activities
Assessments
• Determine patient's/significant other's knowledge/recognition of energy limitations
• Monitor energy level and tolerance for activity
• Identify the obstacles to activity
• Refer to the *Activity intolerance* diagnosis, p. 4 for other assessments

Select from many nursing activities that help patient achieve outcomes →

Patient/Family Teaching
• Develop a realistic plan for adapting to patient's limitations
• Explore with patient the specific consequences of inactivity
• Instruct patient/family to notify primary care provider if fatigue is persistent

In this text, all NANDA defining characteristics have been included. NANDA no longer designates defining characteristics as "major," "minor," and "critical." This simplification was made in order to support: (a) the development of electronic nursing diagnosis databases, (b) diagnosis development, and (c) classification work.

Related Factors

The related factors imply a connection with the nursing diagnosis. Such factors may be described as "related to," "antecedent to," "associated with," or "contributing to" the diagnosis. Related factors indicate what should change for the patient to return to optimal health, and therefore help the nurse to select effective nursing interventions. As an example, for the diagnosis *Activity intolerance*, the nursing activities for a patient whose related factor is arrhythmias would be quite different from those needed for a patient whose related factor is chronic pain.

Risk Factors

Risk factors will be found only in the "risk for" (potential) nursing diagnoses. The risk factors are similar to related factors and defining characteristics in the development of the care plan. They describe events and behaviors that put the patient at risk and suggest interventions to protect the patient. As an example, an elderly patient might be diagnosed with *Risk for trauma*, and exhibit the following risk factors: weakness, poor vision, balancing difficulties, slippery floors, and unanchored rugs. As an etiology, this cluster of risk factors suggests the need for interventions to prevent falls.

Suggestions for Use

For problematic labels, clarifying comments are included, along with suggestions for using the diagnosis appropriately or differentiating it from similar diagnoses.

Suggested Alternative Diagnoses

Suggested alternative diagnoses are other nursing diagnoses that may be considered when identifying the patient's problem. If a review of the definition and defining characteristics indicates that they only partially match the patient data, the nurse may consider the suggested alternative diagnoses as options. This is particularly helpful for the nurse unfamiliar with the nuances of each nursing diagnosis.

NOC Suggested Outcomes

For each NANDA diagnosis, this text lists the NOC "Suggested Outcomes"—those that the Iowa Outcomes Project has identified as most likely to be monitored in patients with that diagnosis. NOC outcomes are neutral concepts reflecting patient states or behaviors (e.g., memory, coping, rest). These nurse-sensitive patient outcomes are not goals, but the nurse can use them along with their indicators to set goals for a specific patient. Indicators are more specific behaviors that are used to measure or rate the patient outcome.

Goal Statements/Evaluation Criteria

Each nursing diagnosis also includes examples of patient goals/evaluation criteria that were developed by using NOC outcomes, outcome indicators, and measuring scales. Goals are statements of patient/family behaviors that are measurable or observable. For example, to evaluate a client outcome of Cognitive Orientation, the nurse might use these indicators:

Identifies self (often)

Identifies significant other (sometimes)

Identifies current place (often)

Use as few or as many patient outcomes and sample goals as necessary. If more are needed, refer to the *Nursing Outcomes Classification (NOC)* manual (1997).

Patient goals, like all components of the care planning process, are dynamic. Therefore, they change frequently. Specific, individualized patient goal statements are critical because they are used to evaluate patient responses to care and the success of the nursing care plan.

The nurse should be realistic when constructing patient goal statements, because partial behavior change may be the only attainable goal. With shortened length of hospital stay, nurses in the community setting may help patients to achieve goals/outcomes after they are discharged from the hospital. At time of discharge, the nurse may initiate discussion with the patient to determine patient/family goals still requiring completion, with referral to appropriate community resources.

Always specify a target date and documentation interval for patient goals. The target date is the estimated date by which the outcome will be accomplished. The date is flexible and individualized to the patient. The documentation interval designates how often documentation should occur for each outcome. This interval should be determined during initial assessment and may be changed as patient nears completion of a goal. For example, in the care plan for *Fatigue,* the documentation interval for the goal, "Maintains adequate nutrition" could be specified as "t.i.d." This would mean that documentation must occur at least three times daily, after meals, until the outcome is accomplished.

NIC Priority Interventions

The Nursing Interventions Classification categorizes nursing activities using standardized language. "Priority interventions" are the research-based interventions developed by the Iowa Intervention Project team as the treatments of choice for a particular nursing diagnosis (NIC, 1996). They are the most obvious interventions to effect problem resolution, but this does not mean that they are the only interventions to be used. A variety of interventions should always be considered. In NIC terminology, "interventions" are broad, general category labels. These category labels were linked to the NANDA diagnosis labels through a systematic process drawing upon the judgments of experts in nursing practice and research.

Nursing Activities

In NIC terminology, the specific, detailed actions taken by the nurse (eg, taking vital signs, monitoring intake and output) are called activities. The NIC Priority Interventions direct the nurse to review first the nursing activities related to those interventions. Other specific nursing activities can be found in the *Nursing Interventions Classification (NIC)* handbook (1996). Following is an example of how the NIC priority interventions can guide care planning for the nursing diagnosis *Fatigue:*

1. In the care plan for *Fatigue,* note that the NIC Priority Intervention is "Energy Management." The definition of this intervention is shown as: "Regulating energy use to treat or prevent fatigue and optimize function."

2. Look in the "Nursing Activities" section for the specific activities that would accomplish "Energy Management"—that is, those that specifically focus on regulating energy and treating/preventing fatigue, such as the following examples:

- Plan activities with patient/family that minimize fatigue. Plan may include setting small, realistic, attainable goals for patient that decrease fatigue.

- Encourage patient to report activities that increase fatigue.
- Discuss with patient/family ways to modify home environment to maintain usual activities and to minimize fatigue.
- Teach organization and time management techniques to reduce fatigue (NIC).

3. Finally, review the rest of the nursing activities for *Fatigue.* There may be activities in addition to those for Energy Management that would be helpful, depending on the client's problem etiologies and individual needs.

You will be able to find effective nursing activities to deal with your patient's fatigue by using Steps 1, 2, and 3. However, you may wish to compare your chosen nursing actions to the research-based interventions and activities listed in the *1996 Nursing Interventions Classification* (NIC) handbook. In the NIC handbook under the intervention label Energy Management, there are other specific nursing activities that accomplish Energy Management. Following are three examples:

- Plan activities for periods when the patient has the most energy
- Encourage an afternoon nap, if appropriate
- Assist patient to schedule rest periods

In addition to the Priority Interventions, the NIC handbook lists other nursing interventions to address *Fatigue,* for example: Exercise Promotion and Sleep Enhancement. The nursing activities for those interventions might also be used.

Nursing orders/activities should address the etiology of the patient's nursing diagnosis. From the activities listed for each care plan, choose those that apply to the patient's condition. Alter standardized nursing activities to make them specific to the patient. In certain instances, "q ___" or "specify plan" is included in the nursing activity as a reminder to individualize the nursing orders. As the patient's condition changes, other activities may be added, changed, or deleted. Frequent updating of this portion of the care plan is essential.

Clinical Conditions Guide to Nursing Diagnoses and Collaborative Problems

The second part of this handbook is organized to help nurses focus their assessments when the patient's medical condition is known but the appropriate nursing diagnoses have not yet been established. In this section, medical, surgical, psychiatric, perinatal, and pediatric conditions are listed with associated collaborative problems and nursing diagnoses.

Nursing Diagnoses

The nursing diagnoses listed are those that most logically occur when the particular medical condition is present. Of course, a patient with one of the medical conditions will not have all of the nursing diagnoses listed. Select only those nursing diagnoses that are confirmed by assessment data. Furthermore, these lists should not be considered exhaustive. It is quite possible that a client with a particular medical condition will have nursing diagnoses that are not on the list. Because they represent unique human responses, nursing diagnoses cannot be predicted on the basis of medical condition alone.

Multidisciplinary (Collaborative) Problems

Multidisciplinary problems, on the other hand, are associated with specific medical conditions. According to Carpenito (1997), collaborative problems are the physiological complications, associated with a particular medical condition, that nurses cannot treat independently. The nurse's responsibility is to monitor the patient in order to detect the onset of collaborative problems, and to use both physician-prescribed and nursing-prescribed interventions to prevent or minimize the complication. Because there are a limited number of physiological complications possible for a particular disease, the same collaborative problems tend to be present any time a particular disease or treatment is present; that is, each disease or treatment has particular complications that are always associated with it.

Before making an individualized nursing diagnosis care plan, the nurse should identify the patient's collaborative problems. These will guide the common assessments and preventive care that all patients with that medical diagnosis should receive— much like a critical pathway. Collaborative problems are included for each condition listed in the "Clinical Conditions Guide to Nursing Diagnoses and Collaborative Problems" beginning on page 525. Also refer to Appendices D ["Multidisciplinary (Collaborative) Problems Associated with Diseases and Other Physiologic Disorders"], Appendix E ["Multidisciplinary (Collaborative) Problems Associated with Tests and Treatments"], and Appendix F ["Multidisciplinary (Collaborative) Problems Associated with Surgical Treatments], on pp. 635–644, 645, and 646–648, respectively.

The list of clinical conditions does not include rare disease conditions, so for unusual diseases it may be necessary to refer to a more general title. For example, the patient's medical diagnosis may be scleroderma. Since this condition occurs infrequently, the nurse should look under the general title "Autoimmune Disorders" and review the nursing diagnoses listed there.

How to Create a Nursing Diagnosis Care Plan

The following example shows how to use this book to create an individualized care plan for a patient.

Situation: Mrs. B, a 75-year-old female, has been admitted to a surgical unit from the recovery room following a hip pinning. Her history indicates that Mrs. B lives alone in an apartment. Her husband died 10 years ago. She has many friends and is involved in community affairs at the local senior center. She loves to walk and to ride a bicycle. Her current hospital admission is a result of falling off her bicycle. Mrs. B's postoperative medical orders include the following:

Foley catheter to gravity drainage

$D_5 2\%$ NaCl with KCl 20 mEq to be infused over 8 hours

Morphine sulfate 1–2 mg, IV push, q15 minutes until comfortable to a maximum of 10 mg in 1 hour

Morphine sulfate 6–8 mg, IM q3–4 hours, prn pain

Phenergan 25 mg IM q4–6 hours, prn nausea

CBC and electrolytes tomorrow in am

Overhead trapeze to bed

Turn patient from back to unaffected side q1–2 hours

Pressure-reducing mattress overlay to bed to relieve pressure to bony prominences

Ambulate with assistance in am and then qid

Assessment

4:00 pm—The nurse's initial assessment following return from the recovery room indicates that the patient is sleeping comfortably, vital signs are within normal limits, and the operative dressing is dry and intact. Foley catheter is draining clear, amber urine. The IV is infusing at the prescribed rate; skin is warm and dry.

5:30 pm—The nurse enters Mrs. B's room to check her vital signs and finds Mrs. B attempting to climb out of bed "because I have to go to the bathroom." The nurse reminds Mrs. B that she is in the hospital and has a Foley catheter in place. Mrs. B's responses indicate that she is disoriented to place and time.

Diagnosis

From her assessment of Mrs. B., the nurse identifies the cues of altered mobility, disorientation, pain medication, and change in environment. These seem to match the defining characteristics for a nursing diagnosis of *Risk for injury*. The definition of *Risk for injury* is "a state in which the individual is at risk of injury as a result of environmental conditions interacting with the individual's adaptive and defensive resources." The nurse considers suggested alternative diagnoses to see if a better diagnosis can be found. She looks at the definition and defining characteristics for *Sensory/perceptual alterations, Altered peripheral tissue perfusion, Risk for trauma,* and *Risk for impaired skin integrity.* After reviewing the alternatives, the nurse decides to use the broad nursing diagnosis, *Risk for injury* related to altered mobility, disorientation, pain medication, and change in environment.

NOC Suggested Outcomes

In order to focus her goal statements, the nurse begins with the NOC Suggested Outcomes for *Risk for injury:* Parenting (Social Safety), Risk Control, and Safety Behavior (Fall Prevention). After reading the outcome definitions and referring to the NOC handbook, the nurse determines that Safety Behavior (Fall Prevention) is probably the only outcome needed for Mrs. B's care plan.

Goal Statements/Evaluation Criteria

Goals: The nurse chooses and modifies the following goals from the listed sample goals and NOC indicators:

Use of restraints as needed (totally adequate)

Agitation and restlessness controlled (moderately adequate)

Patient will avoid physical injury (totally adequate)

The goals are observable and appropriate for Mrs. B's situation. The documentation interval for the goals could be q 4 hours, and the target date could be 1–2 days after surgery, except for the last goal, for which it should be "at all times." The target date should be stated as an actual date (eg, 1/30). The documentation interval and target date should be reviewed at least daily to evaluate appropriateness.

Evaluation: The nurse would collect data about the first two goals in order to evaluate progress in controlling Mrs. B.'s risk factors. Status of the last goal will indicate whether interventions were successful in preventing the potential problem, *Risk for injury.*

Nursing Interventions and Activities

Next, the nurse selects nursing interventions. The NIC priority interventions are: Electronic Fetal Monitoring, Fall Prevention,

Labor Induction, Latex Precautions, and Malignant Hyperthermia Precautions. The nurse determines that only Fall Prevention applies to Mrs. B.

The NIC interventions provide direction for choosing nursing activities, but they are general. In order to write individualized nursing orders for Mrs. B., the nurse selects the following from the list of nursing activities:

Identify characteristics of the environment that may increase potential for falls (NIC).

Reorient patient to reality and immediate environment when necessary.

Place articles within easy reach of patient (NIC).

Provide the dependent patient with a means of summoning help (eg, bell or call light) when caregiver is not present (NIC).

The listed activities are adequate to address Mrs. B's problem for the present. If they were not, the nurse would have referred to the NIC manual for interventions in addition to the Priority Interventions (eg, Surveillance or Physical Restraint).

All of the aforementioned nursing orders could be part of Mrs. B's care plan. Once an intervention or activity is no longer applicable, the nurse deletes it from the care plan. New activities should be added as needed. This example demonstrates the process used to develop a care plan for one nursing diagnosis. Other nursing diagnoses might also be appropriate for Mrs. B.

Creating a Critical Path

Explained very simply, creating a critical path is a matter of combining the care plans from nursing, medical, and other services, and imposing a timeline upon the combined plan. All care and treatments are shown on the plan, and care is organized by days, weeks, or even hours and minutes, for example:

Day 1	**Day 2**	**Day 3**
Outcomes	Outcomes	Outcomes
Nursing orders	Nursing orders	Nursing orders
Medical orders	Medical orders	Medical orders

The timeline of a critical path is different for each institution, depending on the patient population. In some hospitals a hernia repair might mean an overnight stay (and therefore a two-day critical path); in others it might be an outpatient procedure, with the critical path broken up into hourly segments. Therefore, standardized times cannot be given for the interventions on the nursing diagnosis care plans in this book. However, the care plans can be used when creating critical paths, the same as they are used in creating nursing diagnosis care plans.

1. Determine the nursing diagnoses your patient population (eg, herniorrhaphy patients) typically has preoperatively and postoperatively—or on day 1, day 2, and so on. Refer to the Clinical Conditions Guide to Nursing Diagnoses and Collaborative Problems for ideas as needed.

2. Choose patient goals and nursing activities for each day (or hour), just as you would for a traditional nursing care plan. The difference is that instead of a single care plan for a nursing diagnosis, you will have, essentially, a care plan for each day of the patient's stay in the institution. Refer to the figure below.

Critical Pathways for Client Following Laparoscopic Cholecystectomy

	Date _____ PREOPERATIVE	Date _____ 1st 24 hrs. following surgery
Daily outcomes	Client will verbalize understanding of preoperative teaching, including turning ...	Client will • be afebrile • have a dry, clean wound with well-approximated ...
Tests and treatments	CBC Urinalysis Baseline physical assessment	Vital signs and O_2 saturation, neurovascular assessment, dressing and ...
Knowledge deficit	Orient to room and surroundings. Include family in teaching	Reorient to room and postoperative routine, Include family in teaching
Psychosocial	Assess anxiety related to pending surgery	Assess level of anxiety Encourage verbalization ...
Diet	NPO Baseline nutritional assessment	Advance to clear liquids ...
Activity	OOB ad lib until premedicated for surgery	Provide safety precautions. Bathroom privileges ...
Medications	NPO except ordered medications	IM or PO analgesics Antibiotics if ordered
Transfer/ discharge plans	Assess discharge plans and support system.	Probable discharge within 24 hours of surgery

Nursing Diagnoses— with Outcomes and Interventions

Diagnostic labels, definitions, and defining characteristics are based primarily on the North American Nursing Diagnosis Association (NANDA) taxonomy. The first number following the label locates the diagnosis in the NANDA taxonomy. The second number indicates the year the diagnosis was accepted or revised. Suggested alternative diagnoses are provided for most labels. Consider those if a label does not fit the patient data satisfactorily. The author's discussion and recommendations for using certain diagnoses are identified by the heading "Suggestions for Use."

Individualizing Client Goals/Evaluation Criteria

"NOC Suggested Outcomes" and indicators presented under "Goals/Evaluation Criteria" are quoted verbatim from the Nursing Outcomes Classification (NOC). To help you create goals using standardized language, examples of such goals are given. To individualize these and the "Other Examples" provided in the text, add patient-specific target dates and evaluation and documentation intervals. If you do not find goals appropriate to your patient, refer to the *NOC* manual for outcome indicators and scales to develop other goals, as needed. To save space, some indicators have been combined into one goal; however, NOC lists them separately, and they must be evaluated separately.

Individualizing Nursing Activities

"NIC Priority Interventions" are quoted verbatim from the Nursing Interventions Classification (NIC). Selected nursing activities are also written in standardized language. Choose only those activities that address patient problems and etiologies. Individualize nursing activities to meet the unique needs of each patient (eg, by adding times of and frequencies for nursing activities, including more specific details). If you do not find the exact activities you need, refer to the *NIC* manual for other interventions and activities.

Activity Intolerance
(6.1.1.2) (1982)

Definition: A state in which an individual has insufficient physiological or psychological energy to endure or complete required or desired daily activities

Defining Characteristics

Subjective
Exertional discomfort or dyspnea
Verbal report of fatigue or weakness

Objective
Abnormal heart rate or blood pressure in response to activity
ECG changes during activity reflecting arrhythmia or ischemia

Related Factors

Bed rest/immobility
Chronic pain
Generalized weakness
Imbalance between oxygen supply and demand
Sedentary lifestyle
NOTE: The preceding factors are from NANDA. They are secondary to a wide variety of pathophysiologies, including cardiac disease (eg, congestive heart failure), respiratory disease (eg, emphysema), renal disease, cancer, anemia, obesity, and infections (eg, mononucleosis).

Suggestions for Use

Do not use this label unless it is possible to increase the patient's endurance. Use *Activity intolerance* only if the patient reports fatigue or weakness *in response to activity*. Medical conditions (eg, heart disease or peripheral arterial disease) often cause *Activity intolerance*. The nurse cannot independently treat medical conditions, so a diagnostic statement such as "*Activity intolerance* related to coronary artery disease" is not useful.

Activity intolerance often creates other problems, such as *Self-care deficit*, *Social isolation*, or *Ineffective breastfeeding*, and you can use it most effectively as the etiology of these other problems. Specify *Activity intolerance* by levels of endurance, as follows (Gordon, 1994, p. 110):

Level I: Walks regular pace on level ground but becomes more short of breath than normal when climbing one or more flights of stairs

Level II: Walks one city block 500 feet on level or climbs one flight of stairs slowly without stopping

Level III: Walks no more than 50 feet on level without stopping and is unable to climb one flight of stairs without stopping

Level IV: Dyspnea and fatigue at rest

The following is an example of such a diagnostic statement: *Self-care deficit (total) related to Activity intolerance (Level IV).*

Suggested Alternative Diagnoses

Fatigue (Activity intolerance is relieved by rest. Fatigue is not.)
Self-care deficit

NOC Suggested Outcomes

Endurance: Extent that energy enables a person's activity

Energy Conservation: Extent of active management of energy to initiate and sustain activity

Self-Care: Activities of Daily Living (ADL): Ability to perform the most basic physical tasks and personal care activities

Self-Care: Instrumental Activities of Daily Living (IADL): Ability to perform activities needed to function in the home or community

Goals/Evaluation Criteria

Examples Using NOC Language

- Tolerates usual activity, as demonstrated by Endurance, Energy Conservation, and Self-Care: Activities of Daily Living (and IADL)
- Demonstrates **Energy Conservation**, as evidenced by the following indicators (specify 1–5: not at all, to a slight, moderate, great, or very great extent):

    Recognizes energy limitations
    Balances activity and rest
    Endurance level adequate for activity

Other Examples

Patient will:
- Identify activities and/or anxiety-producing situations that may contribute to activity intolerance
- Participate in necessary physical activity with appropriate increases in heart rate, respiratory rate, and blood pressure, and monitor patterns within normal limits

- Verbalize understanding of need for oxygen, medications, and/or equipment that may increase tolerance for activities
- Perform ADLs with some assistance (eg, toilets with help ambulating to bathroom)
- Perform home maintenance management with some help (eg, needs weekly cleaning help)

NIC Priority Interventions

Activity Therapy: Prescription of and assistance with specific physical, cognitive, social, and spiritual activities to increase the range, frequency, or duration of an individual's (or group's) activity

Energy Management: Regulating energy use to treat or prevent fatigue and optimize function

Nursing Activities

Assessments

- Assess emotional, social, and spiritual response to activity
- Evaluate patient's motivation and desire to increase activity
- *(NIC) Energy Management:*

  Determine causes of fatigue (eg, treatments, pain, and medications)

  Monitor cardiorespiratory response to activity (eg, tachycardia, other dysrhythmias, dyspnea, diaphoresis, pallor, hemodynamic pressures, and respiratory rate)

  Monitor patient's oxygen response (eg, pulse rate, cardiac rhythm, and respiratory rate) to self-care activities

  Monitor nutritional intake to ensure adequate energy resources

  Monitor/record patient's sleep pattern and number of sleep hours

Patient/Family Teaching

  Instruct patient/family in:

- Use of equipment, such as oxygen, during activities
- Use of relaxation techniques (eg, distraction, visualization) during activities
- *(NIC) Energy Management:*

  Teach patient and significant other techniques of self-care that will minimize oxygen consumption (eg, self-monitoring and pacing techniques for performance of activities of daily living)

  Teach activity organization and time management techniques to prevent fatigue

Collaborative Activities
- Administer pain medications prior to activity
- Collaborate with occupational, physical, and/or recreational therapists to plan and monitor an activity program, as appropriate
- Refer to home health to obtain services of a home care aide, as needed
- Refer to dietitian for meal planning to increase intake of high-energy foods

Other
- Avoid scheduling care activities during rest periods
- Help patient to change position gradually, dangle, sit, stand, and ambulate, as tolerated
- Plan activities with patient/family that promote independence and endurance. For example:

  Encourage alternate periods of rest and activity

  Keep frequently used objects within easy reach

  Provide positive reinforcement for increased activity

  Set small, realistic, attainable goals for patient that increase independence and self-esteem
- Plan care for the infant/child to minimize the oxygen needs of the body:

  Anticipate needs for food, water, comfort, holding, and stimulation, to prevent unnecessary crying

  Avoid environments low in oxygen concentration (eg, high altitudes, unpressurized airplanes)

  Minimize anxiety and stress

  Prevent hyperthermia and hypothermia

  Prevent infection

  Provide adequate rest
- *(NIC) Energy Management*:

  Assist patient to identify preferences for activity

  Plan activities for periods when the patient has the most energy

  Assist with regular physical activities (eg, ambulation, transfers, turning, and personal care) as needed

  Limit environmental stimuli (eg, light and noise) to facilitate relaxation

  Assist patient to self-monitor by developing and using a written record of calorie intake and energy expenditure, as appropriate

Activity Intolerance, Risk for
(6.1.1.3) (1982)

Definition: A state in which an individual is at risk of experiencing insufficient physiological or psychological energy to endure or complete required or desired daily activities

Risk Factors

Subjective
History of previous intolerance
Inexperience with the activity

Objective
Deconditioned status
Presence of circulatory/respiratory problems

Suggestions for Use

Discriminate among Risk for activity intolerance, Fatigue, and Self-care deficit. See "Activity intolerance," Suggestions for Use, pp. 2–3

Suggested Alternative Diagnoses

Fatigue, risk for
Self-care deficit, risk for

NOC Suggested Outcomes

Cardiac Pump Effectiveness: Extent to which blood is ejected from the left ventricle per minute to support systemic perfusion pressure

Circulation Status: Extent to which blood flows unobstructed, uni-directionally, and at an appropriate pressure through large vessels of the systemic and pulmonary circuits

Coping: Activities to manage stressors that tax an individual's resources

Energy Conservation: Extent of active management of energy to initiate and sustain activity

Respiratory Status: Gas Exchange: Alveolar exchange of CO_2 or O_2 to maintain arterial blood gas concentration

Respiratory Status: Ventilation: Movement of air in and out of the lungs

Goals/Evaluation Criteria

Examples Using NOC Language

- Tolerates usual activity, as demonstrated by: Endurance, Energy Conservation, and Self-Care: Activities of Daily Living (and IADL)
- Demonstrates **Energy Conservation**, as evidenced by the following indicators (specify 1–5: not at all, to a slight, moderate, great, or very great extent):

    Recognizes energy limitations

    Balances activity and rest

    Endurance level adequate for activity

Other Examples

Patient will:

- Identify activities and/or anxiety-producing situations that may contribute to activity intolerance
- Participate in necessary physical activity with appropriate increases in heart rate, respiratory rate, and blood pressure, and monitor such patterns within normal limits
- Report freedom from dyspnea, difficulty breathing, and fatigue with daily activities
- Make lifestyle changes necessary to conserve energy

NIC Priority Interventions

Emotional Support: Provision of reassurance, acceptance, and encouragement during times of stress

Energy Management: Regulation of energy use to treat or prevent fatigue and optimize function

Nursing Activities

Assessments

- Determine patient's/significant other's knowledge/recognition of energy limitations
- Monitor energy level and tolerance for activity
- Identify the obstacles to activity
- Refer to the *Activity intolerance* diagnosis, p. 4 for other assessments

Patient/Family Teaching

- Develop a realistic plan for adapting to patient's limitations
- Explore with patient the specific consequences of inactivity
- Instruct patient/family to notify primary care provider if fatigue is persistent

- *(NIC) Energy Management:*
  Teach patient and significant other techniques of self-care that
      will minimize oxygen consumption (eg, self-monitoring and
      pacing techniques for performance of activities of daily living)
  Teach activity organization and time management techniques to
      prevent fatigue

Other

- Enlist family in efforts to support and encourage the patient's
  completion of activities
- Provide decision-making (and other) support during periods of
  illness or high stress

Adaptive Capacity: Intracranial, Decreased (1.7.1) (1994)

Definition: A clinical state in which intracranial fluid dynamic
mechanisms that normally compensate for increases in
intracranial volumes are compromised, resulting in repeated
disproportionate increases in intracranial pressure (ICP) in
response to a variety of noxious and non-noxious stimuli

Defining Characteristics

Objective
Baseline ICP ≥10 mm Hg
Disproportionate increase in ICP following single environmental or
    nursing maneuver stimulus
Elevated P_2 ICP waveform
Repeated increases in ICP of > 10 mm Hg for more than 5 minutes
    following any of a variety of external stimuli
Volume-pressure response test variation (volume-pressure ratio
    > 2, pressure-volume index < 10)
Wide-amplitude ICP waveform

Related Factors

Brain injuries
Decreased cerebral perfusion pressure ≤ 50–60 mm Hg
Sustained increase in ICP ≥ 10–15 mm Hg
Systemic hypotension with intracranial hypertension

Suggestions for Use

This diagnosis requires both medical and nursing interventions. Most of the nursing care will be dictated by agency protocols. Therefore, this diagnosis may be better stated as a collaborative problem (Potential Complication of head injury: Increased intracranial pressure).

Suggested Alternative Diagnoses

Tissue perfusion, altered (cerebral)

NOC Suggested Outcomes

Electrolyte and Acid-Base Balance: Balance of electrolytes and non-electrolytes in the intracellular and extracellular compartments of the body

Fluid Balance: Balance of water in the the intracellular and extracellular compartments of the body

Neurological Status: Extent to which the peripheral and central nervous systems receive, process, and respond to internal and external stimuli

Neurological Status: Consciousness: Extent to which an individual arouses, orients, and attends to the environment

Goals/Evaluation Criteria

NOTE: The following outcomes cannot be produced by independent nursing activities.

Examples Using NOC Language

- Demonstrates increased *Intracranial adaptive capacity*, as demonstrated by Electrolyte and Acid-Base Balance, Fluid Balance, Neurological Status, and Neurological Status: Consciousness
- Demonstrates **Neurological Status**, as evidenced by the following indicators (specify 1–5: extremely, substantially, moderately, mildly, or not compromised):

    Pupil size and reactivity

    Seizure activity not present

    Headaches not present

    Breathing pattern

    Neurological status: consciousness

    Neurological status: cranial sensory/motor function

    Neurological status: autonomic

Other Examples

- Cerebral perfusion pressure will be ≥ 70 mm Hg (in adults)
- ICP will stabilize at four or less episodes of abnormal waveforms in 24 hours

NIC Priority Interventions

Cerebral Edema Management: Limitation of secondary cerebral injury resulting from swelling of brain tissue

Cerebral Perfusion Promotion: Promotion of adequate perfusion and limitation of complications for a patient experiencing or at risk for inadequate cerebral perfusion

Intracranial Pressure (ICP) Monitoring: Measurement and interpretation of patient data to regulate intracranial pressure

Neurologic Monitoring: Collection and analysis of patient data to prevent or minimize neurologic complications

Nursing Activities

Assessments

- Monitor ICP and cerebral perfusion pressure (CPP) continuously with alarm settings on
- Monitor neurologic status at regular intervals (eg, vital signs; pupil size, shape, reaction to light, equality; consciousness/mental status; response to painful stimuli; ability to follow commands; symmetry of motor response; reflexes such as Babinski's, blink, cough, gag)
- Note events that trigger changes in the ICP waveform (eg, position change, suctioning)
- Determine baseline for vital signs and cardiac rhythm, and monitor for changes during and after activity
- *(NIC) Intracranial Pressure (ICP) Monitoring:*
  Monitor pressure tubing for bubbles
  Monitor amount/rate of cerebrospinal fluid drainage
  Monitor intake and output
  Monitor insertion site for infection
  Monitor temperature and WBC count
  Check patient for nuchal rigidity

Patient/Family Teaching

- Teach caregiver about signs that will indicate increased ICP (eg, changes in eye coordination, increased seizure activity, restlessness, changes in speech). **NOTE:** Changes are specific to the patient, depending on the disability (eg, trauma, hydrocephalus) underlying the increased ICP.

- Teach caregiver the specific situations that trigger ICP in the client (eg, pain, anxiety); discuss appropriate interventions

Collaborative Activities

- Initiate agency protocols for lowering ICP (eg, plan may include ventriculostomy to drain cerebrospinal fluid)
- Follow protocols to maintain systemic blood pressure adequate to keep CPP at ≥ 70 mm Hg
- *(NIC) Intracranial Pressure (ICP) Monitoring:*

  Notify physician for elevated ICP that does not respond to treatment protocols

  Administer pharmacologic agents to maintain ICP within specified range

  Administer antibiotics

  Maintain controlled hyperventilation, as ordered

Other

- Do not use the knee gatch and avoid 90-degree hip flexion
- Stop any activity (eg, suctioning) that triggers *Decreased intracranial adaptive capacity*
- Limit the duration of procedures and care activities; allow time for baseline ICP to recover between noxious activities such as suctioning
- For patients who are performing Valsalva's maneuver, if they can follow directions, instruct them to exhale through their mouths
- Use gentle touching and talking
- Suction only if necessary—not prophylactically
- If suctioning is needed, preoxygenate, do not hyperventilate, and use only one or two catheter passes; administer intratracheal lidocaine, per protocol, to minimize coughing
- Allow family to visit
- *(NIC) Intracranial Pressure (ICP) Monitoring:*

  Calibrate and level the transducer

  Restrain patient, as needed

  Change transducer/flush system

  Change and/or reinforce insertion site dressing, as necessary

  Position the patient with head elevated 30 to 45 degrees and with neck in a neutral position [support with sandbags, small pillows, or rolled towels]

  Minimize environmental stimuli [eg, noise, painful procedures]

Space nursing care to minimize ICP elevation
Maintain systemic arterial pressure within specified range

Adjustment, Impaired
(5.1.1.1.1) (1986, 1998)

Definition: An inability to modify lifestyle/behavior in a manner consistent with a change in health status

Defining Characteristics

Subjective
Denial of health status change
Failure to achieve optimal sense of control

Objective
Demonstration of nonacceptance of health status change
Failure to take actions that would prevent further health problems

Related Factors

Absence of social support for changed beliefs and practices
Disability or health status change requiring change in lifestyle
Failure to intend to change behavior
Intense emotional state
Lack of motivation to change behaviors
Low state of optimism
Multiple stressors
Negative attitudes toward health behavior

Suggestions for Use

This diagnosis is not specific enough to be clinically useful. If you use it, add clarifying phrases (eg, *Impaired adjustment: Inability to resolve anger over illness*). When possible, use a different diagnostic label that identifies the specific way in which adjustment is impaired (eg, *Anxiety, Ineffective management of therapeutic regimen*).

Suggested Alternative Diagnoses

The following are examples of other diagnoses you might consider. Almost every NANDA label indicates some type of "impaired adjustment."

Coping, individual, ineffective
Grieving, dysfunctional

NOC Suggested Outcomes

Acceptance: Health Status: Reconciliation to health circumstances

Coping: Actions to manage stressors that tax an individual's resources

Grief Resolution: Adjustment to actual or impending loss

Health-Seeking Behavior: Actions to promote optimal wellness, recovery, and rehabilitation

Participation: Health Care Decisions: Personal involvement in selecting and evaluating health care options

Psychosocial Adjustment: Life Change: Psychosocial adaptation of an individual to a life change

Treatment Behavior: Illness or Injury: Personal actions to palliate or eliminate pathology

Goals/Evaluation Criteria

Examples Using NOC Language

- Demonstrates adjustment to changes in health status as evidenced by Acceptance: Health Status, Coping, Grief Resolution, Health-Seeking Behavior, Participation: Health Care Decisions, Psychosocial Adjustment: Life Change, and Treatment Behavior: Illness or Injury
- Demonstrates **Acceptance: Health Status**, as evidenced by the following indicators (specify 1–5: none, limited, moderate, substantial, or extensive):
    Relinquishment of previous concept of health
    Pursuit of information
    Demonstration of positive self-regard
    Health-related decision making

Other Examples

Patient will:
- Verbalize acceptance of changes in health status
- Verbalize feelings about the required lifestyle/behavior changes
- Begin to make lifestyle/behavior changes
- Identify priorities for own health outcomes
- Demonstrate decreased anxiety and fear in independent activities
- Comply with prescribed treatments

NIC Priority Interventions

Coping Enhancement: Assisting a patient to adapt to perceived stressors, changes, or threats which interfere with meeting life demands and roles

Nursing Activities

Assessments

- Assess patient's need for social support
- Assess amount/quality of social support available
- *(NIC) Coping Enhancement:*

    Appraise patient's adjustment to changes in body image, as indicated

    Appraise the impact of the patient's life situation on roles and relationships

    Evaluate the patient's decision-making ability

Collaborative Activities

- Refer patient to community agencies and/or support groups
- Include patient/family in a multidisciplinary conference to establish a plan of care. For example:

    Identify obstacles that hinder lifestyle/behavior changes

    Identify personal strengths that will facilitate goal achievement

    Review necessary lifestyle/behavior changes and select one as an initial goal

Other

- Provide a nonjudgmental environment in which patient/family can share concerns/anxieties/fears
- *(NIC) Coping Enhancement:*

    Assist the patient to identify available support systems [to learn new ways to cope and to decrease isolation and fear]

    Appraise and discuss alternative responses to situation

Airway Clearance, Ineffective
(1.5.1.2) (1980, 1996, 1998)

Definition: Inability to clear secretions or obstructions from the respiratory tract to maintain a clear airway

Defining Characteristics

Subjective
Dyspnea
Objective
Adventitious breath sounds (eg, rales, crackles, rhonchi, wheezes)
Changes in respiratory rate and rhythm
Ineffective or absent cough
Cyanosis
Difficulty vocalizing
Diminished breath sounds
Orthopnea
Restlessness
Sputum
Wide-eyed [look]

Related Factors

Environmental: Smoking, smoke inhalation, secondhand smoke

Obstructed Airway: Airway spasm, retained secretions, excessive mucus, presence of artificial airway, foreign body in airway, secretions in the bronchi, exudate in the alveoli

Physiological: Neuromuscular dysfunction, hyperplasia of the bronchial walls, chronic obstructive pulmonary disease, infection, asthma, allergic airways, trauma

Suggestions for Use

Use the key defining characteristics in Table 1 to discriminate carefully among this label and the two alternative respiratory diagnoses. If cough and gag reflexes are ineffective or absent secondary to anesthesia, use *Risk for aspiration* instead of *Ineffective airway clearance* in order to focus on preventing aspiration rather than teaching effective coughing.

Table 1

Nursing Diagnosis	Present	Not Present
Impaired Gas Exchange	Abnormal blood gases Hypoxia Changes in mental status	Ineffective cough Cough
Ineffective Breathing Pattern	"Appearance" of the patient's breathing: nasal flaring, use of accessory muscles, pursed-lip breathing	Tachycardia, restlessness Ineffective cough
	Abnormal blood gases	Obstruction or aspiration
Ineffective Airway Clearance	Cough, ineffective cough	Abnormal blood gases
	Changes in rate or depth of respirations	
	Usual cause is increased or tenacious secretions or obstruction (eg, aspiration)	

Suggested Alternative Diagnoses

Aspiration, risk for
Breathing pattern, ineffective
Gas exchange, impaired

NOC Suggested Outcomes

Respiratory Status: Gas Exchange: Alveolar exchange of CO_2 or O_2 to maintain arterial blood gas concentration

Respiratory Status: Ventilation: Movement of air in and out of the lungs

Symptom Control Behavior: Personal actions to minimize perceived adverse changes in physical and emotional functioning

Treatment Behaviors: Illness or Injury: Personal actions to palliate or eliminate pathology

Goals/Evaluation Criteria

Examples Using NOC Language

- Demonstrates effective airway clearance, as evidenced by Respiratory Status: Gas Exchange and Ventilation not compromised, Symptom Control Behavior consistently demonstrated, and Treatment Behaviors: Illness or Injury consistently demonstrated
- Demonstrates **Respiratory Status: Gas Exchange**, as evidenced by the following indicators (specify 1–5: extremely, substantially, moderately, mildly, or not compromised):

    Ease of breathing

    Restlessness, cyanosis, and dyspnea not present

    O_2 saturation within normal limits

    Chest x-ray findings in expected range

Other Examples

Patient will:

- Have a patent airway
- Expectorate secretions effectively
- Have respiratory rate and rhythm within normal range
- Have pulmonary function within normal limits
- Be able to describe plan for care at home

NIC Priority Interventions

Airway Management: Facilitation of patency of air passages

Airway Suctioning: Removal of airway secretions by inserting a suction catheter into the patient's oral airway and/or trachea

Nursing Activities

Assessments

- Assess and document the following:

    Effectiveness of oxygen administration and other treatments

    Effectiveness of prescribed medications

    Trends in arterial blood gases

- Auscultate anterior and posterior chest for decreased or absent ventilation and presence of adventitious sounds
- *(NIC) Airway Suctioning*

    Determine the need for oral and/or tracheal suctioning

    Monitor patient's oxygen status (SaO_2 and SvO_2 levels) and hemodynamic status (MAP [mean arterial pressure] level and cardiac rhythms) immediately before, during, and after suctioning

    Note type and amount of secretions obtained

Patient/Family Teaching

- Explain proper use of supportive equipment (eg, oxygen, suction, spirometer, inhalers, intermittent positive pressure breathing [IPPB])
- Inform patient and family that smoking is prohibited in room
- Instruct patient and family in plan for care at home (eg, medications, hydration, nebulization, equipment, postural drainage, signs and symptoms of complications, community resources)
- Instruct patient in coughing and deep-breathing techniques to facilitate removal of secretions
- Teach patient/family the significance of changes in sputum, such as color, character, amount, and odor
- *(NIC) Airway Suctioning:*
  Instruct the patient and/or family how to suction the airway, as appropriate

Collaborative Activities

- Confer with respiratory therapist, as needed
- Consult with physician concerning need for percussion and/or supportive equipment
- Administer humidified air/oxygen according to agency policies
- Perform/assist with aerosol, ultrasonic nebulizer, and other pulmonary treatments according to agency policies and protocols
- Notify physician of abnormal blood gases

Other

- Encourage physical activity to promote movement of secretions
- If patient unable to ambulate, turn patient from side to side at least q2h
- Inform patient before initiating procedures, to lower anxiety and increase sense of control
- Suction the nasopharynx/oropharynx to remove secretions q _____
- Perform endotracheal or nasotracheal suctioning, as appropriate. (Hyperoxygenate with ambu bag before and after suctioning ET tube or tracheostomy.)
- Maintain adequate hydration to decrease viscosity of secretions

Anxiety
(9.3.1) (1973, 1982, 1998)

Definition: A vague, uneasy feeling of discomfort or dread accompanied by an autonomic response; the source is often nonspecific or unknown to the individual; a feeling of apprehension caused by anticipation of danger. It is an alerting signal that warns of impending danger and enables the individual to take measures to deal with the threat.

Defining Characteristics

Behavioral
Diminished productivity
Expressed concerns due to change in life events
Extraneous movement (eg, foot shuffling, hand/arm movements)
Fidgeting
Glancing about
Insomnia
Poor eye contact
Restlessness
Scanning and vigilance

Affective
Anguish
Anxious
Apprehension
Distressed
Fearful
Feelings of inadequacy
Focus on self
Increased wariness
Irritability
Jittery
Overexcited
Painful and persistent increased helplessness
Rattled
Regretful
Scared
Uncertainty
Worried

Physiological

Insomnia

Shakiness

Trembling/hand tremors

Voice quivering

Parasympathetic

Abdominal pain

Decreased blood pressure

Decreased pulse

Diarrhea

Faintness

Fatigue

Nausea

Sleep disturbance

Tingling in extremities

Urinary frequency

Urinary hesitancy

Urinary urgency

Sympathetic

Anorexia

Cardiovascular excitation

Dry mouth

Facial flushing

Facial tension

Heart pounding

Increased blood pressure

Increased perspiration

Increased pulse

Increased reflexes

Increased respiration

Increased tension

Pupil dilation

Respiratory difficulties

Superficial vasoconstriction

Twitching

Weakness

Cognitive

Awareness of physiologic symptoms

Blocking of thought

Confusion

Decreased perceptual field

Difficulty concentrating

Diminished ability to problem solve
Diminished learning ability
Expressed concerns due to changes in life events
Fear of unspecific consequences
Focus on self
Forgetfulness
Impaired attention
Preoccupation
Rumination
Tendency to blame others

Related Factors

Exposure to toxins
Familial association/heredity
Interpersonal transmission/contagion
Situational/maturational crises
Stress
Substance abuse
Threat of death
Threat to or change in economic status
Threat to or change in role status and/or function
Threat to or change in environment
Threat to or change in health status
Threat to or change in interaction patterns
Threat to self-concept
Unconscious conflict about essential values/goals of life
Unmet needs

Suggestions for Use

Anxiety should be differentiated from *Fear* because the nursing actions may be different. When a patient is fearful, the nurse tries to remove the source of the fear or help the patient deal with the specific fear. When a patient is anxious, the nurse helps identify the cause of anxiety; however, when the source of anxiety cannot be identified, the nurse helps the patient explore and express anxious feelings.

Fear and *Anxiety* present diagnostic difficulty because they are not mutually exclusive. A person who is afraid is usually anxious as well. Impending surgery may be the etiology for *Fear*, but most of the feelings about surgery relate to *Anxiety*. Because the etiology (surgery) cannot be changed, nursing interventions should focus on supporting patient coping mechanisms for managing *Anxiety* (Carpenito 1997b, pp. 126–127).

Many of the same signs and symptoms are present in both *Fear* and *Anxiety:* increased heart and respiratory rate, dilated pupils, diaphoresis, muscle tension, and fatigue. The following comparisons in Table 2 may be helpful:

Table 2

	Anxiety	**Fear**
Physiologic Manifestations	Stimulation of the parasympathetic nervous system with increased gastrointestinal activity	Sympathetic response only; decreased gastrointestinal activity
Type of Threat	Usually psychologic (eg, to self-image); vague, nonspecific	Often physical (eg, to safety); specific, identifiable
Feeling	Vague, uneasy feeling	Feeling of dread, apprehension
Source of Feeling	Unknown by the person; unconscious	Known by the person

Because the level of anxiety influences the nursing activities, indicate in the diagnostic statement whether anxiety is moderate, severe, or panic-level. Panic may require collaborative interventions, such as medications. Mild anxiety is not a problem, because it is a normal condition present in all human beings. Diagnose *Anxiety* only for patients who require special nursing interventions. Mild anxiety before surgery is a normal, healthy response.

Mild anxiety: Present in day-to-day living; increases alertness and perceptual fields; motivates learning and growth

Moderate anxiety: Narrows perceptual fields; focus is on immediate concerns, with inattention to other communications and details

Severe anxiety: Very narrow focus on specific detail; all behavior is geared toward getting relief

Panic: The person loses control and feels dread and terror. A state of disorganization causes increased physical activity, distorted perceptions and relationships, and loss of rational thought. Panic can lead to exhaustion and death (Stuart and Sundeen 1995).

Suggested Alternative Diagnoses

Decisional conflict

Fear

Individual coping, ineffective

NOC Suggested Outcomes

Aggression Control: Ability to restrain assaultive, combative, or destructive behavior toward others

Anxiety Control: Ability to eliminate or reduce feelings of apprehension and tension from an unidentifiable source

Coping: Actions to manage stressors that tax an individual's resources

Impulse Control: Ability to self-restrain compulsive or impulsive behaviors

Self-Mutilation Restraint: Ability to refrain from intentional self-inflicted injury (nonlethal)

Social Interaction Skills: An individual's use of effective interaction behaviors

Goals/Evaluation Criteria

Examples Using NOC Language

- *Anxiety* relieved, as evidenced by consistently demonstrating Aggression Control, Anxiety Control, Coping, Impulse Control, Self-Mutilation Restraint, and substantially effective Social Interaction Skills
- Demonstrates **Anxiety Control**, as evidenced by the following indicators (specify 1–5: never, rarely, sometimes, often, or consistently demonstrated):
    Plans coping strategies for stressful situations
    Maintains role performance
    Reports absence of sensory perceptual disorders
    Reports absence of physical manifestations of anxiety
    Behavioral manifestations of anxiety absent

Other Examples

Patient will:

- Continue necessary activities even though anxiety persists
- Demonstrate ability to focus on new knowledge and skills
- Identify symptoms that are indicators of own anxiety
- Not demonstrate aggressive behaviors
- Communicate needs and negative feelings appropriately

NIC Priority Interventions

Anxiety Reduction: Minimizing apprehension, dread, foreboding, or uneasiness related to an unidentified source of anticipated danger

Nursing Activities

Assessments

- Assess and document patient's level of anxiety q _____
- Explore with patient techniques that have, and have not, reduced anxiety in the past.
- *(NIC) Anxiety Reduction:* Determine patient's decision-making ability

Patient/Family Teaching

- Develop teaching plan with realistic goals, including need for repetition, encouragement, and praise of the tasks learned
- *(NIC) Anxiety Reduction*:
  Provide factual information concerning diagnosis, treatment, and prognosis
  Instruct patient on the use of relaxation techniques
  Explain all procedures, including sensations likely to be experienced during the procedure

Collaborative Activities

- *(NIC) Anxiety Reduction*: Administer medications to reduce anxiety, as appropriate

Other

- Encourage patient to verbalize thoughts and feelings to externalize anxiety
- Help patient to focus on the present situation as a means of identifying coping mechanisms needed to reduce anxiety
- Provide diversion through television, radio, games, and occupational therapies to reduce anxiety and expand focus
- Provide positive reinforcement when patient is able to continue activities of daily living and other activities despite anxiety
- Reassure patient by touch and empathetic verbal and nonverbal exchanges, encourage patient to express anger and irritation, and allow patient to cry
- Reduce excessive stimulation by providing a quiet environment, limited contact with others if necessary, and limited use of caffeine and other stimulants

- Suggest alternative therapies for reducing anxiety that are acceptable to patient
- *(NIC) Anxiety Reduction:*
  Use a calm, reassuring approach
  Clearly state expectations for patient's behavior
  Stay with patient [eg, during procedures] to promote safety and reduce fear
  Administer back rub/neck rub, as appropriate
  Keep treatment equipment out of sight
  Help patient identify situations that precipitate anxiety
  Encourage parents to stay with child, as appropriate

Anxiety, Death
(9.3.1.1) (1998)

Definition: The apprehension, worry, or fear related to death or dying

Defining Characteristics

Subjective

Anticipated pain related to dying

Concern about meeting one's creator or feeling doubtful about the existence of a god or higher being

Concerns of overworking the caregiver as terminal illness incapacitates self

Deep sadness

Denial of one's own mortality or impending death

Fear of delayed demise

Fear of developing a terminal illness

Fear of leaving family alone after death

Fear of loss of physical and/or mental abilities when dying

Fear of premature death because it prevents the accomplishment of important life goals

Fear of the process of dying

Negative death images or unpleasant thoughts about any event related to death or dying

Powerlessness over issues related to dying

Total loss of control over any aspect of one's own death

Worrying about being the cause of others' grief and suffering

Worrying about the impact of one's own death on significant others

Related Factors

To be developed

Suggestions for Use

Always use the most specific label. For example, if a dying patient's anxiety is related to death or dying, use *Death anxiety*. If not, use the broader label, *Anxiety*.

Suggested Alternative Diagnoses

Anxiety
Sorrow, chronic
Spiritual distress

NOC Suggested Outcomes

Not yet developed

Goals/Evaluation Criteria

Patient will:
- Maintain psychologic comfort during the process of dying
- Verbalize feelings (eg, anger, sorrow, or loss) and thoughts with staff and/or significant others
- Identify areas of personal control
- Express positive feelings about relationships with significant others
- Accept limitations and seek help as needed

NIC Priority Interventions

To be developed

Nursing Activities

Assessments
- Monitor for signs and symptoms of anxiety (eg, vital signs, appetite, sleep patterns, concentration level)
- Assess support provided by significant others
- Monitor for expressions of hopelessness or powerlessness (eg, "I can't")
- Determine sources of anxiety (eg, fear of pain, body malfunction, humiliation, abandonment, nonbeing, negative impact on survivors)

Patient/Family Teaching

- Provide information about the patient's illness and prognosis
- Provide honest and direct answers to the patient's questions about the dying process

Collaborative Activities

- Refer to home care or hospice care, as appropriate
- Arrange access to clergy or spiritual advisors as patient wishes
- Connect patient and family with appropriate support groups

Other

- Support spiritual needs without imposing own beliefs on patient
- Use therapeutic communication skills to build trusting relationship and facilitate expression of patient needs
- Listen attentively
- Offer support for difficult feelings without offering false reassurance or too much advice
- Encourage patient to express feelings with significant others
- Help patient to identify areas of personal control; offer choices and options to the extent of the patient's ability
- Spend time with patient to deter fear of being alone
- Assist patient to reminisce and review personal life positively
- Identify and support the patient's usual coping strategies
- Provide for physical comfort and security

Aspiration, Risk for
(1.6.1.4) (1988)

Definition: The state in which an individual is at risk for entry of gastrointestinal secretions, oropharyngeal secretions, or solids or fluids into tracheobronchial passages

Risk Factors

Objective

Decreased gastrointestinal motility

Delayed gastric emptying [eg, secondary to ileus or intestinal obstruction]

Depressed cough and gag reflexes

Facial/oral/neck surgery or trauma

Gastrointestinal tubes

Hindered elevation of upper body

Impaired swallowing
Incomplete lower esophageal sphincter
Increased gastric residual
Increased intragastric pressure
Medication administration
Presence of tracheostomy or endotracheal tube
Reduced level of consciousness [eg, secondary to anesthesia, head injury, cerebrovascular accident, seizures]
Tube feedings
Wired jaws

Suggestions for Use

Always use the most specific label for which the patient has the necessary defining characteristics. Do not use *Risk for injury* if the patient has the defining characteristics or risk factors for *Risk for aspiration*

Suggested Alternative Diagnoses

Airway clearance, ineffective
Injury, risk for
Self-care deficit: feeding
Swallowing, impaired

NOC Suggested Outcomes

Cognitive Ability: Ability to execute complex mental processes
Immobility Consequences: Physiological: Compromise in physiologic functioning due to impaired physical mobility
Neurological Status: Extent to which the peripheral and central nervous systems receive, process, and respond to internal and external stimuli

Goals/Evaluation Criteria

Examples Using NOC Language

- Will not aspirate, as evidenced by uncompromised Cognitive Ability and Neurological Status and no Physiological Immobility Consequences
- Will demonstrate **Cognitive Ability,** as evidenced by the following indicators (specify 1–5: extremely, substantially, moderately, mildly, or not compromised):
    Attentiveness, concentration, and orientation
    Information processing
    Immediate, recent, and remote memory

Other Examples

Patient will:

- Demonstrate improved swallowing
- Tolerate oral intake and secretions without aspiration
- Tolerate enteral feedings without aspiration
- Have clear lung sounds and patent airway
- Maintain adequate muscle strength and tone

NIC Priority Interventions

Aspiration Precautions: Prevention or minimization of risk factors in the patient at risk for aspiration

Nursing Activities

Assessments

- Check gastric residual prior to feeding and giving medications
- Monitor for signs of aspiration during feedings: coughing, choking, drooling
- Verify placement of enteral tube prior to feeding and giving medications
- Evaluate family's comfort level with feeding, suctioning, positioning, and so forth
- *(NIC) Aspiration Precautions:*

  Monitor level of consciousness, cough reflex, gag reflex, and swallowing ability

  Monitor pulmonary status [eg, before and after feeding and before and after giving medication]

Patient/Family Teaching

- Instruct family in feeding/swallowing techniques
- Instruct family in use of suction for removal of secretions
- Review with patient/family signs and symptoms of aspiration and preventive measures
- Help family to create an emergency plan in case patient aspirates at home

Collaborative Activities

- Report any change in color of lung secretions that resembles food or feeding intake
- Request occupational therapy consultation
- *(NIC) Aspiration Precautions:* Suggest speech pathology consult as appropriate

Other

- Allow patient time to swallow
- Have a suction catheter available at the bedside and suction during meals, as needed
- Involve the family during patient's ingestion of food and meals
- Provide support and reassurance
- Place the patient in semi- or high-Fowler position when eating, if possible
- Place patients who are unable to sit upright on their sides and elevate the head of the bed as much as possible during and after feedings
- Provide positive reinforcement for attempts to swallow independently
- Use a syringe, if necessary, when feeding the patient
- Vary consistency of foods to identify those foods more easily tolerated
- *(NIC) Aspiration Precautions:*
  Keep head of bed elevated 30 to 45 minutes after feeding
  Cut food into small pieces
  Feed in small amounts
  Avoid liquids or use thickening agent
  Place "dye" in NG [nasogastric] feeding
  Break or crush pills before administration
  Request medication in elixir form
- *For children:*
  Choose age-appropriate toys with no small, removable parts; do not give balloons to small children
  Avoid foods such as nuts, gum, grapes, and small candy
  Teach parents not to prop bottle

Body Image Disturbance
(7.1.1) (1973, 1998)

Definition: Confusion in mental picture of one's physical self

Defining Characteristics

Either (A) or (B) must be present to justify the diagnosis of *Body image disturbance.* The remaining defining characteristics may be used to validate the presence of (A) or (B).

(A) Verbal response to actual or perceived change in structure or function

(B) Nonverbal response to actual or perceived change in structure or function

Subjective

Depersonalization of [body] part or loss by impersonal pronouns

Emphasis on remaining strengths and heightened achievement

Fear of rejection or of reaction by others

Focus on past strength, function, or appearance

Negative feelings about body (eg, feelings of helplessness, hopelessness, or powerlessness)

Personalization of body part or loss by name

Preoccupation with change or loss

Refusal to verify actual change

Verbalization of change in lifestyle

Objective

Actual change in [body] structure or function

Change in ability to estimate spatial relationship of body to environment

Change in social involvement

Hiding or overexposing body part (intentional or unintentional)

Missing body part

Not looking at body part

Not touching body part

Showing reluctance to touch or look at affected body part

Trauma to nonfunctioning body part

Related Factors

Biophysical [eg, chronic illness, congenital defects, pregnancy]

Cognitive/perceptual [eg, chronic pain]

Cultural or spiritual

Developmental changes

Illness

Psychosocial [eg, eating disorders]

[Situational crisis (specify)]

Trauma or injury

Treatments [eg, surgery, chemotherapy, radiation]

Suggestions for Use

This label is related to *Self-esteem disturbance* but is specific to negative feelings about one's body or body parts. Although *Body image disturbance* is often caused by loss of a body part or actual body changes, the changes in body structure or function can be perceived rather than actual. Patients on prolonged bed rest or who are dependent on machines (eg, dialysis equipment, respirators) may experience distortion of body image. Eating disorders are often related to *Body image disturbance*.

Suggested Alternative Diagnoses

Nutrition: less than body requirements, altered
Nutrition: more than body requirements, altered
Self-esteem disturbance

NOC Suggested Outcomes

Body Image: Positive perception of own appearance and body functions

Child Development: 2 Years: Milestones of physical, cognitive, and psychosocial progression by 2 years of age. **NOTE:** NOC also suggests **Child Development** outcomes for 3, 4, and 5 years; middle childhood (6–11 years); and adolescence (12–17 years), all having the same definition

Distorted Thought Control: Ability to self-restrain disruption in perception, thought processes, and thought content

Grief Resolution: Adjustment to actual or impending loss

Psychosocial Adjustment: Life Change: Psychosocial adaptation of an individual to a life change

Self-Esteem: Personal judgment of self-worth

Goals/Evaluation Criteria

Examples Using NOC Language

- *Body image disturbance* alleviated as demonstrated by Positive Body Image, no delay in Child Development, consistently demonstrated Distorted Thought Control, Grief Resolution (to a great extent), substantial Psychosocial Adjustment: Life Change, and positive Self-Esteem
- Demonstrates **Body Image**, as evidenced by the following indicators (specify 1–5: never, rarely, sometimes, often, or consistently positive):

    Congruence between body reality, body ideal, and body presentation

    Satisfaction with body appearance and function

    Willingness to touch affected body part

Other Examples

Patient will:
- Identify personal strengths

- Acknowledge impact of situation on existing personal relationships and lifestyle
- Acknowledge the actual change in body appearance
- Describe actual change in body function
- Express willingness to use suggested resources after discharge
- Maintain close social interaction and personal relationships

NIC Priority Interventions

Body Image Enhancement: Improving a patient's conscious and unconscious perceptions and attitudes toward his/her body

Nursing Activities

Assessments

- Assess and document patient's verbal and nonverbal responses to his/her body
- *(NIC) Body Image Enhancement:*
  Determine how child responds to parents' reactions, as appropriate
  Determine patient's body image expectations based on developmental stage
  Determine whether perceived dislike for certain physical characteristics creates a dysfunctional social paralysis for teenagers and other high-risk groups
  Determine whether a recent physical change has been incorporated into patient's body image
  Identify the significance of the patient's culture, religion, race, gender, and age on body image
  Monitor frequency of statements of self-criticism

Patient/Family Teaching

- *(NIC) Body Image Enhancement:* Teach parents the importance of their responses to the child's body changes and future adjustment, as appropriate

Collaborative Activities

- Refer to social services department for planning care with patient/family
- Offer to make initial phone call to appropriate community resources for patient/family

Other

- Actively listen to patient/family and acknowledge reality of concerns about treatments, progress, and prognosis
- Encourage patient/family to air feelings and to grieve
- Assist patient/family to identify coping mechanisms and personal strengths and acknowledge limitations
- Provide care in a nonjudgmental manner, maintaining the patient's privacy and dignity
- Encourage patient to:
    Maintain usual daily grooming routine
    Verbalize concerns about close personal relationships
    Verbalize consequences of physical and emotional changes
        that have influenced self-concept
- *(NIC) Body Image Enhancement:*
    Identify means of reducing the impact of any disfigurement
        through clothing, wigs, or cosmetics, as appropriate.
    Facilitate contact with individuals with similar changes in body
        image
    Use self-picture drawing as a mechanism for evaluating a child's
        body image perceptions
    Instruct children about the functions of the various body parts,
        as appropriate
    Use self-disclosure exercises with groups of teenagers or others
        distraught over normal physical attributes

Body Temperature, Risk for Altered
(1.2.2.1) (1986)

Definition: The state in which the individual is at risk for failure to maintain body temperature within normal range

Risk Factors

Objective
Altered metabolic rate
Dehydration
Exposure to extremes in environmental temperatures
Extremes of age
Extremes of weight
Illness or trauma affecting temperature regulation
[Immaturity of newborn's temperature-regulating system]
[Inability to perspire]

Inactivity
Inappropriate clothing for environmental temperature
[Low birth weight (neonate)]
Medications causing vasoconstriction or vasodilation
Sedation
Vigorous activity

Suggestions for Use

If the patient is at risk for both *Hypothermia* and *Hyperthermia,* then *Risk for altered body temperature* is the appropriate diagnosis. If the patient is at risk for only an elevation in temperature, use *Risk for hyperthermia;* if at risk for only decreased body temperature, use *Risk for hypothermia.*

Suggested Alternative Diagnoses

Hyperthermia
Hypothermia
Thermoregulation, ineffective

NOC Suggested Outcomes

Hydration: Amount of water in the intracellular and extracellular compartments of the body
Infection Status: Presence and extent of infection

Goals/Evaluation Criteria

Examples Using NOC Language

- Exhibits **Hydration**, as evidenced by the following indicators (specify 1–5: extremely, substantially, moderately, mildly, or not compromised):
    Skin hydration
    Neonate: No lethargy
    Moist mucous membranes
    Sunken eyes not present
    Perspiration ability

Other Examples

Patient will:
- Describe adaptive measures to minimize fluctuations in body temperature
- Report early signs/symptoms of hypothermia/hyperthermia
- Maintain body temperature within normal range

NIC Priority Interventions

Temperature Regulation: Attaining and/or maintaining body temperature within a normal range

Temperature Regulation: Intraoperative: Attaining and/or maintaining desired intraoperative body temperature

Vital Signs Monitoring: Collection and analysis of cardiovascular, respiratory, and body temperature data to determine and prevent complications

Nursing Activities

Assessments

- Evaluate home environment for factors that may alter body temperature
- Assess for early signs and symptoms of hypothermia/ hyperthermia
- *(NIC) Temperature Regulation:*
  Monitor temperature at least every 2 h, as appropriate
  Monitor for and report signs and symptoms of hypothermia and hyperthermia
  Monitor newborn's temperature until stabilized
  Wrap infant immediately after birth to prevent heat loss

Patient/Family Teaching

- Instruct patient/family in measures to minimize temperature fluctuations:

    For Hyperthermia
    Drink adequate fluids
    Limit activity on hot days
    Lose weight, if obese
    Maintain stable environmental temperature
    Remove excess clothing

    For Hypothermia
    Bathe in warm room, away from drafts
    Increase activity
    Limit alcohol intake
    Maintain adequate nourishment
    Maintain stable environmental temperature
    Wear adequate clothing

- Instruct patient/family to recognize and report early signs and symptoms of hypothermia/hyperthermia:

    For Hyperthermia Dry skin, headache, increased pulse,

increased temperature, irritability, temperature above 37.8C or 100F, weakness

For Hypothermia Apathy; cold, hard abdomen that feels like marble; disorientation/confusion; drowsiness; hypertension; hypoglycemia; impaired ability to think; reduced pulse and respirations; skin hard and cold to touch; temperature of less than 95F

Collaborative Activities

- Report to physician if adequate hydration cannot be maintained
- *(NIC) Temperature Regulation:* Administer antipyretic medication, as appropriate

Other

- Dry and swaddle infant (or place skin-to-skin with mother) immediately after birth to prevent heat loss by evaporation
- *(NIC) Temperature Regulation:* Adjust environmental temperature to patient needs.

Breastfeeding, Effective
(6.5.1.3) (1990)

Definition: The state in which a mother-infant dyad/family exhibits adequate proficiency and satisfaction with breastfeeding process.

Defining Characteristics

Subjective

Contentment of infant after feeding

Maternal verbalization of satisfaction with the breastfeeding process

Objective

Ability of mother to position infant at breast to promote a successful latch-on response

Adequate infant elimination patterns for age

Appropriate infant weight pattern for age

Eagerness of infant to nurse

Effective mother-infant communication patterns [eg, infant cues, maternal interpretation or response]

Regular and sustained suckling/swallowing at breast

Signs and/or symptoms of oxytocin release [letdown or milk ejection reflex]

Related Factors

Basic breastfeeding knowledge
Infant gestational age greater than 34 weeks
Maternal confidence
Normal breast structure
Normal infant oral structure
Supportive source

Suggestions for Use

This is a wellness diagnosis. It represents a clinical judgment that breastfeeding is progressing satisfactorily and that there are no risk factors for *Ineffective breastfeeding.* During the first few days after childbirth, the nursing focus is to eliminate risk factors that might cause *Ineffective breastfeeding.* It is probably too soon, during that time, to conclude that there are no problems or risk factors, so a better choice might be *Risk for ineffective breast-feeding.*

Suggested Alternative Diagnoses

Ineffective breastfeeding, risk for

NOC Suggested Outcomes

Breastfeeding Establishment: Infant: Proper attachment of an infant to and sucking from the mother's breast for nourishment during the first 2–3 weeks

Breastfeeding Establishment: Maternal: Maternal establishment of proper attachment of an infant to and sucking from the breast for nourishment during the first 2–3 weeks

Breastfeeding Maintenance: Continued nourishment of an infant through breastfeeding

Breastfeeding Weaning: Process leading to the eventual discontinuation of breastfeeding

Goals/Evaluation Criteria

Examples Using NOC Language

See "Ineffective Breastfeeding," pp. 42–43.

Other Examples

- Mother and infant will establish and maintain breastfeeding for as long as desired
- Infant will demonstrate correct:
    Alignment and areolar grasp

Latching-on technique and tongue placement

Suck and audible swallow

- Mother will:

    Recognize early hunger cues

    State satisfaction with breastfeeding

    Experience no nipple tenderness

    Verbalize knowledge of signs of decreased milk supply

    Explain how to safely collect and store breast milk

NIC Priority Interventions

Breastfeeding Assistance: Preparing a new mother to breastfeed her infant

Nursing Activities

Early Postpartum

Assessments

- Observe for correct breastfeeding technique
- *(NIC) Breastfeeding Assistance:*

    Monitor infant's ability to suck

    Monitor infant's ability to grasp the nipple correctly (ie, "latch-on" skills)

    Monitor skin integrity of nipples

    Monitor letdown reflex

Patient/Family Teaching

- Discuss breastfeeding schedule, usually a "demand" time every $1^1/_2$ to 3 hours
- Instruct mother in usual breastfeeding norms (eg, increased frequency of nursing in first weeks of life, baby's elimination patterns, uterine contractions during nursing)
- Provide anticipatory guidance for potential problems such as maternal fatigue; breast engorgement; sore, cracked nipples; multiple births
- Discuss ways to enhance milk supply:

    Drink plenty of fluids

    Get enough rest (eg, between feedings)

    Nurse frequently

    Use alternate breast at start of each feeding
- *(NIC) Breastfeeding Assistance:*

    Assist parents in identifying infant arousal cues as opportunities to practice breastfeeding

    Encourage mother not to restrict infant sucking time

Inform mother of pump options available if needed to maintain lactation

Encourage use of comfortable, cotton, supportive nursing bra

Provide written materials to reinforce instructions at home

Collaborative Activities

- Make referrals to appropriate community resources, such as La Leche League, other nursing mothers, lactation consultant

Other

- Promote maternal confidence by providing positive feedback
- Provide opportunity to breastfeed within 1–2 hours after birth

Home Care

Assessments

- Assess breastfeeding technique within first 5–7 days after birth
- Confirm infant's elimination pattern
- Explore mother's breastfeeding plans, eg, duration, return to work, introduction of solid foods, weaning; provide anticipatory guidance

Patient/Family Teaching

- Discuss mother's need to check with physician prior to taking any medication while breastfeeding
- Provide instruction regarding breast engorgement, cracked/ sore nipples, manual expression, infant appetite spurts, supplemental feedings

Collaborative Activities

- Encourage mother to enlist/request available resources for assistance (eg, family, public health nurse, pediatrician, La Leche League, Nursing Mothers' Council)

Other

- Discuss impact of breastfeeding on family dynamics
- Discuss setting priorities that delegate meal preparation, increase mother's rest, and minimize care of the house
- Promote maternal confidence by providing encouragement, praise, and reassurance

Breastfeeding, Ineffective
(6.5.1.2) (1988)

Definition: The state in which mother, infant, or child experiences
dissatisfaction or difficulty with the breastfeeding process

Defining Characteristics

Subjective
Perceived inadequate milk supply
Unsatisfactory breastfeeding process [as stated by mother]

Objective
Actual inadequate milk supply
Arching and crying at the breast
Fussiness and crying within the first hour after breastfeeding
Inability of infant to latch onto maternal breast correctly
Insufficient emptying of each breast per feeding
Insufficient opportunity for suckling at the breast
No observable signs of oxytocin release
Nonsustained suckling at the breast
Observable signs of inadequate infant intake
Persistence of sore nipples beyond the first week of breastfeeding
Resistance to latching on
Unresponsiveness to other comfort measures

Related Factors

Inadequate sucking reflex in infant
Infant anomaly
Infant receiving supplemental feedings with artificial nipple
Interruption in breastfeeding
Knowledge deficit
Maternal anxiety or ambivalence
Maternal breast anomaly
Nonsupportive partner/family
Prematurity
Previous breast surgery
Previous history of breastfeeding failure

Suggestions for Use

This diagnosis focuses on the mother's satisfaction with the
breastfeeding process and includes an actual or perceived inade-

quate milk supply. The comparisons in Table 3 may be helpful in determining a diagnosis.

Table 3

Diagnosis	Cues (Defining Characteristics)
Ineffective breastfeeding	Dissatisfaction with feeding process
Ineffective infant feeding pattern	Inability of infant to suck or poorly coordinated suck-swallow response
Interrupted breastfeeding	Mother wishes to maintain lactation but unable to put baby to breast for some feedings (eg, illness or working)

Suggested Alternative Diagnoses

Breastfeeding, interrupted
Infant feeding pattern, ineffective

NOC Suggested Outcomes

Breastfeeding Establishment: Infant: Proper attachment of an infant to and sucking from the mother's breast for nourishment during the first 2–3 weeks

Breastfeeding Establishment: Maternal: Maternal establishment of proper attachment of an infant to and sucking from the breast for nourishment during the first 2–3 weeks

Breastfeeding Maintenance: Continued nourishment of an infant through breastfeeding

Breastfeeding Weaning: Process leading to the eventual discontinuation of breastfeeding

Knowledge: Breastfeeding: Extent of understanding conveyed about lactation and nourishment of infant through breastfeeding

Goals/Evaluation Criteria

Examples Using NOC Language

- Mother and infant will experience *Effective breastfeeding* as demonstrated by Knowledge: Breastfeeding; Breastfeeding Establishment: Infant/Maternal; Breastfeeding Maintenance; and Breastfeeding Weaning

- Infant will demonstrate **Breastfeeding Establishment: Infant,** as evidenced by the following indicators (specify 1–5: not, slightly, moderately, substantially, or totally adequate):

    Proper alignment and latch on

    Proper areolar grasp and compression

    Correct suck and tongue placement

    Audible swallow

    Minimum eight feedings per day (on demand)

    Age-appropriate weight gain

    Infant contentment after feeding

Other Examples

Mother will:

- Maintain effective breastfeeding for as long as desired
- Describe increasing confidence with breastfeeding
- Recognize early hunger cues
- Indicate satisfaction with breastfeeding
- Not experience nipple tenderness
- Recognize signs of decreased milk supply

NIC Priority Interventions

Lactation Counseling: Use of an interactive helping process to assist in maintenance of successful breastfeeding

Nursing Activities

Assessments

- Assess infant's ability to latch on and suck effectively
- *(NIC) Lactation Counseling:*

    Evaluate newborn suck/swallow pattern

    Determine mother's desire and motivation to breastfeed

    Evaluate mother's understanding of infant's feeding cues (eg, rooting, sucking, and alertness)

    Monitor maternal skill with latching infant onto the nipple

    Monitor skin integrity of nipples

    Evaluate understanding of plugged milk ducts and mastitis

    Monitor ability to correctly relieve breast congestion

Patient/Family Teaching

- Instruct mother in breastfeeding techniques that increase her skill in feeding infant. Consider relaxation techniques, comfortable positioning, stimulation of rooting reflex, establishment of infant alert state before attempting to feed, stimulation of infant to continue to feed, and alternation of breasts.

- Instruct mother in breast-pumping techniques to maintain milk supply during interruptions or delays in infant sucking reflex
- Instruct mother in need for adequate rest and intake of fluids
- *(NIC) Lactation Counseling:*
  Provide information about advantages and disadvantages of breastfeeding
  Discuss alternative methods of feeding
  Correct misconceptions, misinformation, and inaccuracies about breastfeeding
  Demonstrate suck training, as appropriate
  Instruct about infant stool and urination patterns, as appropriate
  Recommend nipple care, as needed
  Instruct on signs of problems to report to health care practitioner
  Discuss signs of readiness to wean

Collaborative Activities

- Refer to appropriate community resources, such as La Leche League and Public Health Department

Other

- Have mother express enough milk to relieve engorgement, allowing nipples to evert
- Increase number of nursings on demand for a crying, wakeful infant
- Increase number of scheduled nursings for the sleepy infant of low birth weight
- Offer food and fluids to mother during day and evening prior to breastfeeding times
- Provide privacy for mother and infant
- Recognize "time-out" behaviors in premature infant
- Schedule rest periods, as needed
- Reinforce successful behaviors
- *(NIC) Lactation Counseling:*
  Provide support of mother's decisions
  Encourage continued lactation on return to work or school

Breastfeeding, Interrupted
(6.5.1.2.1) (1992)

Definition: A break in the continuity of the breastfeeding process as a result of inability or inadvisability to put baby to breast for feeding

Defining Characteristics

Subjective

Maternal desire to maintain lactation and provide (or eventually provide) her breast milk for her infant's nutritional needs

Objective

Infant does not receive nourishment at the breast for some or all of feedings

Lack of knowledge regarding expression and storage of breast milk

Separation of mother and infant

Related Factors

Abrupt weaning of infant

Contraindications to breastfeeding

[Engorgement]

Maternal employment [obligations outside the home]

Maternal medications that are contraindicated for the infant

Maternal or infant illness

Prematurity

[Sore/cracked nipples]

Suggestions for Use

Because this diagnosis represents a situation rather than a response, there is little the nurse can do to correct the interruption (eg, the need for the mother to work). Therefore, this label might function best as an etiology (eg, *Risk for ineffective breastfeeding related to Interrupted breastfeeding secondary to mother's employment*). Also see "Suggestions for Use" for "Ineffective Breastfeeding," on pp. 41–42.

Suggested Alternative Diagnoses

Breastfeeding, ineffective

Infant feeding pattern, ineffective

NOC Suggested Outcomes

Breastfeeding Establishment: Infant: Proper attachment of an infant to and sucking from the mother's breast for nourishment during the first 2–3 weeks of life

Breastfeeding Establishment: Maternal: Maternal establishment of proper attachment of an infant to and sucking from the breast for nourishment during the first 2–3 weeks

Breastfeeding Maintenance: Continued nourishment of an infant through breastfeeding

Knowledge: Breastfeeding: Extent of understanding conveyed about lactation and nourishment of infant through breastfeeding

Parent-Infant Attachment: Behaviors which demonstrate an enduring affectionate bond between a parent and infant

Goals/Evaluation Criteria

Examples Using NOC Language

- Mother and baby will not experience *Interrupted breastfeeding*, as evidenced by substantial Breastfeeding Knowledge, Establishment and Maintenance of Breastfeeding, and consistently demonstrated Parent-Infant Attachment.
- Mother and baby will demonstrate **Breastfeeding Maintenance**, as evidenced by the following indicators (specify 1–5: not, slightly, moderately, substantially, or totally adequate):

    Infant growth and development in normal range
    Recognition of signs of decreased milk supply
    Mother's continuation of lactation on return to work or school
    Mother's ability to safely collect and store breast milk, if desired
    Care provider's ability to safely thaw, warm and feed stored breastmilk

Other Examples

- Mother and/or infant will maintain effective breastfeeding for as long as desired

Mother will:

- Choose and demonstrate preferred technique for expression of milk
- Describe safe storage techniques for expressed milk

Baby will:

- Receive mother's milk
- Gain _____ grams/day or _____ grams/week

NIC Priority Interventions

Bottle Feeding: Preparation and administration of fluids to an infant via a bottle

Emotional Support: Provision of reassurance, acceptance, and encouragement during times of stress

Lactation Counseling: Use of an interactive helping process to assist in maintenance of successful breastfeeding

Nursing Activities

Assessments

- Assess family's ability to support lactation/breastfeeding plan and cope with lifestyle changes
- Assess mother's desire and motivation to continue breastfeeding
- Confirm readiness for transition to breast after interruption (eg, infant's stability when outside the isolette, infant's coordination of sucking/swallowing/breathing, mother's willingness to try)
- Consider a feeding flow sheet to facilitate assessment: Document infant's state, oxygen needs, positioning, time at breast, total nursing time, daily weight, stool pattern
- *(NIC) Bottle Feeding:*

  Determine water source used to dilute concentrated or powdered formula

  Determine fluoride content of water used to dilute concentrated or powdered formula and refer for fluoride supplementation, if indicated

  Monitor infant weight, as appropriate

Patient/Family Teaching

- Assist working mother to maintain lactation by including the following teaching:

  Provide information about lactation and breast-milk expression (with manual and electric pump), collection, and storage

  Display/demonstrate variety of breast pumps, providing information about costs, effectiveness, and availability of each

  Educate infant caretaker on topics such as storage and thawing of breastmilk and avoidance of bottle feedings in the 2 hours prior to mother's return home

  Provide information to enhance milk volume on topics such as adequate rest, regular expression of milk, increase in mother's intake of fluid, especially toward the end of the work week

  Instruct on how to relactate, as appropriate

- *(NIC) Bottle Feeding:* Caution parent or caregiver about using microwave oven to warm formula

Other

- Assist mother in setting realistic goals for herself
- Encourage continued feeding of breast milk on return to work or school
- Assist mother and premature infant with transition to breast:
    Encourage skin-to-skin contact for mother and infant, using cover blanket over infant to maintain body temperature
    Help infant open mouth wider
    Position baby with one hand supporting head, leaving the other hand free to manipulate breast; ear, shoulder, and hips of infant should be aligned so that mother's nipples do not become sore
    Provide privacy
- Assist working mother to maintain lactation and effective breastfeeding:
    A few days before mother's return to work, introduce baby to bottle in different situations: someone other than mother presents bottle, mother is not present, baby is hungry, in a different place than usual place for breastfeeding
    Develop schedule for expression and storage of milk at work
    Establish support network to ensure that mother has help with day-to-day lactation/breastfeeding problems as they occur
    Provide anticipatory guidance for potential problems (eg, engorgement, pain, leaking, diminished milk production, feelings of disappointment/anger, depression, guilt, inadequacy)
    Allow infant, once latched on, to nurse until sucking and swallowing stop; switch baby to other breast and repeat until suck/swallow stops, then switch back. Time at breast will be longer than at bottle, but not to the point of infant's exhaustion.
- If abrupt weaning is necessary, assist mother to:
    Introduce bottle feeding
    Manage breast discomfort
    Verbalize feelings about sudden change in plans

Breathing Pattern, Ineffective
(1.5.1.3) (1980, 1996, 1998)

Definition: Inspiration and/or expiration that does not provide adequate ventilation

Defining Characteristics

Subjective

Dyspnea

Shortness of breath

Objective

Altered chest excursion

Assumption of three-point position

Decreased inspiratory/expiratory pressure

Decreased minute ventilation

Decreased vital capacity

Depth of breathing (adults V_T 500 mL at rest, infants 6–8 mL/k)

Increased anterior-posterior diameter

Nasal flaring

Orthopnea

Prolonged expiration phases

Pursed-lip breathing

Respiratory rate (adults ages 14 or older <11–24 [breaths per minute], infants 25–60, ages 1–4 <20–30, ages 5–14 <15–25)

Timing ratio

Use of accessory muscles to breathe

Related Factors

Anxiety

Body position

Bony deformity

Chest wall deformity

Decreased energy/fatigue

Hyperventilation

Hypoventilation syndrome

Musculoskeletal impairment

Neurological immaturity

Neuromuscular dysfunction

Obesity

Pain

Perception/cognitive impairment

Respiratory muscle fatigue
Spinal cord injury

Suggestions for Use

Do not use this label if the condition cannot be treated by independent nursing actions. Consider, too, that *Ineffective breathing pattern* may be a symptom of another more useful diagnosis, such as *Anxiety*; or it may be the etiology of another diagnosis, such as *Activity intolerance.* Differentiate carefully among this and the suggested alternative diagnoses. Also see "Suggestions for Use" for "Airway Clearance, Ineffective," pp. 15–16.

Suggested Alternative Diagnoses

Activity intolerance
Airway clearance, ineffective
Gas exchange, impaired

NOC Suggested Outcomes

Respiratory Status: Ventilation: Movement of air in and out of the lungs
Vital Signs Status: Temperature, pulse, respiration, and blood pressure within expected range for the individual

Goals/Evaluation Criteria

Examples Using NOC Language

- Demonstrates effective breathing patterns, as evidenced by uncompromised Respiratory Status: Ventilation and Vital Signs Status
- Demonstrates uncompromised **Respiratory Status: Ventilation,** as evidenced by the following indicators (specify 1–5: extremely, substantially, moderately, mildly, or not compromised):
    Depth of inspiration and ease of breathing
    Chest expansion symmetric
    Accessory muscle use not present
    Adventitious breath sounds not present
    Shortness of breath not present

Other Examples

Patient will:
- Demonstrate optimal breathing while on mechanical ventilator
- Have respiratory rate and rhythm within normal limits
- Have pulmonary function within normal limits for patient

- Request breathing assistance when needed
- Be able to describe plan for care at home

NIC Priority Interventions

Airway Management: Facilitation of patency of air passages
Respiratory Monitoring: Collection and analysis of patient data to ensure airway patency and adequate gas exchange

Nursing Activities

Assessments

- Monitor for pallor and cyanosis
- Monitor effect of medications on respiratory status
- Determine location and extent of crepitus over rib cage
- Assess need for airway insertion
- Observe and document bilateral chest expansion of patient on ventilator
- *(NIC) Respiratory Monitoring:*
  Monitor rate, rhythm, depth, and effort of respirations
  Note chest movement, watching for symmetry, use of accessory muscles, and supraclavicular and intercostal muscle retractions
  Monitor for noisy respirations, such as crowing or snoring
  Monitor breathing patterns: bradypnea; tachypnea; hyperventilation; Kussmaul's respirations; Cheyne-Stokes respirations; and apneustic, Biot, and ataxic patterns
  Note location of trachea
  Auscultate breath sounds, noting areas of decreased/absent ventilation and presence of adventitious sounds
  Monitor for increased restlessness, anxiety, and air hunger
  Note changes in SaO_2, SvO_2, end-tidal CO_2, and arterial blood gas (ABG) values, as appropriate

Patient/Family Teaching

- Inform patient and family about relaxation techniques to improve breathing pattern. Specify techniques.
- Discuss the plan for care at home, including medications, supportive equipment, signs and symptoms of reportable complications, community resources
- Teach how to cough effectively
- Inform patient/family that smoking is prohibited in room
- Instruct patient/family that they should notify the nurse at onset of ineffective breathing pattern

Collaborative Activities

- Confer with respiratory therapist to ensure adequate functioning of mechanical ventilator
- Report changes in sensorium, breath sounds, respiratory pattern, ABGs, sputum, and so on, as needed or per protocols
- Administer medications (eg, bronchodilators) per order or protocols
- Administer ultrasonic nebulizer treatments and humidified air or oxygen per order or agency protocols
- Give pain medications to allow optimal respiratory pattern. Specify schedule.

Other

- Correlate and document all assessment data (eg, patient sensorium, breath sounds, respiratory pattern, ABGs, sputum, effect of medications)
- Help patient to use incentive spirometer, as needed
- Reassure patient during periods of respiratory distress
- Encourage slow abdominal breathing during periods of respiratory distress
- Suction as needed to remove secretions
- Have patient turn, cough, and deep breathe q _____
- Inform patient before beginning intended procedures, to lower anxiety and increase sense of control
- Maintain low-flow oxygen by nasal cannula, mask, hood, or tent. Specify flow rate.
- Position patient for optimal breathing. Specify position.
- Synchronize patient's breathing pattern with ventilator rate

Cardiac Output, Decreased
(1.4.2.1) (1975,1996)

Definition: A state in which the blood pumped by the heart is inadequate to meet the metabolic demands of the body

Defining Characteristics

Subjective
Chest pain
Dyspnea
Fatigue
Paroxysmal nocturnal dyspnea

Shortness of breath

Vertigo

Weakness

Objective

Abnormal chest x-ray (pulmonary vascular congestion)

Abnormal cardiac enzymes

Altered mental states

Arrhythmias

Cold, clammy skin

Cough

Decreased cardiac output by thermodilution method

Decreased peripheral pulses

ECG changes

Edema

Ejection fraction < 40 percent

Elevated pulmonary artery pressures

Increased heart rate

Increased respiratory rate

Jugular vein distention

Mixed venous oxygen (SaO_2)

Oliguria

Orthopnea

Rales

Restlessness

S_3 or S_4 [heart sounds]

Skin color changes

Use of accessory muscles

Variations in blood pressure readings

Weight gain

Wheezing

Related Factors

To be developed by NANDA. The following are non-NANDA factors:

Cardiac anomaly (specify)

Drug toxicity

Dysfunctional electrical conduction

Hypovolemia

Increased ventricular workload

Ventricular damage

Ventricular ischemia

Ventricular restriction

Suggestions for Use

This label does not suggest independent nursing actions. The nurse can neither conclusively diagnose nor definitively treat this problem. For patients with physiologic decreased cardiac output, you may find it more useful to use a label that represents a human response to this pathophysiology (eg, *Activity intolerance related to Decreased cardiac output*). If the patient is at risk of developing complications, write them as collaborative problems (eg, Potential Complication of myocardial infarction: Cardiogenic shock).

Suggested Alternative Diagnoses

Activity intolerance
Self-care deficit

NOC Suggested Outcomes

Cardiac Pump Effectiveness: Extent to which blood is ejected from the left ventricle per minute to support systemic perfusion pressure

Circulation Status: Extent to which blood flows unobstructed, unidirectionally, and at an appropriate pressure through large vessels of the systemic and pulmonary circuits

Tissue Perfusion: Abdominal Organs: Extent to which blood flows through the small vessels of the abdominal viscera and maintains organ function

Tissue Perfusion: Peripheral: Extent to which blood flows through the small vessels of the extremities and maintains tissue function

Vital Signs Status: Temperature, pulse, respiration, and blood pressure within expected range for the individual

Goals/Evaluation Criteria

Examples Using NOC Language

- Demonstrates satisfactory cardiac output, as evidenced by Cardiac Pump Effectiveness, Circulation Status, Tissue Perfusion (Abdominal Organs), and Tissue Perfusion (Peripheral)
- Demonstrates **Circulation Status**, as evidenced by the following indicators (specify 1–5: extremely, substantially, moderately, mildly, or not compromised):

    Systolic, diastolic, and mean BP in expected range [IER]
    Heart rate IER

Central venous pressure and pulmonary wedge pressure IER
Orthostatic hypotension not present
Blood gases IER
Adventitious breath sounds not present
Neck vein distention not present
Peripheral edema not present
Ascites not present
Peripheral pulses strong and symmetric
Cognitive status IER

Other Examples

Patient will:

- Have cardiac index and ejection fraction within normal limits
- Have urine output, urine specific gravity, blood urea nitrogen (BUN), and plasma creatinine within normal limits
- Have normal skin color
- Demonstrate increasing tolerance for physical activity
- Describe the required diet, medications, activity, and limitations
- Identify reportable signs and symptoms of worsening condition

NIC Priority Interventions

Cardiac Care: Limitation of complications resulting from an imbalance between myocardial oxygen supply and demand for a patient with symptoms of impaired cardiac function

Cardiac Care, Acute: Limitation of complications for a patient recently experiencing an episode of an imbalance between myocardial oxygen supply and demand resulting in impaired cardiac function

Circulatory Care: Mechanical Assist Device: Temporary support of the circulation through the use of mechanical devices or pumps

Hemodynamic Regulation: Optimization of heart rate, preload, afterload, and contractility

Shock Management: Cardiac: Promotion of adequate tissue perfusion for a patient with severely compromised pumping function of the heart

Nursing Activities

Assessments

- Assess and document blood pressure, presence of cyanosis, respiratory status, and mental status

- Monitor for signs of fluid overload (eg, dependent edema, weight gain)
- Assess patient's activity tolerance by noting onset of shortness of breath, pain, palpitations, or dizziness
- Evaluate patient's responses to oxygen therapy
- *(NIC) Hemodynamic Regulation:*
  Monitor pacemaker functioning, if appropriate
  Monitor peripheral pulses, capillary refill, and temperature and color of extremities
  Monitor intake/output, urine output, and patient weight, as appropriate
  Monitor systemic and pulmonary vascular resistance, as appropriate
  Auscultate lung sounds for crackles or other adventitious sounds
  Monitor and document heart rate, rhythm, and pulses

Patient/Family Teaching

- Explain purpose of administering oxygen per nasal cannula or mask
- Instruct regarding maintenance of accurate intake and output
- Teach use, dose, frequency, and side effects of medications
- Teach to report and describe palpitations and pain onset, duration, precipitating factors, site, quality, and intensity
- Instruct patient/family in plan for care at home, including activity limitations, diet restrictions, and use of therapeutic equipment
- Provide information on stress-reduction techniques such as biofeedback, progressive muscle relaxation, meditation, and exercise

Collaborative Activities

- Confer with physician regarding parameters for administering/withholding blood pressure medications
- Administer and titrate antiarrhythmic, inotropic, nitroglycerin, and vasodilator medications to maintain contractility, preload, and afterload per medical order or protocols
- Administer anticoagulants to prevent peripheral thrombus formation, per order or protocol
- Promote afterload reduction (eg, with intraaortic balloon pumping) per medical order or protocol

Other

- Change patient's position to flat or Trendelenburg when blood pressure is in a range lower than normal for patient
- For sudden, severe, or prolonged hypotension, establish intravenous access for administration of intravenous fluids and/or medications to raise blood pressure
- Correlate effects of laboratory values, oxygen, medications, activity, anxiety, and/or pain on the dysrhythmia
- Do not take rectal temperatures
- Turn patient every 2 hours or maintain other appropriate/ required activity to decrease peripheral circulation stasis
- *(NIC) Hemodynamic Regulation:*
  Minimize/eliminate environmental stressors
  Insert urinary catheter, if appropriate

Caregiver Role Strain
(3.2.2.1) (1992, 1998)

Definition: A caregiver's felt or exhibited difficulty in performing the family caregiver role

Defining Characteristics

Subjective

Apprehension about care receiver's care when caregiver is ill or deceased

Apprehension about possible institutionalization of care receiver

Apprehension about the future regarding care receiver's health and the caregiver's ability to provide care

Preoccupation with care routine

Objective

Altered caregiver health status (eg, hypertension, cardiovascular disease, diabetes, headaches, gastrointestinal upset, weight change, rash)

Altered caregiving activities

Difficulty performing required activities

Inability to complete caregiving tasks

Other Possible Defining Characteristics (Non-NANDA)

Feels loss because the care receiver is a different person than before caregiving began or, in the case of a child, that the care receiver was never the child the caregiver expected

Feels family conflict around issues of providing care

Feels stress or nervousness in his/her relationship with the care receiver

Feels depressed

Related Factors/Risk Factors

Resources
Caregiver not developmentally ready for caregiver role

Lack of respite or recreational resources

Lack of support from significant others

Inadequate transportation, equipment for providing care, or community services

Insufficient information or finances

Roles and Relationships
Change in relationship

History of family dysfunction

History of marginal family coping

Unrealistic expectations of caregiver by care receiver

Social
Alienation from family, friends, and coworkers

Insufficient recreation

Individual
Illness chronicity

Instability of care receiver's health

Problem behaviors

Psychological or cognitive problems in care receiver

Caregiver
24-hour care responsibility

Addiction or codependency

Amount of activities

Inability to fulfill one's own or other's expectations

Marginal caregiver's coping patterns

Ongoing changes in activities

Psychological or cognitive problems

Unpredictability of care situation

Unrealistic expectations of self

Situational

Caregiver's competing role commitments

Complexity/amount of caregiving tasks

Family/caregiver isolation

Inadequate physical environment for providing care (eg, housing, transportation, community services, equipment)

Inexperience with caregiving

Presence of abuse or violence

Physiological

Addiction or codependency of care receiver

Caregiver health impairment

Discharge of family member with significant home care needs

Illness severity of the care receiver

Increasing care needs and/or dependency

Unpredictable illness course or instability in the care receiver's health

Suggestions for Use

Caregiver role strain focuses on the burden of the individual caregiver who has had to assume the care of a family member. The family diagnoses (*Family coping* and *Altered family processes*) focus on the family system and the manner in which family functioning has been altered by a stressor. The stressor in those diagnoses is not necessarily the need to care for a family member.

Suggested Alternative Diagnoses

Coping: family, ineffective, compromised

Coping: family, ineffective, disabling

Family processes, altered

Management of therapeutic regimen: families, ineffective

NOC Suggested Outcomes

Caregiver Emotional Health: Feelings, attitudes, and emotions of a family care provider while caring for a family member or significant other over an extended period of time

Caregiver Home Care Readiness: Preparedness to assume responsibility for the health care of a family member or significant other in the home

Caregiver Lifestyle Disruption: Disturbances in the lifestyle of a family member due to caregiving

Caregiver-Patient Relationship: Positive interactions and connections between the caregiver and care recipient

Caregiver Performance: Direct Care: Provision by family care provider of appropriate personal and health care for a family member or significant other

Caregiver Performance: Indirect Care: Arrangement and oversight of appropriate care for a family member or significant other

Caregiver Physical Health: Physical well-being of a family care provider while caring for a family member or significant other over an extended period of time

Caregiver Stressors: The extent of biopsychosocial pressure on a family care provider caring for a family member or significant other over an extended period of time

Caregiver Well-Being: Primary care provider's satisfaction with health and life circumstances

Caregiving Endurance Potential: Factors that promote family care provider continuance over an extended period of time

Risk Control: Actions to eliminate or reduce actual, personal, and modifiable health threats

Role Performance: Congruence of an individual's role behavior with role expectations

Goals/Evaluation Criteria

Examples Using NOC Language

- Demonstrates **Caregiver Emotional Health**, as evidenced by the following indicators (specify 1–5: extremely, substantially, moderately, mildly, or not compromised):

  Free of anger, resentfulness, guilt, depression, frustration, perceived burden, and ambivalence concerning situation

  Satisfaction with life

  Sense of control and self-esteem

  Perceived spiritual well-being

Other Examples

Caregiver will:
- Verbalize knowledge of treatment regimen and procedures, follow-up care, and emergency care
- Verbalize knowledge of how to obtain and operate needed equipment
- Express willingness to assume caregiving role
- Ensure provision of appropriate level of care
- Balance competing family and personal needs
- Identify and use personal strengths, social supports, and community resources

NIC Priority Interventions

Caregiver Support: Provision of the necessary information, advocacy, and support to facilitate primary patient care by someone other than a health care professional

Nursing Activities

Assessments

- Assess care receiver for signs of emotional and/or physical neglect or abuse
- Assess caregiver for signs of increasing role strain (eg, depression, anxiety, increased use/abuse of alcohol/ drugs, frustration, helplessness, sleeplessness, lowered morale, physical and/or emotional exhaustion, and personal health problems)
- *(NIC) Caregiver Support:*
  Determine caregiver's level of knowledge
  Determine caregiver's acceptance of role
  Monitor family interaction problems related to care of patient

Patient/Family Teaching

- Acknowledge and teach that the work of the caregiver is both physical and mental and includes (Bowers 1987):
  Anticipatory caregiving (making decisions based on possible future needs of care receiver, eg, place of residence)
  Instrumental caregiving (direct, hands-on care)
  Preventive caregiving (taking action to prevent illness, injury, or complications, eg, altering the physical environment, preparing meals)
  Protective caregiving (protecting care receiver from threats to self-image, identity, and change in relationship with caregiver)
  Supervisory caregiving (arranging for and monitoring care, eg, making appointments, arranging transportation)
- Facilitate coping and adjustment by teaching caregiver and care receiver how to (Chilman, Nunnally & Cox, 1988):
  Deal with pain, incapacitation, and illness-related symptoms
  Deal with hospital environment and disease-related treatments/procedures
  Establish and maintain workable relationships with the health care team

- *(NIC) Caregiver Support:*
  Teach caregiver stress management techniques
  Educate caregiver about the grieving process

Collaborative Activities

- Refer as needed for counseling and support during times of stress or crisis
- Refer for necessary assistance with preventive, supervisory, and instrumental caregiving (eg, Visiting Nurse Association, respite care, hospice care, day treatment, secondary caregivers)
- Report to authorities signs of care receiver physical/emotional neglect or abuse

Other

- Arrange for parent(s) of chronically ill child to receive training in areas of child development and education and compliance-related behavior problems
- Assist caregiver to identify problems or concerns with caregiving (eg, lack of knowledge/skill/emotional readiness for caregiving, lack of social support, financial burden, disruptive behavior, increasing need for physical care)
- Develop a plan of care with caregiver that identifies coping mechanisms, personal strengths, social supports, and acknowledged limitations. Consider including the following:
  Assistance with household tasks
  Family therapy
  Self-help and mutual support groups for information, advocacy, and emotional support
- Explore with caregiver the possibility of institutional care (now or in the future) and feelings associated with institutionalization
- Explore with caregiver/care receiver past and current closeness, shared activities, and confiding in one another as indications of emotional investment and commitment to the caregiver role
- Facilitate family's adjustment to illness of family member by assisting them to (Chilman, Nunnally, & Cox, 1988):
  Develop flexibility regarding future goals
  Grieve for the loss of pre-illness family identity
  Maintain a sense of mastery over their lives
  Move toward acceptance of changes
  Pull together during short-term crisis

- *(NIC) Caregiver Support:*
  Accept expressions of negative emotion
  Act for caregiver if overburdening becomes apparent

Caregiver Role Strain, Risk for
(3.2.2.2) (1992)

Definition: A caregiver is vulnerable for felt difficulty in performing the family caregiver role

Risk Factors

Objective

Addiction or codependency

Care receiver exhibits deviant, bizarre behavior

Caregiver health impairment

Caregiver is female

Caregiver is not developmentally ready for caregiver role (eg, a young adult needing to provide care for middle aged)

Caregiver is spouse

Caregiver's competing role commitments

Complexity/amount of caregiving tasks

Developmental delay or retardation of the care receiver or caregiver

Discharge of family member with significant home care needs

Duration of caregiving required

Family/caregiver isolation

Illness severity of the care receiver

Inadequate physical environment for providing care (eg, housing, transportation, community services, equipment)

Inexperience with caregiving

Lack of respite and recreation for caregiver

Marginal caregiver's coping patterns

Marginal family adaptation or dysfunction prior to the caregiving situation

Past history of poor relationship between caregiver and care receiver

Premature birth/congenital defect

Presence of abuse or violence

Presence of situational stressors which normally affect families (eg, significant loss, disaster or crisis; economic vulnerability; major life events)

Psychological or cognitive problems in care receiver

Unpredictable illness course or instability in the care receiver's health

Suggestions for Use

See "Caregiver Role Strain," p. 59.

Suggested Alternative Diagnoses

Coping: family, ineffective, compromised

Coping: family, ineffective, disabling

Family processes, altered

Management of therapeutic regimen: families, ineffective

NOC Suggested Outcomes

See "Caregiver Role Strain," pp. 59–60.

Goals/Evaluation Criteria

See "Caregiver Role Strain," p. 60.

NIC Priority Interventions

Caregiver Support: Provision of the necessary information, advocacy, and support to facilitate primary patient care by someone other than a health care professional

Nursing Activities

Assessments

- Assess caregiver's level of knowledge of medical/care regimen
- Determine caregiver's desire for and acceptance of role
- See "Assessments" for "Caregiver Role Strain", on p. 61.

Patient/Family Teaching

- See "Patient/Family Teaching" for "Caregiver Role Strain", on pp. 61–62.

Collaborative Activities

- See "Collaborative Activities" for "Caregiver Role Strain", on p. 62.

Other

- See "Other" activities for "Caregiver Role Strain", on pp. 62–63.

Communication, Impaired Verbal
(2.1.1.1) (1973, 1998)

Definition: The state in which an individual experiences a decreased, delayed, or absent ability to receive, process, transmit, and use a system of symbols—anything that has meaning (ie, transmits meaning)

Defining Characteristics

Objective

Absence of eye contact or difficulty in selective attending

Difficulty expressing thoughts verbally (eg, aphasia, dysphasia, apraxia, dyslexia)

Difficulty forming words or sentences (eg, aphonia, dyslalia, dysarthria)

Difficulty in comprehending and maintaining the usual communication pattern

Disorientation in the three spheres of time, space, person

Does not or cannot speak

Dyspnea

Inability or difficulty in use of facial or body expressions

Inappropriate verbalization

Partial or total visual deficit

Slurring

Speaks or verbalizes with difficulty

Stuttering

Unable to speak dominant language

Willful refusal to speak

Related Factors

Absence of significant others

Alteration of central nervous system

Alteration of self-esteem or self-concept

Altered perceptions

Anatomical defect (eg, cleft palate, alteration of the neuromuscular visual system, auditory system, or phonatory apparatus)

Brain tumor

Cultural difference

Decrease in circulation to brain

Differences related to developmental age

Emotional conditions

Environmental barriers
Lack of information
Physical barrier (eg, tracheostomy, intubation)
Physiological conditions
Psychological barriers (eg, psychosis, lack of stimuli)
Side effects of medications
Stress
Weakening of the musculoskeletal system

Suggestions for Use

Use this label for those who want to communicate but who have difficulty doing so. If communication problems are caused by psychiatric illness or coping difficulties, a diagnosis of *Fear* or *Anxiety* may be more appropriate (Carpenito 1997b, p. 53). Note that communication problems may be receptive (ie, difficulty hearing) as well as expressive (ie, difficulty speaking).

Suggested Alternative Diagnoses

Anxiety
Coping: defensive
Fear
Self-esteem disturbance
Sensory/perceptual alterations: visual, auditory
Thought processes, altered

NOC Suggested Outcomes

Communication Ability: Ability to receive, interpret, and express spoken, written, and nonverbal messages

Communication: Expressive Ability: Ability to express and interpret verbal and/or nonverbal messages

Communication: Receptive Ability: Ability to receive and interpret verbal and/or nonverbal messages

Goals/Evaluation Criteria

Examples Using NOC Language:

• Demonstrates **Communication Ability**, as evidenced by the following indicators (specify 1–5: extremely, substantially, moderately, mildly, or not compromised):

    Use of written, spoken, or nonverbal language
    Use of sign language
    Use of pictures and drawings

Acknowledgment of messages received

Exchange [of] messages with others

Other Examples

Patient will:

- Communicate needs to staff and family with minimal frustration
- Communicate satisfaction with alternative means of communication

NIC Priority Interventions

Active Listening: Attending closely to and attaching significance to a patient's verbal and nonverbal messages

Communication Enhancement, Hearing Deficit: Assistance in accepting and learning alternate methods for living with diminished hearing

Communication Enhancement, Speech Deficit: Assistance in accepting and learning alternate methods for living with impaired speech

Nursing Activities

Assessments

- Assess and document patient's:

    Primary language

    Ability to speak, hear, write, read, and understand

    Ability to establish communication with staff and family

    Response to touch, spatial distance, culture, and male/female roles that may influence communication

Patient/Family Teaching

- Explain to patient why he or she cannot speak or understand, as appropriate
- Explain to hearing-impaired patient that sounds will be heard differently with use of a hearing aid
- *(NIC) Communication Enhancement: Speech Deficit:*

    Instruct patient and family on use of speech aids (eg, tracheal-esophageal prosthesis and artificial larynx)

    Teach esophageal speech, as appropriate.

Collaborative Activities

- Consult with physician regarding need for speech therapy
- Help patient/family to locate resources for hearing aids

- *(NIC) Communication Enhancement: Speech Deficit:*
  Use interpreter, as necessary
  Reinforce need for follow-up with speech pathologist after discharge

Other

- Help patient to locate a telephone for the hearing impaired
- Encourage attendance at group meetings for interpersonal contact. Specify group.
- Encourage frequent family visits to provide stimulation for communication
- Encourage patient to communicate slowly and to repeat requests
- Give frequent positive reinforcement to patient efforts to communicate
- Encourage self-expression in any manner that provides information to staff/family
- Establish one-to-one contact with patient q _____
- Use flash cards, pad/pencil, gestures, pictures, foreign language vocabulary lists, computer, and so forth, to facilitate optimal two-way communication
- Speak slowly, distinctly, and quietly, facing the patient
- When speaking to a patient with hearing impairment, be sure your mouth is visible; do not smoke, talk with a full mouth, or chew gum
- Obtain hearing-impaired patient's attention by touching
- Give clear and simple directions; avoid overwhelming choices that may add to the patient's confusion. For example, take patient by the arm, saying, "Walk with me now."
- Involve patient and family in developing a communication plan
- Provide care in a relaxed, unhurried, nonjudgmental manner
- Provide continuity in nursing assignment to establish trust and reduce frustration
- Reassure patient that frustration and anger are acceptable and expected
- Use family/significant person or hospital translator, as appropriate. Specify name, phone number, and relationship in care plan.
- *(NIC) Communication Enhancement: Speech Deficit:*
  Refrain from shouting at patient with communication disorders
  Carry on one-way conversations, as appropriate
  Listen attentively

Confusion, Acute
(8.2.2) (1994)

Definition: The abrupt onset of a cluster of global, transient changes and disturbances in attention, cognition, psychomotor activity, level of consciousness, and/or sleep/wake cycle

Defining Characteristics

Subjective

Lack of motivation to initiate and/or follow through with goal-directed or purposeful behavior

Misperceptions

Objective

Fluctuation in cognition

Fluctuation in sleep/wake cycle

Fluctuation in level of consciousness

Fluctuation in psychomotor activity

Increased agitation or restlessness

Hallucinations

Related Factors

Alcohol abuse

Delirium

Dementia

Over 60 years of age

Drug abuse

Suggestions for Use

"Confusion" may be used to describe a variety of cognitive impairments. It may be difficult to determine whether *Confusion* is acute or chronic. Therefore, until careful assessment and analysis have been done, it may be necessary to use the more general non-NANDA term *Confusion. Acute confusion* develops suddenly. *Chronic confusion* develops over time, and is caused by progressive degenerative changes in the brain. *Altered thought processes* are caused by functional/emotional rather than physiologic disorders.

Suggested Alternative Diagnoses

Confusion (non-NANDA)

Confusion, chronic

Environmental interpretation syndrome, impaired
Thought processes, altered
Tissue perfusion, altered (cerebral)

NOC Suggested Outcomes

Cognitive Ability: Ability to execute complex mental processes

Distorted Thought Control: Ability to self-restrain disruption in perception, thought processes, and thought content

Information Processing: Ability to acquire, organize, and use information

Memory: Ability to cognitively retrieve and report previously stored information

Neurological Status: Consciousness: Extent to which an individual arouses, orients, and attends to the environment

Safety Behavior: Personal: Individual or caregiver efforts to control behaviors that might cause personal injury

Sleep: Extent and pattern of sleep for mental and physical rejuvenation

Goals/Evaluation Criteria

Examples Using NOC Language

- Demonstrates **Cognitive Ability**, as evidenced by the following indicators (specify 1–5: extremely, substantially, moderately, mildly, or not compromised):

    Attentiveness, concentration, and orientation

    Immediate, recent, and remote memory

    Makes appropriate decisions

    Communicates clearly and appropriately for age and ability

Other Examples

Patient will:

- Have decreasing episodes of *Confusion*
- Make lifestyle/behavior changes to alleviate or prevent further episodes of *Confusion*
- Demonstrate decreased restlessness/agitation
- Not respond to hallucinations or delusions
- Demonstrate accurate interpretation of environment
- Organize and process information logically
- Correctly identify common objects and familiar persons
- Read and understand short written statements
- Add and subtract numbers accurately
- Obey verbal instructions/commands

- Retain motor responses to noxious stimuli
- Open eyes to external stimuli
- Be awake at appropriate times
- Have a normal electroencephalogram and electromyogram

NIC Priority Interventions

Delirium Management: Provision of a safe and therapeutic environment for the patient who is experiencing an acute confusional state

Delusion Management: Promoting the comfort, safety, and reality orientation of a patient experiencing false, fixed beliefs that have little or no basis in reality

Nursing Activities

Assessments

- Identify possible causes of delirium (eg, pain, hypoglycemia, infection, medications)
- Monitor neurologic status
- Monitor emotional status
- Obtain baseline history of mental status and any changes
- Perform complete mental status exam
- *(NIC) Delusion Management:*
  Monitor delusions for presence of content that is self-harmful or violent
  Monitor self-care ability

Patient/Family Teaching

- *(NIC) Delusion Management:*
  Educate family and significant others about ways to deal with patient who is experiencing delusions
  Provide illness teaching to patient/significant others, if delusions are illness-based (eg, delirium, schizophrenia, or depression)
  Provide medication teaching to patient/significant others

Collaborative Activities

- *(NIC) Delusion Management:* Administer PRN medications for anxiety or agitation

Other

- Reassure patient with therapeutic communication frequently
- Use touch, as appropriate
- Avoid use of restraints, if possible

- Encourage family/significant others to stay with patient
- Use nursing measures (eg, mouth care, positioning) to promote comfort and sleep
- Continue patient's usual rituals, to limit anxiety
- Give choices but limit options if patient becomes frustrated or confused
- Be sure patient wears an identification bracelet
- Orient patient (eg, to staff, surroundings, and care activities), as needed
- Call the patient by name when beginning an interaction
- Explain routines and procedures slowly, briefly, and in simple terms
- Give patient time to respond when presenting options or new information
- *(NIC) Delusion Management:*
  Focus discussion on the underlying feelings, rather than the content of the delusion ("It appears as if you may be feeling frightened")
  Avoid arguing about false beliefs; state doubt matter-of-factly
  Encourage patient to verbalize delusions to caregivers before acting on them
  Assist with self-care, as needed
  Maintain a safe environment
  Provide for the safety and comfort of patient and others when patient is unable to control behavior (eg, limit setting, area restriction, physical restraint, or seclusion)
  Decrease excessive environmental stimuli, as needed
  Maintain a consistent daily routine
  Assign consistent caregivers on a daily basis

Confusion, Chronic
(8.2.3) (1994)

Definition: An irreversible, long-standing, and/or progressive deterioration of intellect and personality characterized by decreased ability to interpret environmental stimuli [and] decreased capacity for intellectual thought processes and manifested by disturbances of memory, orientation, and behavior

Defining Characteristics

Subjective
Impaired memory (short-term, long-term)
Objective
Altered interpretation/response to stimuli
Altered personality
Clinical evidence of organic impairment
Impaired socialization
No change in level of consciousness
Progressive/long-standing cognitive impairment

Related Factors

Alzheimer's disease
Cerebral vascular accident
Head injury
Korsakoff's psychosis
Multi-infarct dementia

Suggestions for Use

See "Suggestions for Use" for "Confusion, Acute," p. 69. For clients with self-care deficits, be sure to include that diagnostic label in the care plan (eg, *Total self-care deficit related to Chronic confusion*). It is difficult to distinguish between *Chronic confusion* and *Impaired environmental interpretation syndrome*. Research is in progress to clarify this distinction.

Suggested Alternative Diagnoses

Confusion
Confusion, acute
Environmental interpretation syndrome, impaired
Memory, impaired
Self-care deficit (specify)
Thought processes, altered

NOC Suggested Outcomes

Cognitive Ability: Ability to execute complex mental processes
Cognitive Orientation: Ability to identify person, place, and time
Concentration: Ability to focus on a specific stimulus
Decision Making: Ability to choose between two or more alternatives

Distorted Thought Control: Ability to self-restrain disruption in perception, thought processes, and thought content

Identity: Ability to distinguish between self and nonself and to characterize one's essence

Information Processing: Ability to acquire, organize, and use information

Memory: Ability to cognitively retrieve and report previously stored information

Neurological Status: Consciousness: Extent to which an individual arouses, orients, and attends to the environment

Safety Behavior: Personal: Individual or caregiver efforts to control behaviors that might cause personal injury

Sleep: Extent and pattern of sleep for mental and physical rejuvenation

Goals/Evaluation Criteria

Examples Using NOC Language

- Maintains or improves Concentration, Decision Making, Distorted Thought Control, Information Processing, Memory, and Safety Behavior: Personal
- Exhibits minimal deterioration in Cognitive Orientation
- Experiences no loss of Identity
- Neurological Status: Consciousness not compromised
- Demonstrates **Cognitive Ability**, as evidenced by the following indicators (specify 1–5: extremely, substantially, moderately, mildly, or not compromised):

    Attentiveness, concentration, and orientation
    Immediate, recent, and remote memory
    Makes appropriate decisions
    Communicates clearly and appropriately for age and ability.

Other Examples

    Patient will:
- Respond to visual and auditory cues, draw a circle, maintain attention
- Identify relevant information and choose among alternatives
- Interact appropriately with others
- Formulate coherent messages
- Obey simple directions/commands
- Not attend to hallucinations or delusions
- Attend to, perceive, and interpret the environmental stimuli correctly

- Correctly identify objects and people
- Balance activity with rest
- Not be restless or agitated
- Participate to maximum ability in therapeutic milieu and/or activities of daily living
- Not be combative
- Be content and less frustrated by environmental stressors

NIC Priority Interventions

Dementia Management: Provision of a modified environment for the patient who is experiencing a chronic confusional state

Mood Management: Providing for safety and stabilization of a patient who is experiencing dysfunctional mood

Nursing Activities

Assessments

- Obtain information about past and present patterns of behavior (eg, sleep, medication use, elimination, food intake, hygiene, social interaction)
- Assess for signs of depression (eg, insomnia, flat affect, withdrawal, loss of appetite)
- *(NIC) Dementia Management:*
  Monitor cognitive functioning, using a standardized assessment tool [eg, the Mini-Mental State Examination]
  Determine physical, social, and psychologic history of patient before the onset of confusion, usual habits and routines
  Monitor nutrition and weight
  Monitor carefully for physiologic causes of increased confusion that may be acute and reversible

Patient/Family Teaching

- Teach patient/significant others about patient's medications
- Explain the effect of the patient's illness on his/her mood (eg, depression, premenstrual syndrome)

Collaborative Activities

- Administer mood-stabilizing medications
- Refer to social services department for referral to day-care programs, Meals-on-Wheels, respite care, and so on.

Other

- If client experiences delusions or hallucinations, refer to "Nursing Activities" in "Confusion, Acute," pp. 71–72.

- In early dementia, when the main symptoms are those of *Impaired memory*, refer to "Nursing Activities" for "Impaired Memory," pp. 274–276
- Provide opportunity for physical activity
- Alternate activity with scheduled quiet times/activities (eg, an hour in a recliner or chair, quiet music) at least twice a day to allow for resolution of anxiety and tension
- Provide appropriate outlets for patient's feelings (eg, art therapy and physical exercise)
- Assist with reality orientation (eg, provide clocks, calendars, personal items, seasonal decorations)
- For geriatric patients, promote reminiscence and life review (eg, ask questions about client's work and family, such as "Looking back, what was really important to you?")
- Keep environment as quiet as possible (eg, avoid buzzers, alarms, and overhead paging systems)
- *(NIC) Dementia Management:*

  Include family members in planning, providing, and evaluating care, to the extent desired

  Provide a low-stimulation environment (eg, quiet, soothing music; nonvivid and simple, familiar patterns in décor; performance expectations that do not exceed cognitive-processing ability; and dining in small groups)

  Identify and remove potential dangers in environment for patient

  Place identification bracelet on patient

  Prepare for interaction with eye contact and touch, as appropriate

  Address the patient distinctly by name when initiating interaction and speak slowly

  Introduce self when initiating contact

  Give one simple direction at a time [and repeat as necessary (eg, "Follow me," or "Sit on the chair," or "Put on your slippers")]

  Use distraction, rather than confrontation, to manage behavior

  Provide patient a general orientation to the season of the year by using appropriate cues (eg, holiday decorations, seasonal decorations and activities, and access to contained, out-of-doors area)

  Label familiar photos with names of the individuals

  Limit number of choices patient has to make, so not to cause anxiety

Avoid use of physical restraints

Assist with self-care, as needed. [Specify methods.]

Provide boundaries, such as red or yellow tape on the floor, when low-stimulus units are not available

Constipation
(1.3.1.1) (1975, 1998)

Definition: A decrease in a person's normal frequency of defecation accompanied by difficult or incomplete passage of stool and/or passage of excessively hard, dry stool

Defining Characteristics

Subjective

Abdominal pain

Abdominal tenderness with or without palpable muscle resistance

Anorexia

Feeling of rectal fullness or pressure

Generalized fatigue

Headache

Increased abdominal pressure

Indigestion

Nausea

Pain with defecation

Objective

Atypical presentations in older adults (eg, change in mental status, urinary incontinence, unexplained falls, elevated body temperature)

Bright red blood with stool

Change in abdominal growling (borborygmi)

Change in bowel pattern

Dark or black or tarry stool

Decreased frequency

Decreased volume of stool

Distended abdomen

Dry, hard, formed stools

Hypoactive or hyperactive bowel sounds

Oozing liquid stool

Palpable abdominal mass

Palpable rectal mass

Percussed abdominal dullness

Presence of soft pastelike stool in rectum
Severe flatus
Straining with defecation
Unable to pass stool
Vomiting

Related Factors

Functional

Abdominal muscle weakness
Habitual denial/ignoring of urge to defecate
Inadequate toileting (eg, timeliness, positioning for defecation, privacy)
Insufficient physical activity
Irregular defecation habits
Recent environmental changes

Psychologic

Depression
Emotional stress
Mental confusion

Pharmacologic

Aluminum-containing antacids
Anticholinergics
Anticonvulsants
Antidepressants
Antilipemic agents
Bismuth salts
Calcium carbonate
Calcium channel blockers
Diuretics
Iron salts
Laxative overdose
Nonsteroidal anti-inflammatory agents
Opiates
Phenothiazides
Sedatives
Sympathomimetics

Mechanical

Electrolyte imbalance
Hemorrhoids
Megacolon (Hirschsprung's disease)
Neurological impairment

Obesity
Postsurgical obstruction
Pregnancy
Prostate enlargement
Rectal abscess or ulcer
Rectal anal fissures
Rectal anal stricture
Rectal prolapse
Rectocele
Tumors

Physiologic

Change in usual foods and eating patterns
Decreased motility of gastrointestinal tract
Dehydration
Inadequate dentition or oral hygiene
Insufficient fiber intake
Insufficient fluid intake
Poor eating habits

Suggested Alternative Diagnoses

Constipation, perceived
Constipation, risk for

NOC Suggested Outcomes

Bowel Elimination: Ability of the gastrointestinal tract to form and
evacuate stool effectively

Goals/Evaluation Criteria

Examples Using NOC Language

- *Constipation* alleviated, as indicated by **Bowel Elimination**
  (specify 1–5: extremely, substantially, moderately, mildly, or not
  compromised):
    Elimination pattern in expected range; stool soft and formed
    Passes stool without aids
    Ingests adequate fluids and fiber
    Exercises adequate amount

Other Examples

  Patient will:
- Demonstrate knowledge of bowel regimen necessary to over-
  come the side effects of medications
- Report the passage of stool with a reduction of pain and straining

NIC Priority Interventions

Constipation/Impaction Management: Prevention and alleviation of constipation/impaction

Nursing Activities

Assessments

- Gather baseline data on bowel regimen, activity, medications and patient's usual pattern
- Assess and document:

    Color and consistency of first stool postoperatively

    Frequency, color, and consistency of stool q _____

    Passage of flatus

    Presence of impaction

    Presence or absence of bowel sounds and abdominal distention in all four quadrants

- *(NIC) Constipation/Impaction Management:*

    Monitor for signs and symptoms of bowel rupture and/or peritonitis

    Identify factors (eg, medications, bed rest, and diet) that may cause or contribute to constipation

Patient/Family Teaching

- Inform patient of possibility of medication-induced constipation
- Instruct patient in bowel elimination aids that will promote optimal bowel pattern at home
- Teach patient the effects of diet (eg, fluids and fiber) on elimination
- Instruct patient in consequences of long-term laxative use
- Stress the avoidance of straining during defecation to prevent change in vital signs, dizziness, or bleeding
- *(NIC) Constipation/Impaction Management:*

    Explain etiology of problem and rationale for actions to patient

    Teach patient/family how to keep a food diary

Collaborative Activities

- Consult with dietitian for increase in fiber and fluids in diet
- Request a physician's order for elimination aids, such as dietary bran, stool softeners, enemas, and laxatives
- *(NIC) Constipation/Impaction Management:*

    Consult with physician about a decrease/increase in frequency of bowel sounds

Consult with physician if signs and symptoms of constipation or impaction persist

Other

- Encourage patient to request pain medication prior to defecation to facilitate painless passage of stool
- Encourage optimal activity to stimulate patient's bowel elimination
- Provide privacy and safety for patient during bowel elimination
- Provide care in an accepting, nonjudgmental manner
- Provide fluids of patient's choice. Specify: _____.

Constipation, Perceived
(1.3.1.1.1) (1988)

Definition: The state in which an individual makes a self-diagnosis of constipation and ensures a daily bowel movement through the use of laxatives, enemas, and suppositories

Defining Characteristics

Subjective

Expectation of a daily bowel movement

Expected passage of stool at same time every day

Objective

Overuse of laxatives, enemas, and suppositories [to induce a daily bowel movement]

Related Factors

Cultural/family health beliefs

Faulty appraisal [of normal bowel function]

Impaired thought processes

Suggestions for Use

None

Suggested Alternative Diagnoses

Constipation

Constipation, risk for

NOC Suggested Outcomes

Bowel Elimination: Ability of the gastrointestinal tract to form and evacuate stool effectively

Health Beliefs: Personal convictions that influence health behaviors

Health Beliefs: Perceived Threat: Personal conviction that a health problem is serious and has potential negative consequences for lifestyle

Goals/Evaluation Criteria

Examples Using NOC Language

- *Perceived constipation* alleviated, as indicated by Bowel Elimination and Health Beliefs.
- Demonstrates **Bowel Elimination**, as evidenced by the following indicators (specify 1–5: extremely, substantially, moderately, mildly, or not compromised):

    Elimination pattern in expected range

    Passes stool without aids

    Abuse of aids not present

    Ingests adequate fluids and fiber

Other Examples

Patient will:

- Verbalize understanding of need to decrease use of laxatives, enemas, and suppositories
- Describe dietary regimen that will more naturally regulate bowel function

NIC Priority Interventions

Bowel Management: Establishment and maintenance of a regular pattern of bowel elimination

Nursing Activities

Assessments

- Assess patient's expectation of normal bowel function
- Observe, document, and report requests for laxatives, enemas, and/or suppositories
- *(NIC) Bowel Management:*

    Monitor bowel movements, including frequency, consistency, shape, volume, and color, as appropriate

    Note preexistent bowel problems, bowel routine, and use of laxatives

Patient/Family Teaching
- Instruct patient and family in diet, fluid intake, activity, exercise, and the consequence of overuse of laxatives, enemas, and suppositories

Collaborative Activities
- Initiate a multidisciplinary care conference involving the patient/family to encourage positive behaviors (eg, change in diet)

Other
- Assist patient to identify realistic use of laxatives, enemas, and suppositories
- Provide positive feedback to patient when behavior change occurs
- *(NIC) Bowel Management:* Encourage decreased gas-forming food intake, as appropriate

Constipation, Risk for
(1.3.1.4) (1998)

Definition: At risk for a decrease in a person's normal frequency of defecation accompanied by difficult or incomplete passage of stool and/or passage of excessively hard, dry stool

Risk Factors

Functional
Abdominal muscle weakness
Habitual denial/ignoring of urge to defecate
Inadequate toileting (eg, timeliness, positioning for defecation, privacy)
Insufficient physical activity
Irregular defecation habits
Recent environmental changes

Psychological
Depression
Emotional stress
Mental confusion

Physiological
Change in usual foods and eating patterns
Decreased motility of gastrointestinal tract

Dehydration
Inadequate dentition or oral hygiene
Insufficient fiber intake
Insufficient fluid intake
Poor eating habits

Pharmacological

Aluminum-containing antacids
Anticholinergics
Anticonvulsants
Antidepressants
Antilipemic agents
Bismuth salts
Calcium carbonate
Calcium channel blockers
Diuretics
Iron salts
Laxative overuse
Nonsteroidal anti-inflammatory agents
Opiates
Phenothiazines
Sedatives
Sympathomimetics

Mechanical

Electrolyte imbalance
Hemorrhoids
Megacolon (Hirschsprung's disease)
Neurological impairment
Obesity
Postsurgical obstruction
Pregnancy
Prostate enlargement
Rectal abscess or ulcer
Rectal anal fissures
Rectal anal stricture
Rectal prolapse
Rectocele
Tumors

Suggested Alternative Diagnoses

None

NOC Suggested Outcomes

To be developed

Goals/Evaluation Criteria

The patient will:
- Demonstrate knowledge of bowel regimen necessary to overcome the side effects of medications
- Describe dietary requirements (eg, fluids and fiber) necessary to maintain usual bowel pattern
- Pass stool of usual consistency and frequency for patient
- Report the passage of stool with no pain or straining

NIC Priority Interventions

To be developed

Nursing Activities

Assessments

- Gather baseline data on bowel regimen, activity, and medications
- Assess and document postoperatively:
    Color and consistency of first stool
    Passage of flatus
    Presence or absence of bowel sounds and abdominal distention

Patient/Family Teaching

- Inform patient of possibility of medication-induced constipation
- Explain the effects of fluids and fiber in preventing constipation
- Instruct patient in consequences of long-term laxative use

Collaborative Activities

- Refer to dietitian, as needed, to increase fiber and fluids in diet

Other

- Encourage optimal activity to stimulate bowel elimination
- Provide privacy and safety for patient during bowel elimination
- Provide fluids of patient's choice. Specify fluids.

Coping: Community, Ineffective
(5.1.3.2) (1994, 1998)

Definition: A pattern of community activities for adaptation and problem solving that is unsatisfactory for meeting the demands or needs of the community

Defining Characteristics

Subjective

Community does not meet its own expectations

Expressed community powerlessness

Expressed vulnerability

Objective

Deficits in community participation

Excessive community conflicts

High illness rates

Increased social problems (eg, homicides, vandalism, arson, terrorism, robbery, infanticide, abuse, divorce, unemployment, poverty, militancy, mental illness)

Stressors perceived as excessive

Related Factors

Deficits in community social support services and resources

Inadequate resources for problem solving

Ineffective or nonexistent community systems (eg, lack of emergency medical system, transportation system, or disaster planning systems)

Natural or man-made disasters

Suggestions for Use

This diagnosis is most useful for community health nurses who focus on the health of groups (eg, unwed mothers, all the people in a county, patients with diabetes).

Suggested Alternative Diagnoses

Coping: community, potential for enhanced

Management of therapeutic regimen: community, ineffective

NOC Suggested Outcomes

To be developed

Goals/Evaluation Criteria

The community:
- Develops improved communication among its members
- Implements effective problem-solving strategies
- Develops group cohesiveness
- Expresses the power to manage change and improve community functioning

NIC Priority Interventions

Environmental Management: Community: Monitoring and influencing of the physical, social, cultural, economic, and political conditions that affect the health of groups and communities

Health Policy Monitoring: Surveillance and influence of government and organization regulations, rules, and standards that affect nursing systems and practices to ensure quality care of patients

Nursing Activities

Assessments

- Assess/identify causative or risk factors affecting the community's ability to adapt/cope effectively (eg, lack of information about available resources)
- Assess the effects of health policies and standards on nursing practice, patient outcomes, and health care costs
- Determine the availability of resources and the extent to which they are being used
- *(NIC) Environmental Management: Community:*
  Initiate screening for health risks from the environment
  Monitor status of known health risks

Teaching

- Help to identify and mobilize available resources/supports (eg, emergency aid from the Red Cross)
- Inform policy makers of projected effects of policies on patient welfare
- Inform health care consumers of current and proposed changes in health policies and standards and potential effects on health
- *(NIC) Environmental Management: Community:* Conduct educational programs for targeted risk groups [eg, teenage pregnancy]

Collaborative Activities

- *(NIC) Environmental Management: Community:*

  Participate in multidisciplinary teams to identify threats to safety in the community

  Coordinate services to at-risk groups and communities

  Work with environmental groups to secure appropriate governmental regulations

  Collaborate in the development of community action programs

Other

- Participate in lobbying for changes in health policies and standards to improve health care
- Arrange opportunities for community members to meet and discuss the situation (eg, civic organizations, church groups, town meetings)
- Assist community members to become aware of conflicts that prevent them from working together (eg, anger, mistrust)
- Determine ways of disseminating information to the community (eg, radio and television reports, flyers, meetings)
- Help write grant proposals to obtain funding for programs needed to improve community coping
- Advocate for the community (eg, write letters to government agencies and newspapers)
- *(NIC) Environmental Management: Community:* Encourage neighborhoods to become active participants in community safety

Coping: Community, Potential for Enhanced (5.1.3.1) (1994)

Definition: A pattern of community activities for adaptation and problem solving that is satisfactory for meeting the demands or needs of the community but can be improved for management of current and future problems/stressors

Defining Characteristics

Objective

Active planning by community for predicted stressors

Active problem solving by community when faced with issues

Agreement that community is responsible for stress management

Deficits in one or more characteristics that indicate effective coping
Positive communication among community members
Positive communication between community/aggregates and the larger community
Programs [available] for recreation and relaxation
Resources sufficient for managing stressors

Related Factors

Community has a sense of power to manage stressors
Resources available for problem solving
Social supports available

Suggestions for Use

This diagnosis can be used for a community that is meeting its basic needs for a clean environment, food, shelter, and safety, and wishes to focus on higher levels of functioning, such as wellness promotion. When external threats (eg, floods, epidemics) occur in such a community, they pose risk factors; as long as the community continues to adapt, *Risk for ineffective community coping* should be used. If the threat produces defining characteristics (symptoms) in the community, use *Ineffective community coping.*

Suggested Alternative Diagnoses

Coping: community, ineffective
Coping: community, risk for ineffective

NOC Suggested Outcomes

To be developed

Goals/Evaluation Criteria

The community:
- Has a plan in place to deal with problems and stressors
- Accesses or develops programs designed to improve the well-being of specific groups within the population (eg, weight-control programs, retirement-planning programs)
- Continues to enhance present methods of communication and problem solving
- Expresses the power to manage change and improve community functioning

NIC Priority Interventions

Environmental Management, Community: Monitoring and influencing of the physical, social, cultural, economic, and political conditions that affect the health of groups and communities

Health Education: Developing and providing instruction and learning experiences to facilitate voluntary adaptation of behavior conducive to health in individuals, families, groups, or communities

Health Policy Monitoring: Surveillance and influence of government and organization regulations, rules, and standards that affect nursing systems and practices to ensure quality care of patients

Nursing Activities

Assessments

- Determine the availability of resources and the extent to which they are being used
- Identify groups that are at high risk for unhealthful behavior
- Identify factors in high-risk groups that may motivate or prevent healthful behavior
- Determine sociocultural and historic context of individual and group health behaviors
- Create and implement processes for regular evaluation of client outcomes during and after completion of program/activities
- Assess the effects of health policies and standards on nursing practice, patient outcomes, and health care costs
- *(NIC) Environmental Management: Community:* Initiate screening for health risks from the environment

Teaching

- Help to identify and mobilize available resources/supports (eg, funding sources, supplies)
- Select learning strategies based on identified characteristics of target population
- Design processes for informing health care consumers of existing and proposed changes in health policies
- Provide educational materials written at an appropriate level for the target group
- *(NIC) Environmental Management: Community:* Conduct educational programs for targeted risk groups [eg, teenage pregnancy]

Collaborative Activities

- Help the community obtain funding for wellness programs (eg, education, smoking prevention)
- *(NIC) Environmental Management: Community:*
  Participate in multidisciplinary teams to identify threats to safety in the community
  Collaborate in the development of community-action programs
  Work with environmental groups to secure appropriate governmental regulations

Other

- Establish a collaborative partnership with the community and explain the role of a community health nurse in wellness promotion
- Lobby/write letters to urge policies that promote health (eg, health education guaranteed as an employee benefit; insurance premium reductions for healthy behaviors/lifestyles)
- Help write grants to obtain funding for wellness programs
- Assist in improving educational levels within the community
- *(NIC) Environmental Management: Community:*
  Promote governmental policy to reduce specified risks
  Encourage neighborhoods to become active participants in community safety
  Coordinate services to at-risk groups and communities

Coping, Defensive
(5.1.1.1.2) (1988)

Definition: The state in which an individual repeatedly projects falsely positive self-evaluation based on a self-protective pattern that defends against underlying perceived threats to positive self-regard

Defining Characteristics

Subjective
Denial of obvious problems/weaknesses
Difficulty in reality-testing perceptions
Projection of blame/responsibility
Rationalizes failures

Objective

Grandiosity

Difficulty in establishing/maintaining relationships

Hostile laughter or ridicule of others

Hypersensitive to slight or criticism

Lack of follow-through or participation in treatment or therapy

Superior attitude toward others

Related Factors

Not yet developed by NANDA. Non-NANDA Related Factors include the following:

Physical illness (specify)

Situational crisis (specify)

Psychologic impairment (specify)

Suggestions for Use

This diagnosis is less specific than *Ineffective denial*, which is actually one of many manifestations of *Defensive coping* (see "Defining Characteristics," pp. 91–92). Use the more specific diagnosis when attempts to cope involve overuse/misuse of denial.

Suggested Alternative Diagnoses

Adjustment, impaired

Communication, impaired verbal

Coping: individual, ineffective

Denial, ineffective

Thought processes, altered

NOC Suggested Outcomes

Acceptance: Health Status: Reconciliation to health circumstances

Child Development: Adolescence (12–17 years): Milestones of physical, cognitive, and psychosocial progression between 12 and 17 years of age

Coping: Actions to manage stressors that tax an individual's resources

Self-Esteem: Personal judgment of self-worth

Social Interaction Skills: An individual's use of effective interaction behaviors

Goals/Evaluation Criteria

Examples Using NOC Language

- Patient will not use *Defensive coping*, as demonstrated by Acceptance: Health Status, effective Coping, positive Self-Esteem and Social Interaction Skills, and/or normal Child Development: Adolescence
- **Coping** indicators include the following (specify 1–5: never, rarely, sometimes, often, or consistently demonstrated):
    Modifies lifestyle, as needed
    Seeks information concerning illness and treatment
    Seeks professional help, as appropriate
    Verbalizes acceptance of situation
    Uses effective coping strategies

Other Examples

Patient will:
- Acknowledge specific problems/conflicts that interfere with social interactions/relationships
- Demonstrate decrease in defensiveness
- Express feelings about changes in health
- Express feelings of self-worth
- Reformulate previous concept of health
- Maintain effective interactions with others

NIC Priority Interventions

Self-Awareness Enhancement: Assisting a patient to explore and understand his/her thoughts, feelings, motivations, and behaviors

Nursing Activities

Assessments

- Assess degree of defensiveness/denial that interferes with self-assessment

Patient/Family Teaching

- Teach alternative behaviors to obtain positive regard through group therapy, individual therapy, role playing, and role modeling

Collaborative Activities

- Refer to appropriate community resources (eg, family/ marriage counseling, substance-abuse groups)

Other
- Assist patient in recognizing negative coping behaviors
- Identify and discuss the subjects, situations, and people that trigger negative coping behaviors
- Include family in treatment, as needed
- Provide feedback in a supportive environment on how behavior is being perceived by others
- Provide reality testing during times of grandiose behavior, denial of obvious problems, and projected blame/responsibility
- *(NIC) Self-Awareness Enhancement:*
  Assist patient to identify the impact of illness on self-concept
  Verbalize patient's denial of reality, as appropriate
  Assist patient to identify life priorities
  Assist patient to identify positive attributes of self

Coping: Family, Ineffective, Compromised (5.1.2.1.2) (1980, 1996)

Definition: A usually supportive primary person (family member or close friend) is providing insufficient, ineffective, or compromised support, comfort, assistance, or encouragement which may be needed by the client to manage or master adaptive tasks related to his or her health challenge

Defining Characteristics

Subjective
Client expresses or confirms a concern or complaint about significant other's response to his or her health problem

Significant person describes or confirms an inadequate understanding or knowledge base, which interferes with effective assistive or supportive behaviors

Significant person describes preoccupation with personal reaction (eg, fear, anticipatory grief, guilt, anxiety) to client's illness, disability, or other situational or developmental crises

Objective
Significant person attempts assistive or supportive behaviors with less-than-satisfactory results

Significant person displays protective behavior disproportionate (too little or too much) to the client's abilities or need for autonomy

Significant person withdraws or enters into limited or temporary personal communication with the client at the time of need

Other Possible Defining Characteristics (Non-NANDA)
Family displays emotional lability
Family displays rigid role boundaries
Family member interferes with necessary medical/nursing actions
Family members are divisive and form unsupportive coalitions
Family verbal interaction with patient is absent or decreased

Related Factors

Developmental crisis of significant person [specify]
Inadequate or incorrect information or understanding by a primary person
Little support provided by client, in turn, for primary person
Prolonged disease or disability progression that exhausts supportive capacity of significant people
Situational crisis of significant person [specify]
Temporary family disorganization and role changes
Temporary preoccupation by a significant person who is trying to manage emotional conflicts and personal suffering and is unable to perceive or act effectively in regard to client's needs

Suggestions for Use

(1) *Caregiver role strain* focuses on the needs of the *caregiving* family member, whereas *Ineffective Family Coping: Compromised* focuses more on the needs of the patient. (2) The distinctions between this diagnosis and *Altered family processes* are not clear. (3) For severe malfunction or for abusive or destructive situations, use *Ineffective family coping: disabling*, which is distinguished by the following defining characteristics:

Denial of existence or severity of illness of a family member
Despair, rejection
Desertion
Abuse (child, spousal, elder)

Suggested Alternative Diagnoses

Caregiver role strain (actual/risk for)
Family coping: ineffective, disabling
Family processes, altered
Management of therapeutic regimen: families, ineffective
Parental role conflict
Parenting, altered

NOC Suggested Outcomes

To be developed

Goals/Evaluation Criteria

Family member(s) will:
- Acknowledge needs of family unit
- Acknowledge needs of patient
- Begin to demonstrate effective interpersonal skills
- Express increased ability to cope with changes in family structure and dynamics
- Express unresolved feelings
- Participate in developing and implementing a treatment plan
- Use more flexible problem-solving strategies

NIC Priority Interventions

Family Involvement: Facilitating family participation in the emotional and physical care of the patient

Family Mobilization: Utilization of family strengths to influence patient's health in a positive direction

Family Support: Promotion of family interests and goals

Nursing Activities

Assessments

- Identify level of patient's self-care deficits and dependency on family
- Assess interaction between patient and family; be alert for potential destructive behaviors
- Assess ability and readiness of family members to learn
- Determine extent to which family members wish to be involved with the patient
- Identify the family's expectations of and for the patient
- Identify family structure and roles
- *(NIC) Family Support:*
  Appraise family's emotional reaction to patient's condition
  Identify nature of spiritual support for family

Patient/Family Teaching

- Discuss the common responses to health challenges (eg, anxiety, dependency, depression)
- Provide information about specific health challenge and necessary coping skills

- Teach the family those skills required for care of patient. Specify skills.
- Teach, role-model, and reinforce communication skills, which may include active listening, reflection, "I" statements, conflict resolution
- *(NIC) Family Support:*
  Teach the medical and nursing plans of care to family
  Provide necessary knowledge of options to family that will assist them to make decisions about patient care

Collaborative Activities

- Explore available hospital resources and support systems with family
- Request social service consultation to help the family determine posthospitalization needs and identify sources of community support
- Initiate a multidisciplinary patient care conference, involving the patient/family in problem solving and facilitation of communication
- *(NIC) Family Support:*
  Provide spiritual resources for family, as appropriate
  Arrange for ongoing respite care, when indicated and desired
  Provide opportunities for peer group support

Other

- Promote an open, trusting relationship with family
- Encourage patient/family to focus on positive aspects of the patient's situation
- Assist family in identifying behaviors that may be hindering prescribed treatment
- Assist family in realistically identifying the needs of patient and family unit
- Assist family with decision making and problem solving
- Encourage family to identify needed role changes to maintain family integrity
- Encourage family to recognize changes in interpersonal relationships
- Explore impact of conflicting values or coping styles on family relationships
- Encourage family to visit and/or care for patient whenever possible; provide privacy to facilitate family interactions
- Provide structure to family interaction. Consider content of interaction, length of visiting time, staff support during visit,

and which family member(s) will visit, based on patient's treatment plan

- *(NIC) Family Support:*
  Foster realistic hope
  Listen to family concerns, feelings, and questions
  Facilitate communication of concerns/feelings between patient
  and family or between family members
  Answer all questions of family members or assist them to get
  answers
  Give care to patient in lieu of family to relieve them and/or when
  family is unable to give care
  Provide feedback for family regarding their coping

Coping: Family, Ineffective, Disabling
(5.1.2.1.1) (1980, 1996)

Definition: Behavior of significant person (family member or other
primary person) that disables his or her own capacities and the
client's capacities to effectively address tasks essential to either
person's adaptation to the health challenge

Defining Characteristics

Subjective
Depression
Distortion of reality of patient's health problem, including extreme
denial about its existence or severity

Objective
Abandonment
Aggression/hostility
Agitation
Carrying on usual routines, disregarding client's needs
Client's development of helplessness, inactive dependence
Decisions and actions by family that are detrimental to economic
or social well-being
Desertion
Disregarding needs
Impaired individualization
Impaired restructuring of a meaningful life for self
Intolerance
Neglectful care of client in regard to basic human needs and/or illness treatment

Neglectful relationships with other family members
Prolonged overconcern for client
Psychosomatic symptoms
Rejection
Taking on illness signs of client

Related Factors

Arbitrary handling of family's resistance to treatment, which tends
to solidify defensiveness as it fails to deal adequately with
underlying anxiety
Dissonant discrepancy of coping styles for dealing with adaptive
tasks by the significant person and client or among significant
people
Highly ambivalent family relationships
Significant person with chronically unexpressed feelings of (hostility, anxiety, guilt, despair, and so on)

Other Possible Defining Characteristics (Non-NANDA)
Emotionally disturbed family member
Substance-abusing family member
Use of violence to manage conflict

Suggestions for Use

This label is appropriate when there is severe malfunction or for
abusive or destructive situations. It represents a more dysfunctional situation than does *Altered family processes* or *Ineffective
family coping: compromised*. The diagnostic label *Caregiver role
strain* focuses on the needs of the caregiving family member,
whereas *Ineffective family coping: disabling* focuses more on the
needs of the patient and/or the family unit. If there is actual violence in the family, the diagnosis might be *"Ineffective family coping: disabling related to use of violence to manage conflict."* When
the abusive behavior is potential rather than actual, the label *Risk
for violence* should be used.

Suggested Alternative Diagnoses

Caregiver role strain (actual/risk for)
Coping: family, ineffective, compromised
Coping: family, ineffective, disabling
Management of therapeutic regimen: families/individual, ineffective
Parenting, altered
Violence: directed at others, risk for

NOC Suggested Outcomes

To be developed

Goals/Evaluation Criteria

Family will:
- Acknowledge needs of family unit
- Acknowledge needs of patient
- Begin to demonstrate effective interpersonal skills
- Demonstrate ability to resolve conflict without violence
- Express unresolved feelings
- Identify and maintain intrafamily sexual boundaries
- Identify conflicting coping styles
- Participate in effective problem solving
- Participate in treatment plan

NIC Priority Interventions

Family Support: Promotion of family interests and goals

Family Therapy: Assisting family members to move their family toward a more productive way of living

Nursing Activities

Also refer to "Nursing Activities" in "Coping: Family, Ineffective, Compromised", pp. 96–98.

Assessments

- Obtain history of family's pattern of behaviors and interactions and changes that have occurred
- Assess interaction between patient and family, being alert for potential destructive behaviors (eg, elder abuse, child abuse)
- Determine physical, emotional, and educational resources of family members
- Assess family members' motivation/desire for resolving areas of dissatisfaction and/or conflict
- *(NIC) Family Support:*
  Determine the psychological burden of prognosis for family
  Identify nature of spiritual support for family

Patient/Family Teaching

- Discuss how violence is a learned behavior and can be transmitted to offspring
- Discuss with family effective ways to demonstrate feelings

Collaborative Activities

- Refer family/individual members to support groups, psychiatric treatment, social services (eg, chemical-dependence programs, Parents United, Incest Survivors Anonymous, child protective services, battered wives' shelters)
- Report indications of physical/sexual abuse as directed by law to appropriate authorities
- *(NIC) Family Support:*
  Provide spiritual resources for family, as appropriate
  Arrange for ongoing respite care, when indicated and desired

Other

- In family discussions, begin with the least emotionally laden subjects
- Assist family in realistically identifying the needs of patient and family unit
- Assist family in recognizing the problem (eg, managing conflict with violence, sexual abuse)
- Encourage family participation in all group meetings
- Encourage family to express concerns and to help plan posthospital care
- Help motivate family to change
- Assist family in finding better ways to handle dysfunctional behavior
- Provide "homework" for family members (eg, a no-television night or eating some meals together)
- Assist family members in clarifying what they expect and need from each other
- *(NIC) Family Support:*
  Foster realistic hope
  Listen to family concerns, feelings, and questions
  Facilitate communication of concerns/feelings between patient and family or between family members
  Answer all questions of family members or assist them to get answers
  Provide feedback for family regarding their coping
  Give care to patient in lieu of family to relieve them and/or when family is unable to give care

Coping: Family, Potential for Growth
(5.1.2.2) (1988)

Definition: Effective managing of adaptive tasks by family member involved with the client's health challenge, who now is exhibiting desire and readiness for enhanced health and growth in regard to self and in relation to the client

Defining Characteristics

Subjective

Individual expressing interest in making contact on a one-to-one basis or on a mutual-aid group basis with another person who has experienced a similar situation

Objective

Family member attempting to describe growth impact of crisis on his or her own values, priorities, goals, or relationships

Family member moving in direction of health promoting and enriching lifestyle that supports and monitors maturational processes, audits and negotiates treatment programs, and chooses experiences that optimize wellness

Related Factors

Needs sufficiently gratified and adaptive tasks effectively addressed to enable goals of self-actualization to surface

Suggestions for Use

Use this diagnosis for a normally functioning family that wishes to preserve and improve family integrity during changes brought about by illness or developmental and situational crises. Such a family might wish to have control over outcomes and/or enhance their quality of life. There is some overlap between this label and the following "Suggested Alternative Diagnoses." Pending further research, use *Altered family processes* and *Health-Seeking behaviors.*

Suggested Alternative Diagnoses

Altered family processes
Health-seeking behaviors

NOC Suggested Outcomes

To be developed

Goals/Evaluation Criteria

(Also refer to "Goals/Evaluation Criteria" for the diagnoses "Altered family processes" and "Health seeking behaviors," on pp. 150 and 193–194, respectively)

Family member(s) will:

- Develop a plan for personal growth.
- Evaluate and change plan as needed.
- Identify and prioritize personal goals.
- Implement plan.

NIC Priority Interventions

Developmental Enhancement: Facilitating or teaching parents/caregivers to facilitate the optimal gross-motor, fine-motor, language, cognitive, social, and emotional growth of preschool and school-age children

Family Support: Promotion of family interests and goals

Normalization Promotion: Assisting parents and other family members of children with chronic illnesses or disabilities in providing normal life experiences for their children and families

Pass Facilitation: Arranging a leave for a patient from a health care facility

Nursing Activities

Assessments

- Assess physical, emotional, and educational resources of the family
- Identify family cultural influences
- Identify any self-care deficits in patient
- Identify family structure and roles
- *(NIC) Family Support:*
  Appraise family's emotional reaction to patient's condition
  Determine the psychological burden of prognosis for family
  Identify nature of spiritual support for family

Patient/Family Teaching

- *(NIC) Family Support:*
  Teach the medical and nursing plans of care to family
  Provide necessary knowledge of options to family that will assist them to make decisions about patient care
  Assist family to acquire necessary knowledge, skills, and equipment to sustain their decision about patient care

Collaborative Activities

- Identify community resources that can be used to enhance the health status of the patient with family members
- *(NIC) Family Support:* Arrange for ongoing respite care, when indicated and desired

Other

- Assist family member(s) in developing a plan for personal growth. Plan may include investigation of employment opportunities, school, support groups, enrichment activities, and exercise
- Provide emotional support and availability to family member(s) during implementation, evaluation, and revision of plan
- Assist family member(s) in identifying and prioritizing personal goals
- Encourage family member(s) to compare initial response to the crisis with current situation and to recognize change
- Provide an opportunity for family member(s) to reflect on impact of patient's illness on family structure and dynamics
- Discuss how strengths and resources can be used to enhance health status of the patient with family members
- *(NIC) Family Support:*

  Assure family that best care possible is being given to patient

  Accept the family's values in a nonjudgmental manner

  Listen to family concerns, feelings, and questions

  Facilitate communication of concerns/feelings between patient and family or between family members

  Answer all questions of family members or assist them to get answers

  Respect and support adaptive coping mechanisms used by family

  Provide feedback for family regarding their coping

  Encourage family decision making in planning long-term patient care affecting family structure and finances

  Advocate for family, as appropriate

  Foster family assertiveness in information seeking, as appropriate

Coping: Individual, Ineffective
(5.1.1.1) (1978, 1998)

Definition: Inability to form a valid appraisal of the stressors, inadequate choices of practiced responses, and/or inability to use available resources

Defining Characteristics

Subjective

Change in usual communication patterns

Fatigue

Verbalization of inability to cope or to ask for help

Objective

Abuse of chemical agents

Decreased use of social support

Destructive behavior toward self and others

High illness rate

Inability to meet basic needs

Inability to meet role expectations

Inadequate problem solving

Lack of goal-directed behavior/resolution of problems, including inability to attend and difficulty with organizing information

Poor concentration

Risk taking

Sleep disturbance

Use of forms of coping that impede adaptive behavior

Other Possible Defining Characteristics (Non-NANDA)

Evidence of physical/psychologic abuse

Expression of unrealistic expectations

High rate of accidents

Inappropriate use of defense mechanisms

Verbal manipulation

Related Factors

Disturbance in pattern of appraisal of threat

Disturbance in pattern of tension release

Gender differences in coping strategies

High degree of threat

Inability to conserve adaptive energies

Inadequate level of confidence in ability to cope

Inadequate level of perception of control

Inadequate opportunity to prepare for stressor

Inadequate resources available

Inadequate social support created by characteristics of relationships

Situational or maturational crises

Uncertainty

Suggestions for Use

Many labels represent failure to cope (eg, *Anxiety, Risk for violence, Hopelessness*). Always use the most specific label that fits the patient's defining characteristics. *Ineffective individual coping* represents a more chronic or long-term pattern than does *Impaired adjustment*. It is also less specific than the label *Defensive coping*.

Suggested Alternative Diagnoses

Adjustment, impaired

Anxiety

Denial, ineffective

Fear

Grieving, dysfunctional

Post-trauma syndrome

Violence, risk for: self-directed or directed at others

NOC Suggested Outcomes

Coping: Actions to manage stressors that tax an individual's resources

Decision Making: Ability to choose between two or more alternatives

Impulse Control: Ability to self-restrain compulsive or impulsive behaviors

Information Processing: Ability to acquire, organize, and use information

Goals/Evaluation Criteria

Examples Using NOC Language

- Demonstrates effective **Coping**, as evidenced by the following indicators (specify 1–5: never, rarely, sometimes, often, or consistently demonstrated):

    Identifies effective [and ineffective] coping patterns

    Seeks information concerning illness and treatment

Employs behaviors to reduce stress
Identifies and uses multiple coping strategies
Reports decrease in negative feelings
- Demonstrates **Impulse Control** by consistently maintain[ing] self-control without supervision
- Demonstrates normal **Information Processing** by consistently exhibit[ing] logical thought processes

Other Examples

Patient will:
- Demonstrate interest in diversional activities
- Identify personal strengths that may promote effective coping
- Weigh and choose among alternatives and consequences
- Initiate conversation
- Participate in activities of daily living
- Participate in decision-making process
- Use verbal and nonverbal expressions applicable to situation
- Verbalize plan for either accepting or changing the situation

NIC Priority Interventions

Coping Enhancement: Assisting a patient to adapt to perceived stressors, changes, or threats which interfere with meeting life demands and roles

Decision-Making Support: Providing information and support for a patient who is making a decision regarding health care

Nursing Activities

Assessments

- Monitor for aggressive behaviors
- Identify the patient's view of own condition and its congruence with the view of health care providers
- *(NIC) Coping Enhancement:*
  Appraise patient's adjustment to changes in body image, as indicated
  Appraise the impact of the patient's life situation on roles and relationships
  Evaluate the patient's decision-making ability
  Explore with the patient previous methods of dealing with life problems
  Determine the risk of the patient's inflicting self-harm

Patient/Family Teaching

- *(NIC) Coping Enhancement:*

    Provide factual information concerning diagnosis, treatment, and prognosis

    Instruct the patient on the use of relaxation techniques, as needed

    Provide appropriate social skills training

Collaborative Activities

- Initiate a patient care conference to review patient's coping mechanisms and to establish a plan of care
- Involve hospital resources in provision of emotional support for patient and family
- Serve as a liaison between patient, other health care providers, and community resources (eg, support groups)

Other

- Assist patient in developing a plan for accepting or changing situation
- Assist patient in identifying personal strengths
- Encourage patient to:

    Be involved in planning care activities

    Initiate conversations with others

    Participate in activity
- Ask family to visit whenever possible
- *(NIC) Coping Enhancement:*

    Encourage patient to identify a realistic description of change in role

    Use a calm, reassuring approach

    Reduce stimuli in the environment that could be misinterpreted as threatening

    Provide an atmosphere of acceptance

    Discourage decision making when the patient is under severe stress

    Foster constructive outlets for anger and hostility

    Explore patient's reasons for self-criticism

    Arrange situations that encourage patient's autonomy

    Assist patient in identifying positive responses from others

    Support the use of appropriate defense mechanisms

    Encourage verbalization of feelings, perceptions, and fears

    Assist the patient to clarify misconceptions

    Assist the patient to identify available support systems

    Appraise and discuss alternative responses to situation

Decisional Conflict (specify)
(5.3.1.1) (1988)

Definition: The state of uncertainty about course of action to be taken when choice among competing actions involves risk, loss, or challenge to personal life values

Defining Characteristics

Subjective

Focusing on self

Questioning personal values and beliefs while attempting a decision

Verbalized feeling of distress while attempting a decision

Verbalized uncertainty about choices

Verbalization of undesired consequences of alternative actions being considered

Objective

Delayed decision making

Physical signs of distress or tension (eg, increased heart rate, increased muscle tension, restlessness)

Vacillation between alternative choices

Related Factors

Lack of experience or interference with decision making

Lack of relevant information

Lack of support system

Multiple or divergent sources of information

Perceived threat to value system

Unclear personal values/beliefs

Suggestions for Use

(1) The role of the nurse is to help clients make logical, informed decisions by providing information and support. The nurse should not try to influence the client to decide in a particular way. (2) Do not assume that clients facing a serious, even life-and-death, decision are conflicted. Such decisions may actually be easy to make in some cases.

Suggested Alternative Diagnoses

Parental role conflict

Management of therapeutic regimen: individual, ineffective

NOC Suggested Outcomes

Decision Making: Ability to choose between two or more alternatives

Information Processing: Ability to acquire, organize, and use information

Participation: Health Care Decisions: Personal involvement in selecting and evaluating health care options

Goals/Evaluation Criteria

Examples Using NOC Language

- *Decisional conflict* will lessen, as demonstrated by Information Processing abilities and Participation: Health Care Decisions
- **Decision Making** will be demonstrated, as evidenced by the following indicators (specify 1–5: never, rarely, sometimes, often, or consistently demonstrated):

    Identifies relevant information

    Recognizes contradiction with others' desires

    Acknowledges relevant legal implications

    Weighs and chooses among alternatives

    Identifies resources necessary to support each alternative

    Acknowledges social context of the situation

Other Examples

Patient will:
- Evaluate available choices in relation to personal values
- Report a decrease in tension or distress
- Exhibit information processing and logical thought processes
- Uses problem solving to achieve chosen outcomes

NIC Priority Interventions

Decision-Making Support: Providing information and support for a patient who is making a decision regarding health care

Nursing Activities

Assessments

- Assess patient's understanding of available choices
- Evaluate patient's level of tension or distress
- *(NIC) Decision-Making Support:* Determine whether there are differences between the patient's view of own condition and the view of health care providers

Patient/Family Teaching

- *(NIC) Decision-Making Support:*
  Inform patient of alternative views of solutions
  Provide information requested by patient

Collaborative Activities

- Use resources (eg, ethics committee) as appropriate.
- *(NIC) Decision-Making Support:*
  Serve as a liaison between patient and other health care providers
  Refer to support groups, as appropriate
  Refer to legal aid, as appropriate
  Facilitate collaborative decision making

Other

- Assist patient in identifying a course of action and adapt as necessary
- *(NIC) Decision-Making Support:*
  Establish communication with patient early in admission
  Facilitate patient's articulation of goals for care
  Facilitate collaborative decision making
  Help patient identify the advantages and disadvantages of each alternative
  Help patient explain decision to others, as needed
  Serve as a liaison between patient and family
  Serve as a liaison between patient and other health care providers
  Respect patient's right to receive or not to receive information

Denial, Ineffective
(5.1.1.1.3) (1988)

Definition: The state of a conscious or unconscious attempt to disavow the knowledge or meaning of an event to reduce anxiety/fear to the detriment of health

Defining Characteristics

Subjective

Displaces fear of impact of the condition
Does not admit fear of death or invalidism
Displays inappropriate affect
Minimizes symptoms
Unable to admit impact of disease in life pattern

Objective

Delays seeking or refuses health care attention to the detriment of health

Displaces source of symptoms to other organs

Does not perceive personal relevance of symptoms or danger

Makes dismissive gestures or comments when speaking of distressing events

Uses home remedies (self-treatment) to relieve symptoms

Related Factors

To be developed

Suggestions for Use

Some denial in response to illness or other crises may be necessary in order for the client to cope with the situation. Such normal denial is gradually replaced by acceptance or changing of the situation, and it does not interfere with the treatment regimen. *Ineffective denial* should be used for clients whose denial persists or interferes with the treatment regimen. For example, a client newly diagnosed with myocardial infarction may respond with denial and, therefore, fail to make changes in lifestyle needed to prevent further heart damage.

Suggested Alternative Diagnoses

Coping: defensive

Family coping: ineffective, compromised

Family coping: ineffective, disabling

Grieving, dysfunctional

Coping: individual, ineffective

Management of therapeutic regimen: individual, ineffective

Noncompliance (specify)

Rape-trauma syndrome: silent reaction

NOC Suggested Outcomes

Acceptance: Health Status: Reconciliation to health circumstances

Anxiety Control: Ability to eliminate or reduce feelings of apprehension and tension from an unidentifiable source

Health Beliefs: Perceived Threat: Personal conviction that a health problem is serious and has potential negative consequences for lifestyle

Symptom Control Behavior: Personal actions to minimize perceived adverse changes in physical and emotional functioning

Goals/Evaluation Criteria

Examples Using NOC Language

- Patient will not use *Ineffective denial*, as evidenced by Health Beliefs (Perceived Threat), Anxiety Control, and Symptom Control Behavior
- Patient will demonstrate **Acceptance: Health Status** as indicated by:

    Relinquishment of previous concept of health

    Recognition of reality of health situation

    Pursuit of information

    Coping with health situation

    Health-related decision making

Other Examples

    Patient will:

- Acknowledge and recognize significance of symptoms
- Report significant symptoms
- Not demonstrate physical and behavioral manifestations of anxiety
- Acknowledge vulnerability to health problem

NIC Priority Interventions

Anxiety Reduction: Minimizing apprehension, dread, foreboding, or uneasiness related to an unidentified source of anticipated danger

Counseling: Use of an interactive helping process focusing on the needs, problems, or feelings of the patient and significant others to enhance or support coping, problem solving, and interpersonal relationships

Nursing Activities

Assessments

- Assess patient's understanding of symptoms/illness
- Determine whether patient's perception of his/her health status is realistic
- (*NIC*) *Anxiety Reduction:*

    Determine patient's decision-making ability

    Identify when level of anxiety changes

Patient Teaching

- Teach recognition of symptoms and desired patient responses

- *(NIC) Anxiety Reduction:* Provide factual information concerning diagnosis, treatment, and prognosis

Collaborative Activities

- Include patient/family in a multidisciplinary conference to develop a plan of action. Plan may include:

  Arranging for follow-up support after discharge

  Meeting with patients in similar situations to learn new ways to cope and to decrease anxiety and fear

Other

- Establish a therapeutic relationship with patient that will allow exploration of denial
- Use every opportunity to reinforce consequences of patient's actions
- Engage patient in discussion about anxiety, fears, symptoms, and impact of illness
- Identify and reinforce patient strengths
- *(NIC) Anxiety Reduction:*

  Seek to understand the patient's perspective of a stressful situation

  Reinforce behavior, as appropriate

  Encourage verbalization of feelings, perceptions, and fears

  Demonstrate empathy, warmth, and genuineness

  Support the use of appropriate defense mechanisms

  Assist patient to articulate a realistic description of an upcoming event

Dentition, Altered
(1.6.2.1.2.3) (1998)

Definition: Disruption in tooth development/eruption patterns or structural integrity of individual teeth

Defining Characteristics

Subjective

Toothache

Objective

Asymmetrical facial expression

Crown or root caries

Erosion of enamel

Excessive calculus

Excessive plaque

Halitosis

Incomplete eruption for age (may be primary or permanent teeth)

Loose teeth

Malocclusion or tooth misalignment

Missing teeth or complete absence

Premature loss of primary teeth

Tooth enamel discoloration

Tooth fracture(s)

Worn-down or abraded teeth

Related Factors

Access or economic barriers to professional care

Barriers to self-care

Bruxism

Chronic use of tobacco, coffee, tea, or red wine

Chronic vomiting

Dietary habits

Excessive intake of fluorides

Excessive use of abrasive cleaning agents

Genetic predisposition

Ineffective oral hygiene

Lack of knowledge regarding dental health

Nutritional deficits

Premature loss of primary teeth

Selected prescription medications

Sensitivity to heat or cold

Suggestions for Use

None

Suggested Alternative Diagnosis

Self-care deficit: bathing/hygiene

NOC Suggested Outcomes

To be developed

Goals/Evaluation Criteria

Patient will:

- Be free from debris and plaque on dental surfaces
- Have firm, well-hydrated, nonbleeding gums of uniform color
- Verbalize feeling of oral cleanliness

- Demonstrate correct brushing and flossing procedures
- Follow sound nutritional practices, such as avoiding sweets between meals
- Have a checkup by a dentist every six months
- Be free from caries, loose teeth, and/or toothaches
- Parent will take child for first dentist visit by age 2
- Child will not experience premature loss of primary teeth

NIC Priority Interventions

To be developed

Nursing Activities

Assessments

- Inspect mouth for loose or missing teeth, color and condition of enamel, number of dental fillings and caries, and tartar at base of teeth
- Observe for halitosis
- Determine client's usual oral hygiene practices
- Assess client's level of knowledge of measures to prevent *Altered dentition* (eg, "How often do you see your dentist?")
- Assess client's access to and resources for dental care
- Assess client's ability to perform oral care (eg, "Do you have any problems caring for your teeth?")
- Assess client's knowledge of oral hygiene practices/routines (eg, brushing method)
- Identify risk factors for *Altered dentition* (eg, clients who are seriously ill, confused, depressed)

Collaborative Activities

- Refer to dental hygienist, dentist, or clinic, as needed

Client Teaching

- Teach parents the importance of caring for the child's primary teeth
- Teach parents to help children brush or inspect their mouths after brushing
- Teach brushing and flossing techniques, as needed
- Explain the causes of dental problems, such as tooth decay
- Teach to avoid heavy use of tobacco, tea, coffee, and red wine, to prevent discoloration
- Teach measures to avoid tooth decay:
    Brush after meals and at bedtime

Ensure adequate intake of calcium, phosphorus, and vitamins A, C, and D

Avoid sweets between meals; take in moderation with meals

Eat cleansing foods, such as raw fruits and vegetables

If water is not fluoridated, take a fluoride supplement daily until at least age 14

Have a dental checkup every six months

Floss teeth daily

Other

- Provide oral hygiene for patients with *Self-care deficit* (eg, thorough brushing and rinsing)
- Help patient establish an oral hygiene schedule after meals and at bedtime. For example:

    Use sulcular technique and soft toothbrush

    Rinse with mouthwash or solution of warm water and salt or baking soda

Development, Risk for Altered
(6.6.1) (1998)

Definition: At risk for delay of 25 percent or more in one or more of the areas of social or self-regulatory behavior or cognitive, language, gross or fine-motor skills

Risk Factors

Prenatal

Genetic or endocrine disorders

Illiteracy

Inadequate nutrition

Infections

Lack of, late, or poor prenatal care

Maternal age < 15 or > 35 years

Poverty

Substance abuse

Unplanned or unwanted pregnancy

Individual

Behavior disorders

Brain damage (eg, hemorrhage in postnatal period, shaken baby, abuse, accident)

Chemotherapy

Chronic illness
Congenital or genetic disorders
Failure to thrive, inadequate nutrition
Foster or adopted child
Hearing impairment or frequent otitis media
Lead poisoning
Natural disaster
Positive drug-screening test
Prematurity
Radiation therapy
Seizures
Substance abuse
Technology-dependent
Vision impairment

Environmental
Poverty
Violence

Caregiver
Abuse
Mental illness
Mental retardation or severe learning disability

Suggestions for Use

(1) This diagnosis is made when one or more risk factors are present and the nursing focus is on preventing developmental delays by eliminating the risk factors. (2) Because development is routinely assessed in nursing care of children, a diagnostic statement is usually not required for that application; such assessment is usually included in pediatric standards of care. (3) This label is not appropriate for a mentally impaired child (eg, *Risk for Altered development related to Down syndrome*). Instead, diagnose the specific functional task that the child is unable to perform (eg, *Feeding self-care deficit, Bowel incontinence*).

Suggested Alternative Diagnoses

Bowel incontinence
Communication, impaired verbal
Coping: family, ineffective, compromised
Coping: family, ineffective, disabling
Growth, risk for altered
Growth and development, altered

Coping: individual, ineffective
Parenting, altered
Self-care deficit (specify)
Urinary incontinence

NOC Suggested Outcomes

To be developed

Goals/Evaluation Criteria

NOTE: This text can only provide examples of developmental milestones. Refer to pediatrics or child development texts for complete discussion of growth and development

- The child will achieve developmental milestones, that is, not experience a delay of 25 percent or more in one or more of the areas of social or self-regulatory behavior or cognitive, language, gross-motor, or fine-motor skills. For example:

  For a 6-month-old: Rolls over, sits with support, grasps and mouths objects

  For a 3-year-old: Demonstrates autonomy, is toilet trained

NIC Priority Interventions

To be developed

Nursing Activities

NOTE: Because this nursing diagnosis is so broad and nonspecific, it is not possible to list every nursing activity here. Refer to age-specific sections in growth and development texts.

Assessments

- Conduct a thorough health assessment (eg, child's history, temperament, culture, family environment, developmental screening) to determine functional level
- Determine caretakers' level of knowledge, resources, support system, and coping skills
- Identify parental future expectations for child (eg, ability to learn, developmental achievements)
- Monitor parent/child interactions (eg, during feedings)
- Assess prenatally for presence of risk factors (eg, poverty, substance abuse)
- Assess for postnatal risk factors (eg, chronic illness, seizures, violence, caregiver mental illness)

Patient/Family Teaching

- Teach parents about normal developmental milestones
- Demonstrate activities that promote development
- Teach ways to provide meaningful stimulation for infants and children
- Teach about age-appropriate behaviors
- Teach about age-appropriate toys and materials

Other

- If risk factors cannot be removed (as in a natural disaster), assist family to find resources and support coping efforts
- Assist patient to achieve next level of development through appropriate mastery of tasks specific to his/her level (refer to growth and development text)
- Establish a therapeutic and trusting relationship with caretakers
- Provide appropriate play activities; encourage activities with other children
- Communicate with patient at appropriate cognitive level of development
- Provide positive rewards or feedback for attempts at self-expression
- Use consistent, structured behavior modification techniques
- Involve patient in self-care and activities of daily living as much as possible
- Encourage parents to expect and require responsible behavior in child

Diarrhea
(1.3.1.2) (1975, 1988)

Definition: Passage of loose, unformed stools

Defining Characteristics

Subjective
Abdominal pain
Cramping
Urgency

Objective
At least three loose liquid stools per day
Hyperactive bowel sounds

Related Factors

Psychological
High stress levels and anxiety

Situational
Adverse effects of medications
Alcohol abuse
Contaminants
Laxative abuse
Radiation
Toxins
Travel
Tube feedings

Physiological
Infectious processes
Inflammation
Irritation
Malabsorption
Parasites

Suggestions for Use

None

Suggested Alternative Diagnosis

Incontinence, Bowel

NOC Suggested Outcomes

Bowel Elimination: Ability of the gastrointestinal tract to form and evacuate stool effectively

Electrolyte and Acid/Base Balance: Balance of electrolytes and nonelectrolytes in the intracellular and extracellular compartments of the body

Fluid Balance: Balance of water in the intracellular and extracellular compartments of the body

Hydration: Amount of water in the intracellular and extracellular compartments of the body

Treatment Behavior: Illness or Injury: Personal actions to palliate or eliminate pathology

Goals/Evaluation Criteria

Examples Using NOC Language

- *Diarrhea* will be controlled/eliminated, as demonstrated by effective Bowel Elimination, Electrolyte and Acid/Base Balance, Fluid Balance, adequate Hydration, and Treatment Behavior (Illness or Injury) to palliate or eliminate the diarrhea
- Demonstrates effective **Bowel Elimination**, as evidenced by the following indicators (specify 1–5: extremely, substantially, moderately, mildly, or not compromised):

  Elimination pattern in expected range

  Diarrhea not present

  Stool free of blood and mucus

  Painful cramps not present

  Bloating not present

Other Examples

Patient will:

- Follow dietary requirements to alleviate diarrhea
- Practice hygiene adequate to prevent skin breakdown
- Verbalize understanding of the causes of her/his diarrhea
- Maintain electrolyte balance within normal limits
- Maintain acid/base balance within normal limits
- Be well hydrated (mucous membranes moist; afebrile; good eyeball turgor; B/P, hematocrit, and urine output within normal limits)

NIC Priority Interventions

Diarrhea Management: Prevention and alleviation of diarrhea

Nursing Activities

Assessments

- Perform guaiac test on stools
- Have patient identify usual bowel pattern
- Monitor laboratory values (electrolytes, CBC), and report abnormalities
- Weigh patient daily
- Assess and document:

  Frequency, color, consistency, and amount (measure) of stool

  Skin turgor and condition of oral mucosa as indicators of dehydration
- *(NIC) Diarrhea Management:*

  Obtain stool for culture and sensitivity, if diarrhea continues

Evaluate medication profile for gastrointestinal side effects

Evaluate recorded intake for nutritional content

Monitor skin in perianal area for irritation and ulceration

Patient/Family Teaching

- Inform patient of possibility of medication-induced diarrhea
- *(NIC) Diarrhea Management:*

  Teach patient appropriate use of antidiarrheal medications

  Instruct patient/family members to record color, volume, frequency, and consistency of stools

  Instruct patient to notify staff of each episode of diarrhea

  Teach patient stress-reduction techniques, as appropriate

Collaborative Activities

- Consult with dietitian for adjustment of diet
- Consult with pediatrician for alternative type of feeding
- *(NIC) Diarrhea Management:* Consult physician if signs and symptoms of diarrhea persist

Other

- Help patient to identify stressors that may contribute to diarrhea
- Provide care in an accepting, nonjudgmental manner
- Provide fluids of patient's choice (specify)
- Provide privacy and safety for patient during bowel elimination
- *(NIC) Diarrhea Management:*

  Perform actions to rest the bowel (eg, NPO or liquid diet)

  Encourage frequent, small feedings and add bulk gradually

Disuse Syndrome, Risk for
(1.6.1.5) (1988)

Definition: A state in which an individual is at risk for deterioration of body systems as the result of prescribed or unavoidable musculoskeletal inactivity. **NOTE:** Complications from immobility can include pressure ulcer, constipation, stasis of pulmonary secretions, thrombosis, urinary tract infection/retention, decreased strength/endurance, orthostatic hypotension, decreased range of joint motion, disorientation, body image disturbance, and powerlessness.

Risk Factors

Subjective
Severe pain

Objective
Altered level of consciousness
Mechanical immobilization
Paralysis
Prescribed immobilization

Suggestions for Use

This label describes the cluster of potential complications of immobility (eg, *Risk for constipation, Risk for impaired skin integrity*). It is a "syndrome diagnosis" under which a number of actual and potential problems are clustered. Therefore, when the risk factor is immobility, it is not necessary to write separate risk diagnoses such as *Risk for impaired skin integrity*. Those more specific labels should be used only if an actual problem develops (eg, actual *Impaired skin integrity related to immobility*), or if the risk factor is something other than immobility (eg, Risk for impaired skin integrity related to malnutrition). Furthermore, this diagnosis should not be written with an etiology. As a syndrome diagnosis, the etiology (disuse) is contained in the label itself.

Even though the NANDA terminology is still "*Risk for disuse syndrome*," Carpenito (1997b, p. 326) recommends that syndrome diagnoses not be written with "risk for," since they include both actual and risk diagnoses. In that case, the diagnosis "*Disuse syndrome*" would be used both for clients with the risk factor of immobility and those with the defining characteristics for actual *Disuse syndrome*.

Suggested Alternative Diagnoses

If an actual problem occurs as a result of immobility or if the etiology of a potential problem is something other than immobility, consider using a more restricted physiological nursing diagnosis, such as one of the following:

Actual or Risk for:
Activity intolerance
Body image disturbance
Breathing pattern, ineffective
Constipation
Physical mobility, impaired

Powerlessness

Sensory/perceptual alterations: all (specify)

Sexuality patterns, altered

Skin integrity, impaired

Swallowing, impaired

Tissue perfusion, altered (peripheral)

Urinary retention

Risk for:

Infection

Injury

Peripheral neuromuscular dysfunction

NOC Suggested Outcomes

Endurance: Extent that energy enables a person's activity

Immobility Consequences: Physiological: Compromise in physiological functioning due to impaired physical mobility

Mobility Level: Ability to move purposefully

Neurological Status: Consciousness: Extent to which an individual arouses, orients, and attends to the environment

Pain Level: Amount of reported or demonstrated pain

Goals/Evaluation Criteria

Examples Using NOC Language

- Risk factors will be controlled and patient will not experience *Disuse syndrome*, as evidenced by outcomes of Endurance, Mobility Level, Neurological Status: Consciousness, and Pain Level

- Patient will demonstrate **Immobility Consequences: Physiological**, as evidenced by the following indicators (specify 1–5: severe, substantial, moderate, slight, or none):

     Constipation, stool impaction, hypoactive bowel, or paralytic ileus

     Decreased nutritional status

     Urinary calculi, urinary retention, or urinary tract infection

     Pressure sore(s)

     Decreased muscle strength or decreased muscle tone

     Bone fracture, impaired joint movement, contracted joints or ankylosed joints

     Orthostatic hypotension

     Venous thrombosis

     Decreased cough effectiveness, decreased vital capacity, or pneumonia

Other Examples

Goals of care for this label are broad. They focus on preventing complications of immobility for all body systems. For example, patient will:

- Be oriented to time, place, and person
- Have adequate peripheral circulation
- Maintain optimal respiratory function (eg, effective cough, no lung congestion, normal vital capacity)
- Maintain satisfactory body image
- Demonstrate concentration and interest in surroundings
- Have laboratory values within normal limits (eg, oxygen, blood glucose, hemoglobin and hematocrit, and serum electrolyte levels)

NIC Priority Interventions

Energy Management: Regulating energy use to treat or prevent fatigue and optimize function

Nursing Activities

NOTE: In addition to the following generic activities, the outcomes and interventions selected for this diagnosis are determined by the affected body system and the degree of disuse. For patient goals and nursing activities specific to each body system, refer to plans for the "Suggested Alternative Diagnoses" listed on pp. 124–125.

Assessments

- Make all assessments indicated in the preceding "Goals/Evaluation Criteria," pp. 125–126.
- *(NIC) Energy Management:*
  Monitor nutritional intake to ensure adequate energy resources
  Monitor patient's oxygen response (eg, pulse rate, cardiac rhythm, and respiratory rate) to self-care or nursing activities
  Determine what and how much activity is required to build endurance

Patient/Family Teaching

- *(NIC) Energy Management:*
  Assist the patient to understand energy conservation principles (eg, the requirement for restricted activity or bed rest)
  Teach activity organization and time-management techniques to prevent fatigue
  Instruct patient/significant other to recognize signs and symptoms of fatigue that require reduction in activity

Collaborative Activities
- Consult with physical therapy for ways to improve mobility
- *(NIC) Energy Management:* Consult with dietitian about ways to increase intake of high-energy foods

Other
- Plan and implement a turning schedule
- *(NIC) Energy Management:*
  Avoid care activities during scheduled rest periods
  Encourage verbalization of feelings about limitations
  Use passive and/or active range-of-motion exercises to relieve muscle tension
  Encourage physical activity (eg, ambulation or performance of activities of daily living) consistent with patient's energy resources
  Assist patient to sit on side of bed ("dangle") if unable to transfer or walk

Diversional Activity Deficit
(6.3.1.1) (1980)

Definition: The state in which an individual experiences decreased stimulation from or decreased interest/engagement in recreational leisure activities

Defining Characteristics

Subjective
Patient's statements regarding: boredom, wish there was something to do, to read, etc.

Objective
Usual hobbies cannot be undertaken in hospital

Other Possible Defining Characteristics (Non-NANDA)
Anger, hostility
Complaints of inability to initiate or continue with usual activity
Disruptive behavior
Flat affect
Increase in daytime sleep periods
Restlessness
Withdrawn behavior

Related Factors

Environmental lack of diversional activity, as in long-term hospitalization

Frequent, lengthy treatments

Other Possible Related Factors (Non-NANDA)
Deficit in social skills
Forced inactivity
Impaired perception of reality
Lack of motivation
Prolonged bed rest

Suggestions for Use

Diversional activity deficit must be diagnosed from the patient's point of view because only the patient can determine whether the activities available are adequate to meet her/his needs.

Suggested Alternative Diagnoses

Adjustment, impaired
Coping: individual, ineffective
Loneliness, risk for
Social interaction, impaired

NOC Suggested Outcomes

Leisure Participation: Use of restful or relaxing activities as needed to promote well-being

Play Participation: Use of activities as needed for enjoyment, entertainment, and development by children

Social Involvement: Frequency of an individual's social interactions with persons, groups, or organizations

Goals/Evaluation Criteria

Examples Using NOC Language

- *Diversional activity deficit* will be relieved, as evidenced by Leisure Participation, Play Participation, and Social Involvement
- Demonstrates **Social Involvement,** as evidenced by the following indicators (specify 1–5: none, limited, moderate, substantial, or extensive):

    Interaction with close friends, neighbors, family members, or members of work group(s)

    Participation as member of church, club member, club officer, or volunteer group member

Other Examples

Patient will:

- Demonstrate socially acceptable behaviors during activities
- Verbalize acceptance of limitations that interfere with usual leisure activities
- Identify options for recreation
- Verbalize satisfaction with leisure activities
- Participate in appropriate play
- Demonstrate/verbalize enjoyment of play

NIC Priority Interventions

Recreation Therapy: Purposeful use of recreation to promote relaxation and enhancement of social skills

Self-Responsibility Facilitation: Encouraging a patient to assume more responsibility for own behavior

Nursing Activities

Assessments

- Assess patient's physical and mental abilities to take part in activities
- Identify patient's interests
- Monitor emotional, physical, and social responses to diversional activity
- *(NIC) Self-Responsibility Facilitation:* Monitor level of responsibility that patient assumes

Collaborative Activities

- Identify resources, such as volunteers and occupational therapists, that could assist patient in recreational/leisure activities

Other

- Introduce and encourage new or alternative leisure-time activities. Specify activities
- Introduce patient to other patients who have successfully dealt with similar situations
- Provide appropriate stimuli, such as music, games, puzzles, visitors, and relaxation therapy, to vary monotonous routines and stimulate thought
- Provide compatible roommate, if possible
- Help patient to choose recreational activities appropriate to capabilities (eg, physical, psychologic, and social)
- Supervise recreational activities, as necessary

- Encourage family, friends, and significant persons to visit
- *(NIC) Self-Responsibility Facilitation:*

  Encourage patient to take as much responsibility for own self-care as possible

  Encourage independence but assist patient when unable to perform

  Assist parents in identifying age-appropriate tasks for which child could be responsible, as appropriate

  Provide positive reinforcement for accepting additional responsibility and/or behavior change

Dysreflexia
(1.2.3.1) (1988)

Definition: The state in which an individual with a spinal cord injury at T7 or above experiences a life-threatening, uninhibited sympathetic response of the nervous system to a noxious stimulus

Defining Characteristics

Subjective

Blurred vision

Chest pain

Headache (a diffuse pain in different portions of the head and not confined to any nerve distribution area)

Metallic taste in mouth

Paresthesia

Objective

Bradycardia (pulse rate of < 60 beats/min [bpm])

Chills

Conjunctival congestion

Diaphoresis above injury

Horner's syndrome (contraction of pupil, partial ptosis of eyelid, enophthalmos, and sometimes loss of sweating over affected side of face)

Nasal congestion

Pallor below injury

Paroxysmal hypertension (sudden periodic elevation of blood pressure, where systolic is > 140 and diastolic is > 90 bpm)

Pilomotor reflex (gooseflesh formation when skin is cooled)

Red splotches on skin (above the injury)

Tachycardia (pulse rate >100 bpm.)

Related Factors

Bladder distention
Bowel distention
Lack of patient and caregiver knowledge
Skin irritation [or skin lesion]

Suggestions for Use

Dysreflexia is a potential problem for the patient with high spinal cord injury. *Dysreflexia* cannot continue as an actual nursing diagnosis. If independent nursing actions do not resolve it, medical treatment becomes necessary. As a rule, *Risk for automatic dysreflexia* is a more useful label than actual *Dysreflexia* because the patient is in a potential state most of the time (Carpenito 1997b, p. 342). The suggested alternative diagnoses represent noxious stimuli that can trigger a sympathetic response in the patient with spinal cord injury. They may be used as actual problems or as the etiology of *Dysreflexia* or *Risk for autonomic dysreflexia*.

Suggested Alternative Diagnoses

Constipation [fecal impaction]
Skin integrity, impaired
Urinary retention

NOC Suggested Outcomes

Neurological Status: Extent to which the peripheral and central nervous systems receive, process, and respond to internal and external stimuli

Vital Signs Status: Temperature, pulse, respiration, and blood pressure within expected range for the individual

Goals/Evaluation Criteria

Examples Using NOC Language

- Patient will not experience *Dysreflexia,* as demonstrated by Neurological Status and Vital Signs Status within expected range for the individual
- Patients will demonstrate satisfactory **Neurological Status,** as evidenced by the following indicators (specify 1–5: extremely, substantially, moderately, mildly, or not compromised):

    Neurological status: consciousness
    Neurological status: central motor control
    Neurological status: cranial sensory/motor function

Neurological status: autonomic
Breathing pattern

Other Examples

Patient will:

- Maintain vital signs in expected range: temperature, apical and radial pulse rates, respiration rate, systolic and diastolic BP
- Demonstrate ability to maintain bowel and bladder routine
- Identify early signs and symptoms of dysreflexia (eg, headache, blurred vision, paresthesia)

NIC Priority Interventions

Dysreflexia Management: Prevention and elimination of stimuli which cause hyperactive reflexes and inappropriate autonomic responses in a patient with a cervical or high thoracic cord lesion

Nursing Activities

Assessments

- Assess patient's knowledge of condition, including history of previous episodes, early signs and symptoms, and bowel and bladder regimen
- Assess skin condition at least daily, noting any reddened areas above level of spinal cord injury
- Obtain baseline temperature, blood pressure, and pulse
- *(NIC) Dysreflexia Management:*

  Identify and minimize stimuli that may precipitate dysreflexia: bladder distention, renal calculi, infection, fecal impaction, rectal examination, suppository insertion, skin breakdown, and constrictive clothing or bed linen

  Monitor for signs and symptoms of autonomic dysreflexia: paroxysmal hypertension, bradycardia, tachycardia, diaphoresis above the level of injury, facial flushing, pallor below the level of injury, headache, nasal congestion, engorgement of temporal and neck vessels, conjunctival congestion, chills without fever, pilomotor erection, and chest pain

Patient/Family Teaching

- Ask patient to report any early signs and symptoms of condition that occur
- *(NIC) Dysreflexia Management:* Instruct patient and family about causes, symptoms, treatment, and prevention of dysreflexia

Collaborative Activities

- *(NIC) Dysreflexia Management:* Administer antihypertensive agents intravenously, as ordered

Other

- If symptoms occur, stop activity and have someone notify physician
- Quickly eliminate noxious stimulus in the following order:
    Bladder: Check catheter for patency, or catheterize patient
    Bowel: If distended, apply anesthetic ointment to rectal area and disimpact. Consider enema or flatus tube.
    Body temperature: Maintain normal body temperature
- *(NIC) Dysreflexia Management:* Identify and minimize stimuli that may precipitate dysreflexia: bladder distention, renal calculi, infection, fecal impaction, rectal examination, suppository insertion, skin breakdown, and constrictive clothing or bed linen
- During onset of crisis, carry out management plan according to *(NIC) Dysreflexia Management:*
    Administer antihypertensive agents intravenously, as ordered
    Stay with patient and monitor status every 3 to 5 minutes if hyperreflexia occurs
    Place head of bed in upright position, as appropriate, if hyperreflexia occurs

Dysreflexia, Risk for Autonomic
(1.2.3.2) (1998)

Definition: A life-threatening uninhibited response of the sympathetic nervous system for an individual with a spinal cord injury or lesion at T8 or above [who has] recovered from spinal shock

Risk Factors

Cardiac/Pulmonary Problems
Pulmonary emboli

Gastrointestinal Problems
Constipation
Distention
Enemas
Esophageal reflux
Gastric ulcers
Gastrointestinal system pathology
Stimulation (eg, digital, instrumentation, surgery)

Neurological Problems
Painful or irritating stimuli below the level of injury

Regulatory Problems
Temperature fluctuations

Reproductive Problems
Ejaculation
Menstruation
Sexual intercourse

Integumentary Problems
Cutaneous stimulations (eg, pressure ulcer, ingrown toenail, dressings, burns, rash)
Heterotrophic bone

Situational Problems
Constrictive clothing
Deep vein thrombosis
Drug reactions (eg, decongestants, sympathomimetics, vasoconstrictors, narcotic withdrawal)
Fractures
Labor and delivery
Ovarian cyst
Positioning
Pregnancy
Range-of-motion exercises
Surgical procedures

Urological Problems
Bladder distention
Epididymitis
Infection
Instrumentation
Spasm
Urethritis

Suggestions for Use

See "Suggestions for Use" for "Dysreflexia" on p. 131.

Suggested Alternative Diagnoses

Constipation [fecal impaction]
Skin integrity, impaired
Urinary retention

NOC Suggested Outcomes

To be developed

NIC Priority Interventions

To be developed

Nursing Activities

Assessments

See "Assessments" for "Dysreflexia," p. 132

Patient/Family Teaching

See "Patient/Family Teaching" for "Dysreflexia," p. 132

Other

- Quickly eliminate any noxious stimulus in the following order:
    Bladder: Check catheter for patency or catheterize patient
    Bowel: If distended, apply anesthetic ointment to rectal area and disimpact; consider enema or flatus tube
    Body temperature: Maintain normal body temperature

Energy Field Disturbance
(1.8) (1994)

Definition: A disruption of the flow of energy surrounding a person's being that results in a disharmony of the body, mind, and/or spirit

Defining Characteristics

Objective
Disruption of the field (vacant/hold/spike/bulge)
Movement (wave/spike/tingling/dense/flowing)
Sounds (tone/words)
Temperature change (warmth/coolness)
Visual changes (image/color)

Related Factors

To be developed

Suggestions for Use

This diagnosis suggests independent but nontraditional nursing interventions, which require specialized instruction and practice. Therefore, it should be used only by nurses who possess such expertise (Krieger 1979, Meehan 1991).

Suggested Alternative Diagnoses

Anxiety

Pain

NOC Suggested Outcomes

Spiritual Well-Being: Personal expressions of connectedness with self, others, higher power, all life, nature, and the universe that transcend and empower the self

Well-Being: An individual's expressed satisfaction with health status

Goals/Evaluation Criteria

Also refer to "Goals/Evaluation Criteria" for "Anxiety" and "Pain," on pp. 23 and 312, respectively.

Examples Using NOC Language

- Demonstrates **Spiritual Well-Being,** as evidenced by the following indicators (specify 1–5: extremely, substantially, moderately, mildly, or not compromised):

    Faith, hope, serenity, love, and forgiveness

    Meaning and purpose in life

Other Examples

Patient will:

- Verbalize relief of symptoms (eg, pain, anxiety) after treatment
- Demonstrate physical evidence of relaxation (eg, decrease in blood pressure, pulse and respiration rates, and muscle tension)
- Indicate satisfaction with psychologic, social, spiritual, physiologic, and cognitive functioning
- Demonstrate adequate coping skills

NIC Priority Interventions

Therapeutic Touch: Directing one's own interpersonal energy to flow through the hands to help or heal another

Nursing Activities

Prior to administering therapeutic touch

- *(NIC) Therapeutic Touch:*

    Center oneself physically and psychologically to purposefully relax tensions

Sit in a relaxed position with body in alignment and hands in lap

Close eyes and breathe evenly and slowly

Attain a sense of inner equilibrium in preparation for directing physical and psychodynamic energies

Assessment

- Position the patient comfortably before beginning assessment
- *NIC (Therapeutic Touch):*

  Place hands 2 or 3 inches from patient's skin

  Move hands slowly and steadily over patient

  Complete total body assessment, typically working from head to toe, front to back

  Note any sign of temperature change, tingling, pressure, electric shock, or pulsation in your hands

  Note objective signs of patient's experience [during and after treatment]: relaxation, slow respirations, peripheral flush, relief of pain, relief of nausea, and increased peristalsis

Treatment

- Provide privacy for the treatment
- Explain the process of therapeutic touch to the patient; obtain verbal permission; discuss findings with patient
- When working in the head area, or for those who may be sensitive to it (eg, the mentally ill, the elderly, premature infants), use therapeutic touch gently and only for short periods of time
- Use actual, hands-on touch/massage, as needed
- Provide a rest period for the patient after the treatment
- *(NIC) Therapeutic Touch:*

  "Unruffle the field" around pressure areas by placing hands with palms away from the body and moving hands away in a sweeping gesture

  Direct energies to the patient's areas of imbalances

  Stop [therapeutic touch] when there are no longer bilateral differences in the patient's [energy] field

Patient/Family Teaching

- Teach therapeutic touch to family members
- Teach the patient deep-breathing exercises to aid in relaxation
- Teach the patient to use guided imagery in conjunction with the therapeutic-touch treatment

Environmental Interpretation Syndrome, Impaired (8.2.1) (1994)

Definition: Consistent lack of orientation to person, place, time, or circumstances over more than three to six months, necessitating a protective environment

Defining Characteristics

Subjective

Consistent disorientation in known and unknown environments

Objective

Chronic confusional states

Loss of occupation or social functioning from memory decline

Inability to follow simple directions, instructions

Inability to reason

Inability to concentrate

Slow in responding to questions

Related Factors

Alcoholism

Dementia (eg, Alzheimer's disease, multi-infarct dementia, Pick's disease, AIDS [-related] dementia)

Depression

Huntington's disease

Parkinson's disease

Suggestions for Use

Because this diagnosis and those in the "Suggested Alternative Diagnoses" overlap, careful analysis of the patient's defining characteristics is needed. This diagnosis is especially difficult to differentiate from *Chronic confusion*. The author prefers to use *Chronic confusion*.

Suggested Alternative Diagnoses

Confusion (non-NANDA)

Confusion, chronic

Injury, risk for

Memory, impaired

Thought processes, altered

Tissue perfusion, altered (cerebral)

NOC Suggested Outcomes

Cognitive Orientation: Ability to identify person, place, and time

Information Processing: Ability to acquire, organize, and use information

Memory: Ability to cognitively retrieve and report previously stored information

Neurological Status: Consciousness: Extent to which an individual arouses, orients, and attends to the environment

Goals/Evaluation Criteria

Examples Using NOC Language

- Maintains or improves Information Processing, Memory, and Cognitive Orientation
- Demonstrates **Neurological Status: Consciousness,** as evidenced by the following indicators (specify 1–5: extremely, substantially, moderately, mildly, or not compromised):

    Opens eyes to external stimuli

    Communication appropriate to situation

    Obeys commands

    Motor responses to noxious stimuli

    Attends to environmental stimuli

Other Examples

Patient will:

- Correctly identify common objects
- Speak coherently
- Identify significant other, place, and day
- Remain free from injury/harm
- Participate to maximum level of independence in activities of daily living
- Be content and less frustrated by environmental stressors

NIC Priority Interventions

Dementia Management: Provision of a modified environment for the patient who is experiencing a chronic confusional state

Environmental Management: Manipulation of the patient's surroundings for therapeutic benefit

Reality Orientation: Promotion of patient's awareness of personal identity, time, and environment

Nursing Activities

Also refer to "Nursing Activities" for "Confusion, Chronic," pp.75–77. In early dementia, when the main symptoms are those of *Impaired memory*, refer to "Nursing Activities" for "Impaired Memory," pp. 274–276.

Assessments

- Determine patient's self-care abilities
- *(NIC) Dementia Management:*

  Identify usual patterns of behavior for such activities as sleep, medication use, elimination, food intake, and self-care

  Monitor cognitive functioning, using a standardized assessment tool

  Identify safety needs of patient based on level of physical and cognitive function and past history of behavior

Patient/Family Teaching

- Teach family/significant others ways to remove safety hazards from the home

Collaborative Activities

- Refer to social services for referral to day-care programs

Other

- Modify physical environment to ensure safety for patient
- Accompany ambulatory patient to activities away from the unit
- Encourage family to bring objects from home
- Promote consistency in caregiver assignment
- Orient patient to person, place, and time
- Limit visitors if patient becomes more agitated or disoriented
- Use a calm, unhurried approach
- *(NIC) Dementia Management:*

  Provide a low-stimulation environment (eg, quiet, soothing music; nonvivid and simple, familiar patterns in décor; performance expectations that do not exceed cognitive-processing ability; and dining in small groups)

  Provide cues—such as current events, seasons, location, and names—to assist orientation

  Address the patient distinctly by name when initiating interaction and speak slowly

  Give one simple direction at a time

Failure to Thrive, Adult
(6.4.2.2) (1998)

Definition: A progressive functional deterioration of a physical and cognitive nature; the individual's ability to live with multi-system diseases, cope with ensuing problems, and manage his/her care are remarkably diminished

Defining Characteristics

Subjective

Altered mood state—expresses feelings of sadness, being low in spirit

Expresses loss of interest in pleasurable outlets, such as food, sex, work, friends, family, hobbies, or entertainment

Verbalizes desire for death

Objective

Anorexia—does not eat meals when offered; states does not have an appetite, not hungry, or "I don't want to eat"

Apathy, as evidenced by lack of observable feeling or emotion in terms of normal activities of daily living and environment

Cognitive decline—decline in mental processing; as evidenced by problems with responding appropriately to environmental stimuli and demonstration of difficulty in reasoning, decision making, judgment, memory and concentration, decreased perception

Decreased participation in activities of daily living that the older person once enjoyed

Decreased social skills/social withdrawal—noticeable decrease from usual past behavior in attempts to form or participate in cooperative and interdependent relationships (eg, decreased verbal communication with staff, family, friends)

Frequent exacerbations of chronic health problems, such as pneumonia or urinary tract infections

Inadequate nutritional intake—eating less than body requirements; consumes minimal to no food at most meals (ie, consumes less than 75 percent of normal requirements at each or most meals)

Physical decline—decline in bodily function; evidence of fatigue, dehydration, incontinence of bowel and bladder

Self-care deficit—no longer looks after or takes charge of physical cleanliness or appearance; difficulty performing simple self-care tasks; neglects home environment and/or financial responsibilities

Weight loss (decreased body mass from baseline weight)—5 percent unintentional weight loss in one month, 10 percent unintentional weight loss in six months

Related Factors
Apathy
Depression
Fatigue

Suggestions for Use
(1) The list of "Related Factors" shown previously appears to be incomplete for this diagnosis. Considering the multisystem and multifunctional nature of the "Defining Characteristics," there are a large number of factors that would cause them. (2) This diagnosis should be used only when several of the "Defining Characteristics" are present and when all are caused by the same related factors. Many of the "Defining Characteristics" are actually other nursing diagnoses (see the following "Suggested Alternative Diagnoses"), and when the patient has only a few of those problems, care planning may be better guided by those more narrowly focused diagnoses.

Suggested Alternative Diagnoses
Anxiety
Confusion, acute/chronic
Coping: individual, ineffective
Fatigue
Fluid volume deficit
Grieving, dysfunctional
Home maintenance management, impaired
Hopelessness
Incontinence, bowel
Incontinence, urinary
Infection, risk for
Injury, risk for
Loneliness, risk for
Memory, impaired
Nutrition: less than body requirements, altered
Powerlessness
Protection, altered
Role performance, altered

Self-care deficit (specify)
Self-esteem disturbance
Sexuality patterns, altered
Social interaction, impaired
Spiritual distress
Thought processes, altered

NOC Suggested Outcomes

To be developed

Goals/Evaluation Criteria

NOTE: Some examples are given, but the specific goals for this diagnosis will depend upon which of the defining characteristics are present. For other goals, refer to "Defining Characteristics" for the preceding "Suggested Alternative Diagnoses" (eg, the goals for *Anxiety* and *Confusion*).

The patient will:

- Regain energy needed to cope with problems resulting from multisystem diseases
- Eat diet adequate to provide for body requirements
- Regain lost weight
- Not experience further cognitive decline
- Participate in decision making
- Restore relationships with significant others
- Perform activities of daily living (eg, bathing, toileting)

NIC Priority Interventions

To be developed

Nursing Activities

Because this diagnosis is so broad, a comprehensive list of nursing activities is not practical. Refer to "Nursing Activities" for the appropriate "Suggested Alternative Diagnoses." For example, if the patient is experiencing anorexia and weight loss, refer to *Altered nutrition: less than body requirements* for nursing activities that improve the patient's nutrition; if the patient is incontinent, refer to *Bowel incontinence* or *Urinary incontinence* for the appropriate nursing activities.

Family Processes: Alcoholism, Altered
(3.2.2.3.1) (1994)

Definition: The state in which the psychosocial, spiritual, and physiologic functions of the family unit are chronically disorganized, leading to conflict, denial of problems, resistance to change, ineffective problem solving, and a series of self-perpetuating crises

Defining Characteristics

Feelings

Abandonment
Anger/suppressed rage
Anxiety/tension/distress
Being different from other people
Being unloved
Confused love and pity
Confusion
Decreased self-esteem/worthlessness
Depression
Dissatisfaction
Emotional control by others
Emotional isolation/loneliness
Failure
Fear
Frustration
Guilt
Hopelessness
Hostility
Hurt
Insecurity
Lack of identity
Lingering resentment
Loss
Mistrust
Misunderstood
Moodiness
Powerlessness
Rejection
Repressed emotions
Responsibility for alcoholic's behavior
Shame/embarrassment
Unhappiness
Vulnerability

Roles and Relationships

Altered role function/disruption of family roles
Chronic family problems
Closed communication systems
Deterioration in family relationships/disturbed family dynamics
Disrupted family rituals
Economic problems
Family denial
Family does not demonstrate respect for individuality and autonomy of its members
Family unable to meet security needs of its members
Inconsistent parenting/low perception of parental support
Ineffective spouse communication/marital problems
Intimacy dysfunction

Lack of cohesiveness

Lack of skills necessary for relationships

Neglected obligations

Pattern of rejection

Reduced ability of family members to relate to each other for mutual growth and maturation

Triangulating of family relationships

Behaviors

Agitation

Alcohol abuse

Blaming

Broken promises

Chaos

Contradictory, paradoxical communication

Controlling communication/ power struggles

Criticizing

Denial of problems

Dependency

Difficulty having fun

Difficulty with intimate relationships

Diminished physical contact

Disturbances in academic performance in children

Disturbances in concentration

Enabling to maintain drinking

Escalating conflict

Expression of anger inappropriately

Failure to accomplish current or past developmental tasks/difficulty with life-cycle transitions

Family special occasions are alcohol centered

Harsh self-judgment

Immaturity

Impaired communication

Inability to adapt to change

Inability to deal with traumatic experiences constructively

Inability to express or accept wide range of feelings

Inability to meet emotional needs of its members

Inability to meet spiritual needs of its members

Inadequate understanding or knowledge of alcoholism

Ineffective problem-solving skills

Isolation

Lack of dealing with conflict

Lack of reliability

Loss of control of drinking

Lying

Manipulation

Nicotine addiction

Orientation toward tension relief rather than achievement of goals

Rationalization/denial of problems

Refusal to get help/inability to accept and receive help appropriately

Seeking approval and affirmation

Self-blaming

Stress-related physical illnesses

Substance abuse other than alcohol

Unresolved grief

Verbal abuse of spouse or parent

Related Factors

Abuse of alcohol
Addictive personality
Biochemical influences
Family history of alcoholism, resistance to treatment
Genetic predisposition
Inadequate coping skills
Lack of problem-solving skills

Suggestions for Use

(1) Note that, by definition, alcohol abuse by a family member *must* be the related factor. Alcohol abuse may be secondary to the other listed related factors. The diagnostic statement "*Altered family processes: alcoholism related to alcohol abuse*" would not be useful because the etiology is merely a repetition of the problem (alcoholism). (2) *Ineffective family coping* may be more useful for describing the alcoholic family. (3) *Altered family processes* cannot be used because it describes a family that has a history of normal functioning.

Suggested Alternative Diagnoses

Coping: family, ineffective, compromised
Coping: family, ineffective, disabling
Violence, risk for: self-directed or directed at others

NOC Suggested Outcomes

Not yet developed

Goals/Evaluation Criteria

Patient/family will:
- Acknowledge that alcoholism is a family illness
- Acknowledge the severity of the threat to the well-being of the family
- Identify destructive behaviors
- Begin to change dysfunctional (eg, codependent) patterns

NIC Priority Interventions

Family Process Maintenance: Minimization of family process disruption effects
Substance Use Treatment: Supportive care of patient/family members with physical and psychosocial problems associated with the use of alcohol or drugs

Nursing Activities

Assessments

- Determine history of drug/alcohol use
- Identify nature of spiritual support for family
- *(NIC) Substance Use Treatment:*
  Identify with patient those factors (eg, genetic, psychological distress, and stress) which contribute to chemical dependency
  Screen patient at frequent intervals for continued substance use, using urine screens or breath analysis, as appropriate
  Determine whether codependent relationships exist in the family

Patient/Family Teaching

- Provide family members with information about alcoholism or help them to find other sources of information
- *(NIC) Substance Use Treatment:* Instruct patient and family about drugs used to treat specific substance used

Collaborative Activities

- *(NIC) Substance Use Treatment:* Identify support groups in the community for long-time substance abuse treatment

Other

- Recognize and accept that resolution of the alcoholism may not be the goal of care
- Emphasize to family members that they must allow the person to be responsible for his/her own drinking and behaviors
- Explore with the family the methods they use to control the alcoholic's behaviors (eg, hiding the alcohol)
- Help family to identify realistic goals for changing family interaction patterns
- Assist family members to focus on changing their responses to the drinking instead of trying to control it
- Facilitate communication among family members
- Give positive feedback for adaptive coping mechanisms used by patient and family
- *(NIC) Substance Use Treatment:*
  Establish a therapeutic relationship with patient [and family]
  Assist patient/family to identify use of denial as a substitute for confronting the problem
  Facilitate support by significant others
  Encourage patient to take control over own behavior
  Help family members recognize that chemical dependency is a family disease

Discuss with patient the effect of associations with other users during leisure or work time

Discuss the effect of substance use on relationships with family, coworkers, and friends

Encourage patient to keep a detailed chart of substance use to evaluate progress

Assist patient to learn alternate methods of coping with stress or emotional distress

Family Processes, Altered
(3.2.2) (1982, 1988)

Definition: A change in family relationships and/or functioning. [The NANDA definition does not necessarily describe a problem. A clearer definition might be: The state in which a family that normally functions effectively experiences dysfunction.]

Defining Characteristics

Subjective
Changes in satisfaction with family
Objective
Changes in [the following factors]:
  Assigned tasks
  Availability for affective responsiveness and intimacy
  Availability for emotional support
  Communication patterns
  Effectiveness in completing assigned tasks
  Expressions of conflict with and/or isolation from community resources
  Expressions of conflict within family
  Mutual support
  Participation in decision making
  Participation in problem solving
  Patterns and rituals
  Power alliances
  Somatic complaints
  Stress-reduction behaviors

Related Factors

Developmental transition and/or crisis
Family roles shift

Informal or formal interaction with community
Modification in family finances
Modification in family social status
Power shift of family members
Shift in health status of a family member
Situational transitions or crises

Suggestions for Use

This label describes a family that normally functions effectively but is experiencing a stressor that alters its functioning. The stressors causing *Altered family processes* tend to be situational or developmental transitions and crises, such as death of a family member, divorce, infidelity, loss of a job, serious illness, or hospitalization of a family member. When the altered family processes are specifically focused, a diagnosis such as *Dysfunctional grieving* or *Parental role conflict* may describe the problem more specifically.

This label is different from *Ineffective family coping: compromised*, in which the family coping problem is caused by a change in the relationship between the family members. The stressor in *Ineffective family coping* is withdrawal of support by a significant other, not necessarily an external stressor such as death or divorce (as in *Altered family processes*). *Compromised family coping* may involve the patient and only one significant other, whereas *Altered family processes* involves the entire family. Likewise, *Caregiver role strain* focus on the individual caregiver rather than the whole family.

Altered family processes describes a family that has the resources for coping effectively with stressors, in contrast with *Ineffective family coping: disabling*, which describes a family that demonstrates destructive behaviors. If stressors are not effectively resolved, *Altered family processes* can progress to *Ineffective family coping*. To differentiate among the suggested alternative diagnoses, carefully examine the defining characteristics and related factors of each.

Suggested Alternative Diagnoses

Caregiver role strain (actual/risk for)
Coping: family, ineffective, compromised
Coping: family, ineffective disabling
Grieving, dysfunctional
Management of therapeutic regimen: families, ineffective
Parental role conflict
Parenting, altered

NOC Suggested Outcomes

To be developed

Goals/Evaluation Criteria

Patient/family will:
- Acknowledge change in family roles
- Identify coping patterns
- Participate in decision-making processes regarding posthospital care
- Function to provide mutual support for each family member

NIC Priority Interventions

Family Integrity Promotion: Promotion of family cohesion and unity

Family Process Maintenance: Minimization of family process disruption effects

Normalization Promotion: Assisting parents and other family members of children with chronic illnesses or disabilities in providing normal life experiences for their children and families

Nursing Activities

Assessments

- Assess interaction between patient and family, being alert for potential destructive behaviors
- Assess child's limitations, so that accommodations can be made to allow child to participate in usual activities
- *(NIC) Family Integrity Promotion:*
  Determine guilt family may feel
  Determine typical family relationships
  Monitor current family relationships
  Determine disruption in typical family processes
  Identify conflicting priorities among family members

Patient/Family Teaching

- Teach the family those skills (eg, time management, treatments) required for care of patient
- Teach family the need to work with the school system to ensure access to appropriate educational opportunities for the chronically ill or disabled child

Collaborative Activities

- Explore available hospital and community resources with family
- Initiate a multidisciplinary patient care conference, involving the patient/family in problem solving and facilitation of communication
- Provide continuity of care by maintaining effective communication between staff members through nurse report and care planning
- Refer family to a financial counselor
- Request social service consultation to help the family determine posthospitalization needs and identify sources of community support (eg, for child care)
- *(NIC) Family Integrity Promotion:* Refer for family therapy, as indicated

Other

- Assist family in identifying behaviors that may be hindering prescribed treatment
- Assist family in identifying personal strengths
- Encourage family to verbalize feelings and concerns
- Encourage family to participate in patient's care and help plan posthospital care
- Provide flexible visiting hours to accommodate family visits
- Preserve family routines and rituals (eg, providing for private meals together or family decision making)
- Provide positive reinforcement for effective use of coping mechanisms
- Help family to focus on the child rather than on the illness or disability
- Encourage opportunities for normal childhood experiences for the chronically ill or disabled child
- *(NIC) Family Integrity Promotion:*
  Provide for family privacy
  Facilitate open communications among family members
  Counsel family members on additional effective coping skills for their own use
  Assist family with conflict resolution

Fatigue
(6.1.1.2.1) (1988, 1998)

Definition: An overwhelming, sustained sense of exhaustion and decreased capacity for physical and mental work at usual level

Defining Characteristics

Subjective
Compromised concentration
Compromised libido
Disinterest in surroundings, introspection
Drowsy
Feelings of guilt for not keeping up with responsibilities
Increased physical complaints
Perceived need for additional energy to accomplish routine tasks
Tired
Verbalization of unremitting and overwhelming lack of energy

Objective
Decreased performance
Inability to maintain usual routines
Inability to restore energy even after sleep
Increase in rest requirements
Lack of energy or inability to maintain usual level of physical activity
Lethargic or listlessness

Related Factors

Psychologic
Anxiety
Boring lifestyle
Depression
Stress

Environmental
Humidity
Lights
Noise
Temperature

Situational
Negative life events
Occupation

Physiologic
Anemia
Disease states
Increased physical exertion
Malnutrition
Poor physical condition
Pregnancy
Sleep deprivation

Other Possible Related Factors (non-NANDA)
Altered body chemistry (eg, caused by medications, drug withdrawal, chemotherapy)
Excessive social and/or role demands
Overwhelming psychologic or emotional demands

Suggestions for Use

Do not use this label to describe temporary tiredness resulting from lack of sleep. *Fatigue* describes a chronic condition. The patient's previous energy levels and capabilities cannot immediately be restored, so the nursing focus is to help the patient find ways to adapt. Discriminate carefully between *Fatigue* and *Activity intolerance*. The energy deficit in *Fatigue* is overwhelming and may exist even when the patient has not performed any activities. *Fatigue* may be the etiology of other nursing diagnoses, such as *Self-care deficit* and *Impaired home maintenance management.* Conversely, other labels, such as *Decreased cardiac output*, may be the etiology of *Fatigue*.

Suggested Alternative Diagnoses

Activity intolerance
Cardiac output, decreased
Self-care deficit
Sleep pattern disturbance

NOC Suggested Outcomes

Concentration: Ability to focus on a specific stimulus
Endurance: Extent that energy enables a person's activity
Energy Conservation: Extent of active management of energy to initiate and sustain activity
Nutritional Status: Energy: Extent to which nutrients provide cellular energy

Goals/Evaluation Criteria

Examples Using NOC Language

- The patient will adapt to *Fatigue*, as evidenced by Concentration, Energy Conservation, Endurance, and Nutritional Status: Energy
- The patient will demonstrates **Energy Conservation,** as evidenced by the following indicators (specify 1–5: not at all; to a slight, moderate, great, or very great extent):

    Endurance level adequate for activity

    Maintains adequate nutrition

    Balances activity and rest

    Uses energy conservation techniques

    Adapts lifestyle to energy level

Other Examples

Patient will:

- Maintain usual social interaction
- Identify psychologic and physical factors that may cause *Fatigue*
- Maintain ability to concentrate
- Attend and respond appropriately to visual, auditory, verbal, tactile, and olfactory cues
- Report that energy is restored after rest

NIC Priority Interventions

Energy Management: Regulating energy use to treat or prevent fatigue and optimize function

Nursing Activities

Assessments

- Determine the effects of *Fatigue* on quality of life
- *(NIC) Energy Management:*

    Monitor patient for evidence of excess physical and emotional fatigue

    Monitor cardiorespiratory response to activity (eg, tachycardia, other dysrhythmias, dyspnea, diaphoresis, pallor, hemodynamic pressures, and respiratory rate)

    Monitor/record patient's sleep pattern and number of sleep hours

    Monitor location and nature of discomfort or pain during movement/activity

    Determine patient's/significant other's perception of causes of *Fatigue*

Monitor nutritional intake to ensure adequate energy resources

Monitor administration and effect of stimulants and depressants

Patient/Family Teaching

- Instruct patient in the relationship of *Fatigue* to disease process/condition.
- *(NIC) Energy Management:*

  Instruct patient/significant other to recognize signs and symptoms of *Fatigue* that require reduction in activity

  Teach activity organization and time-management techniques to prevent fatigue

Collaborative Activities

- Make other practitioners aware of the effects of *Fatigue*
- *(NIC) Energy Management:* Consult with dietitian about ways to increase intake of high-energy foods

Other

- Encourage patient/family to express feelings related to life changes caused by *Fatigue*
- Assist patient in identifying measures that increase concentration. Consider initiating tasks after rest periods and prioritizing necessary tasks
- Discuss with patient/family ways to modify home environment to maintain usual activities and to minimize *Fatigue*
- Encourage limited social interaction at times of higher energy
- Encourage patient to:

  Report activities that increase *Fatigue*

  Report onset of pain that may produce *Fatigue* (severity, location, precipitating factors)
- Plan activities with patient/family that minimize *Fatigue*. Plan may include:

  Assist with activities of daily living (ADLs), as needed. Specify.

  Reduce low-priority activities
- *(NIC) Energy Management:*

  Reduce physical discomforts that could interfere with cognitive function and self-monitoring/regulation of activity

  Assist the patient/significant other to establish realistic activity goals

  Provide calming diversional activities (eg, reading, talking to others) to promote relaxation

  Promote bed rest/activity limitation (eg, increase number of rest periods)

Avoid care activities during scheduled rest periods

Limit environmental stimuli (eg, light and noise) to facilitate relaxation

Limit number of and interruptions by visitors, as appropriate

Fear
(9.3.2) (1980, 1998)

Definition: Fear is anxiety caused by consciously recognized and realistic danger. It is a perceived threat, real or imagined. Operationally, fear is the presence of immediate feeling of apprehension and fright; source known and specific; subjective responses that act as energizers but cannot be observed and objective signs that are the result of the transformation of energy into relief behaviors and responses.

Defining Characteristics

Subjective

Afraid

Alarm

Apprehension

Decreased self-assurance

Dread

Frightened

Horror

Increased tension

Scared

Terrified

Worry

Objective

Attack behavior

Bed-wetting

Concentration on the source [of fear]

Fight behavior—aggression

Flight behavior—withdrawal

Focus on "it" out there

Identifies object of fear

Immediate response to object of fear

Impulsiveness

Increased alertness

Increased heart rate
Jittery
Panic
Physical arousal
Wariness
Wide-eyed

Related Factors

Classical conditioning
Discrepancy
Environmental stimuli
Fear for others
Ideas
Innate releasers
Knowledge deficit
Language barrier
Learned response
Natural/innate origins
Phobic stimulus or phobia
Physical/social conditions
Sensory impairment
Separation from support system in potentially stressful situation

Suggestions for Use

See "Suggestions for Use" for "Anxiety," pp. 21–22

Suggested Alternative Diagnoses

Anxiety
Post-trauma syndrome
Rape-trauma syndrome

NOC Suggested Outcomes

Fear Control: Ability to eliminate or reduce disabling feelings of alarm aroused by an identifiable source

Goals/Evaluation Criteria
Examples Using NOC Language

- The patient will exhibit **Fear Control**, as evidenced by the following indicators (specify 1–5: never, rarely, sometimes, often, or consistently demonstrated):
    Seeks information to reduce fear
    Avoids source of fear when possible

Uses relaxation techniques to reduce fear

Reports decreased duration of episodes

Reports increased length of time between episodes

Maintains control over life

Maintains role performance and social relationships

Controls fear response

Remains productive

NIC Priority Interventions

Anxiety Reduction: Minimizing apprehension, dread, foreboding, or uneasiness related to an unidentified source of anticipated danger

Coping Enhancement: Assisting a patient to adapt to perceived stressors, changes, or threats which interfere with meeting life demands and roles

Security Enhancement: Intensifying a patient's sense of physical and psychologic safety

Nursing Activities

Also refer to "Nursing Activities" for "Anxiety," pp. 24–25

Assessments

- Assess patient's subjective and objective fear responses
- *(NIC) Coping Enhancement:* Appraise the patient's understanding of the disease process

Patient/Family Teaching

- Explain all tests and treatments to patient/family

Collaborative Activities

- Assess need for social service and/or psychiatric intervention
- Encourage a patient-physician discussion of the patient's fear
- Initiate a multidisciplinary patient care conference to develop a plan of care

Other

- Provide frequent, positive reinforcement when patient demonstrates behaviors that may reduce or eliminate fear
- Stay with patient during new situations
- Remove the source of the patient's fear whenever possible
- Convey acceptance of the patient's perception of fear to encourage open communication regarding the source of the fear
- Provide continuity of patient care through patient assignment and use of care plan

- Provide frequent verbal and nonverbal reassurances that may assist in reducing the patient's fear state. Avoid clichés
- Offer pacifier to infant
- Hold or rock child
- Place a night-light in room
- Encourage parent(s) to spend the night at the hospital with a child
- *(NIC) Coping Enhancement:*

   Appraise and discuss alternative responses to situation

   Use a calm, reassuring approach

   Assist the patient in developing an objective appraisal of the event

   Encourage an attitude of realistic hope as a way of dealing with feelings of helplessness

   Discourage decision making when the patient is under severe stress

   Encourage gradual mastery of the situation

   Introduce the patient to persons (or groups) who have successfully undergone the same experience

   Encourage verbalization of feelings, perceptions, and fears

   Reduce stimuli in the environment that could be misinterpreted as threatening

Fluid Volume Deficit
(1.4.1.2.2.1) (1978, 1996)

Definition: The state in which an individual experiences decreased intravascular, interstitial, and/or intracellular fluid. This refers to dehydration—water loss alone without change in sodium.

Defining Characteristics

Subjective

Thirst

Objective

Change in mental state

Decreased blood pressure

Decreased pulse volume/pressure

Decreased skin/tongue turgor

Decreased urine output

Decreased venous filling

Dry skin/mucous membrane
Elevated hematocrit
Increased body temperature
Increased pulse rate
Increased urine concentration
Sudden weight loss (except in third-spacing)
Weakness

Related Factors

Active fluid volume loss
[Excessive continuous consumption of alcohol]
Failure of regulatory mechanisms [as in diabetes insipidus, hyper-
    aldosteronism]
[Inadequate fluid intake secondary to _____]

Suggestions for Use

Use this label for patients experiencing vascular, cellular, or intracellular dehydration. Use the label cautiously, because many fluid balance problems require nurse-physician collaboration. Do not use this label routinely, even as a potential problem, for patients who have a medical order of "NPO." Independent nursing treatments for *Fluid volume deficit* are meant to prevent fluid loss (eg, diaphoresis) and encourage oral fluid intake. For a diagnosis such as *Risk for fluid volume deficit related to NPO order*, there are no independent nursing actions to prevent or treat either side of the diagnostic statement. The treatment of *Fluid volume deficit related to NPO status*, for example, requires a medical order for intravenous therapy.

Do not use *Fluid volume deficit* to describe patients who are, or are at risk for, hemorrhaging or in hypovolemic shock. These situations usually represent collaborative problems.

Incorrect: Risk for fluid volume deficit related to postpartum hemorrhage

Correct: Potential Complication of childbirth: Postpartum hemorrhage

Correct: Risk for postpartum hemorrhage related to uterine atony

The most appropriate use of the *Fluid volume deficit* label is as a diagnosis (either actual or potential) for patients who are not drinking sufficient amounts of oral fluids, especially in the presence of increased fluid loss (eg, diarrhea, vomiting, burns). An actual *Fluid volume deficit* may also be the etiology of other nursing diagnoses, such as *Altered oral mucous membrane*.

Suggested Alternative Diagnoses

Fluid volume deficit, risk for
Fluid volume imbalance, risk for
Oral mucous membrane, altered
Tissue perfusion, altered (renal)

NOC Suggested Outcomes

Electrolyte and Acid-Base Balance: Balance of electrolytes and nonelectrolytes in the intracellular and extracellular compartments of the body

Fluid Balance: Balance of water in the intracellular and extracellular compartments of the body

Hydration: Amount of water in the intracellular and extracellular compartments of the body

Nutritional Status: Food and Fluid Intake: Amount of food and fluid taken into the body over a 24-hour period

Goals/Evaluation Criteria

NOTE: Although some NOC outcomes relate to electrolyte and acid-base balance, the focus of this nursing diagnosis is on *fluid volume*.

Examples Using NOC Language

- *Fluid volume deficit* will be eliminated, as evidenced by Fluid Balance, Electrolyte and Acid-Base Balance, adequate Hydration, and adequate Nutritional Status: Food and Fluid Intake
- **Electrolyte and Acid-Base Balance** will be achieved, as evidenced by the following indicators (specify 1–5: extremely, substantially, moderately, mildly, or not compromised):

    Heart rate and rhythm in expected range
    Respiratory rate and rhythm in expected range
    Mental alertness and cognitive orientation not compromised
    Serum electrolytes (eg, sodium, potassium, calcium, magnesium) within normal limits
    Serum and urine pH within normal limits

Other Examples

Patient will:

- Not have excessively concentrated urine. Specify baseline specific gravity
- Have hemoglobin and hematocrit within normal range for patient

- Have central venous and pulmonary wedge pressures in expected range
- Not experience abnormal thirst
- Have balanced intake and output over 24 hours
- Exhibit good hydration (moist mucous membranes, ability to perspire)
- Have adequate oral and/or intravenous fluid intake

NIC Priority Interventions

Electrolyte Management: Promotion of electrolyte balance and prevention of complications resulting from abnormal or undesired serum electrolyte levels

Fluid Management: Promotion of fluid balance and prevention of complications resulting from abnormal or undesired fluid levels

Fluid Monitoring: Collection and analysis of patient data to regulate fluid balance

Hypovolemia Management: Expansion of intravascular fluid volume in a patient who is volume depleted

Intravenous (IV) Therapy: Administration and monitoring of intravenous fluids and medications

Shock Management, Volume: Promotion of adequate tissue perfusion for a patient with severely compromised intravascular volume

Nursing Activities

NOTE[1]: Some of these activities are specific for patients who are hemorrhaging. Refer to the preceding "Suggestions for Use" before including those activities in your plan of care.

NOTE[2]: Although some of the NIC interventions relate to electrolyte and acid-base balance, the focus of this nursing diagnosis is on *fluid volume*.

Assessments

- Monitor color, amount, and frequency of fluid loss
- Observe especially for loss of fluids high in electrolytes (eg, diarrhea, wound drainage, nasogastric suction, diaphoresis, ileostomy drainage)
- Monitor for bleeding (eg, check all secretions for frank or occult blood)
- Identify contributing factors that may aggravate dehydration (eg, medications, fever, stress, medical orders)

- Review electrolytes, especially sodium, potassium, chloride, and creatinine
- Assess for vertigo or postural hypotension
- Assess orientation to person, place, and time
- *(NIC) Fluid Management:*

  Monitor hydration status (eg, moist mucous membranes, adequacy of pulses, and orthostatic blood pressure)

  Monitor laboratory results relevant to fluid balance (eg, hematocrit, BUN, albumin, total protein, serum osmolality, and urine specific gravity levels)

  Weigh daily and monitor trends

  Count or weigh diapers

  Maintain accurate intake and output record

Patient/Family Teaching

- Instruct patient to inform nurse of thirst.

Collaborative Activities

- Report and document output less than _____ mL
- Report and document output more than _____ mL
- Report electrolyte abnormalities
- *(NIC) Fluid Management:*

  Arrange availability of blood products for transfusion, if necessary

  Administer prescribed nasogastric replacement based on output, as appropriate

  Administer IV therapy, as prescribed

Other

- Provide frequent oral hygiene
- Specify amount of fluids to be ingested in 24 hours, quantifying desired intake during the day, evening, and night shifts
- Ensure that patient is well hydrated preoperatively
- Position in Trendelenburg or elevate patient's legs when hypotensive, unless contraindicated
- *(NIC) Fluid Management:*

  Promote oral intake (eg, provide oral fluids that are the patient's preference, place in easy reach, provide a straw, and provide fresh water), as appropriate

  Insert urinary catheter, if appropriate

  Give fluids, as appropriate

Fluid Volume Deficit, Risk for
(1.4.1.2.2.2) (1978)

Definition: The state in which an individual is at risk of experiencing vascular, cellular, or intracellular dehydration

Risk Factors

Objective
Deviations affecting access to or intake or absorption of fluids (eg, physical immobility)
Excessive losses through normal routes (eg, diarrhea)
Extremes of age
Extremes of weight
Factors influencing fluid needs (eg, hypermetabolic state)
Knowledge deficit related to fluid volume
Loss of fluid through abnormal routes (eg, indwelling tubes)
Medications (eg, diuretics)

Suggestions for Use

Do not use routinely for patients who are NPO. Refer to "Suggestions for Use" for "Fluid Volume Deficit," p. 160

Suggested Alternative Diagnoses

Fluid volume deficit
Fluid volume imbalance, risk for

NOC Suggested Outcomes

Electrolyte and Acid-Base Balance: Balance of electrolytes and nonelectrolytes in the intracellular and extracellular compartments of the body
Fluid Balance: Balance of water in the intracellular and extracellular compartments of the body
Hydration: Amount of water in the intracellular and extracellular compartments of the body
Nutritional Status: Food and Fluid Intake: Amount of food and fluid taken into the body over a 24-hour period

Goals/Evaluation Criteria

Also refer to "Goals/Evaluation Criteria" for "Fluid Volume Deficit," pp. 161–162

Example Using NOC Language

* *Fluid volume deficit* will be prevented, as evidenced by Fluid Balance, Electrolyte and Acid-Base Balance, adequate Hydration, and adequate Nutritional Status: Food and Fluid Intake

NIC Priority Interventions

Autotransfusion: Collection and reinfusion of blood that has been lost intraoperatively or postoperatively from clean wounds

Electrolyte Management: Promotion of electrolyte balance and prevention of complications resulting from abnormal or undesired serum electrolyte levels (eg, serum calcium, potassium, magnesium, sodium, and phosphate)

Fluid Management: Promotion of fluid balance and prevention of complications resulting from abnormal or undesired fluid levels

Fluid Monitoring: Collection and analysis of patient data to regulate fluid balance

Hypovolemia Management: Expansion of intravascular fluid volume in a patient who is volume depleted

Intravenous (IV) Therapy: Administration and monitoring of intravenous fluids and medications

Shock Management, Volume: Promotion of adequate tissue perfusion for a patient with severely compromised intravascular volume

Nursing Activities

NOTE: "Nursing Activities" for *Risk for fluid volume deficit* are essentially the same as those for actual *Fluid volume deficit*, listed on pp. 162–163. Refer to "Suggestions for Use" for "Fluid Volume Deficit," p. 160, before including those activities in your plan of care.

Fluid Volume Excess
(1.4.1.2.1) (1982, 1996)

Definition: The state in which an individual experiences increased isotonic fluid retention

Defining Characteristics

Subjective
Anxiety
Dyspnea or shortness of breath

Objective

Abnormal breath sounds (rales or crackles)

Altered electrolytes

Anasarca

Anxiety

Azotemia

Blood pressure changes

Change in mental status

Change in respiratory pattern

Decreased hemoglobin and hematocrit

Edema

Increased central venous pressure

Intake exceeds output

Jugular vein distention

Oliguria

Orthopnea

Pleural effusion

Positive hepatojugular reflex

Pulmonary congestion

Restlessness

S_3 heart sound

Specific gravity changes

Weight gain over short period

Related Factors

Compromised regulatory mechanism

Excess fluid intake

Excess sodium intake

[Increased fluid intake secondary to hyperglycemia, medications, compulsive water drinking, and so on]

[Insufficient protein secondary to decreased intake or increased losses]

Renal dysfunction, heart failure, sodium retention, immobility, and so on

Suggestions for Use

Do not use this label for conditions that nurses cannot prevent or treat (eg, do not use *Fluid volume excess* to describe renal failure or pulmonary edema—these are medical diagnoses). The main type of *Fluid volume excess* that nurses can treat independently is peripheral, dependent edema, which can be symptomatically relieved by elevating the patient's affected limbs. Edema (a symptom of *Fluid volume excess*) is an important risk factor for *Impaired skin integrity*, which can be addressed by patient teaching and protective measures. If the patient requires medical intervention to resolve the fluid excess, use a collaborative problem such as Potential Complication of renal failure: Generalized edema. *Fluid volume excess* can also be the cause of complications, such as Potential Complication of *Fluid volume excess*: Pulmonary edema.

> *Incorrect: Fluid volume excess related to decreased cardiac output*
> *Correct:* Potential Complication of decreased cardiac output: Fluid volume excess
> *Correct:* Potential Complication of heart failure: Pulmonary edema
> *Correct: Risk for impaired skin integrity related to Fluid volume excess, as manifested by generalized edema*

Suggested Alternative Diagnoses

Cardiac output, decreased
Fluid volume imbalance, risk for
Skin integrity, risk for impaired
Tissue perfusion, altered

NOC Suggested Outcomes

Electrolyte and Acid-Base Balance: Balance of electrolytes and nonelectrolytes in the intracellular and extracellular compartments of the body

Fluid Balance: Balance of water in the intracellular and extracellular compartments of the body

Hydration: Amount of water in the intracellular and extracellular compartments of the body

Goals/Evaluation Criteria

Examples Using NOC Language

- *Fluid volume excess* will be eliminated, as evidenced by Fluid Balance, Electrolyte and Acid-Base Balance, and indicators of adequate Hydration
- **Fluid Balance** will not be compromised (in excess) as evidenced by the following indicators (specify 1–5: extremely, substantially, moderately, mildly, or not compromised):

    24-hour intake and output balanced
    Adventitious breath sounds not present

Body weight stable

Ascites, neck vein distention, and peripheral edema not present

Urine specific gravity within normal limits

Other Examples

Patient will:

- Verbalize understanding of fluid and dietary restrictions
- Verbalize understanding of prescribed medications
- Maintain vital signs within normal limits for patient
- Not experience shortness of breath
- Have hematocrit within normal limits

NIC Priority Interventions

Fluid Management: Promotion of fluid balance and prevention of complications resulting from abnormal or undesired fluid levels

Fluid Monitoring: Collection and analysis of patient data to regulate fluid balance

Nursing Activities

Assessments

- Specify location and degree of peripheral, sacral, and periorbital edema on scale from 1+ to 4+
- Assess for pulmonary and/or cardiovascular complications as indicated by increased respiratory distress, increased pulse rate, increased blood pressure, abnormal heart sounds, and/or abnormal lung sounds
- Assess edematous extremity or body part for impaired circulation and skin integrity
- Assess effects of medications (eg, steroids, diuretics, lithium) on edema
- Regularly monitor abdominal or limb girth
- *(NIC) Fluid Management:*

  Weigh daily and monitor trends

  Maintain accurate intake and output record

  Monitor laboratory results relevant to fluid retention (eg, electrolyte changes, increased specific gravity, increased BUN, decreased hematocrit, and increased urine osmolality levels)

  Monitor for indications of fluid overload/retention (eg, crackles, elevated CVP or pulmonary capillary wedge pressure, edema, neck vein distention, and ascites), as appropriate

Patient/Family Teaching

- Instruct patient regarding causes and resolutions of edema; dietary restrictions; and use, dosage, and side effects of prescribed medications
- *(NIC) Fluid Management:* Instruct patient on nothing by mouth (NPO) status, as appropriate

Collaborative Activities

- Administer dialysis, if indicated
- *(NIC) Fluid Management:*
  Consult physician if signs and symptoms of fluid volume excess persist or worsen
  Administer diuretics, as appropriate

Other

- Change position q _____
- Elevate extremities to increase venous return
- Maintain and allocate patient's fluid restrictions
- *(NIC) Fluid Management:* Distribute the fluid intake over 24 h, as appropriate

Fluid Volume Imbalance, Risk for
(1.4.1.2) (1998)

Definition: A risk of a decrease, increase, or rapid shift from one to the other of intravascular, interstitial, and/or intracellular fluid. This refers to the loss or excess or both of body fluids or replacement fluids

Risk Factors

Scheduled for major invasive procedures
(Other risk factors/defining characteristics to be developed)

Suggestions for Use

This diagnosis was submitted by the Association of Operating Room Nurses and may have specific applications for that setting. It appears that it should be used when a patient is at risk for *both Fluid volume deficit* and *Fluid volume excess.*

Suggested Alternative Diagnoses

Fluid volume deficit, risk for

NOC Suggested Outcomes

To be developed

Goals/Evaluation Criteria

Refer to "Goals/Evaluation Criteria" for "Fluid Volume Deficit," pp. 161–162, and "Fluid Volume Excess," pp. 167–168

NIC Priority Interventions

To be developed

Nursing Activities

Refer to "Nursing Activities" for "Fluid Volume Deficit," pp. 162–163, and "Fluid Volume Excess," pp. 168–169

Gas Exchange, Impaired
(1.5.1.1) (1980, 1996, 1998)

Definition: Excess or deficit in oxygenation and/or carbon dioxide elimination at the alveolar-capillary membrane

Defining Characteristics

Subjective

Dyspnea

Headache upon awakening

Visual disturbance

Objective

Abnormal arterial blood gases

Abnormal arterial pH

Abnormal rate, rhythm, depth of breathing

Abnormal skin color (eg, pale, dusky)

Confusion

Cyanosis (in neonates only)

Decreased carbon dioxide

Diaphoresis

Hypercapnia

Hypercarbia

Hypoxia

Hypoxemia

Irritability

Nasal flaring
Restlessness
Somnolence
Tachycardia

Related Factors

Alveolar-capillary membrane changes
Ventilation-perfusion imbalance

Suggestions for Use

Use this label cautiously. Decreased passage of gases between the alveoli of the lungs and the vascular system can be discovered only by means of a medically prescribed diagnostic test: blood gas analysis. A patient might easily have most of the defining characteristics without actually having impaired alveolar gas exchange. It is better to use a diagnostic statement that describes oxygen-related problems that *can* be diagnosed and treated independently by nurses (eg, *Activity intolerance*). If the patient is *at risk* for *Impaired gas exchange*, write the appropriate collaborative problem (eg, Potential Complication of thrombophlebitis: Pulmonary embolus). See "Suggestions for Use" for "Ineffective Airway Clearance," on pp. 15–16, "Ineffective Breathing Pattern," on p. 50, and "Dysfunctional Ventilatory Weaning Response (DVWR)," on p. 509.

Impaired gas exchange may be associated with a number of medical diagnoses. For example, decreased functional lung tissue may be secondary to chronic lung disease, pneumonia, thoracotomy, atelectasis, respiratory distress syndrome, mass, and diaphragmatic hernia; in addition, decreased pulmonary blood supply may occur secondary to pulmonary hypertension, pulmonary embolus, congestive heart failure, respiratory distress syndrome, and anemia.

Suggested Alternative Diagnoses

Activity intolerance
Airway clearance, ineffective
Breathing pattern, ineffective
Dysfunctional ventilatory weaning response (DVWR)
Spontaneous ventilation, inability to sustain

NOC Suggested Outcomes

Respiratory Status: Gas Exchange: Alveolar exchange of CO_2 or O_2 to maintain arterial blood gas concentrations

Respiratory Status: Ventilation: Movement of air in and out of the lungs

Goals/Evaluation Criteria

Examples Using NOC Language

- *Impaired gas exchange* will be alleviated, as evidenced by uncompromised Respiratory Status: Gas Exchange and Respiratory Status: Ventilation
- **Respiratory Status: Gas Exchange** will not be compromised as evidenced by the following indicators (specify 1–5: extremely, substantially, moderately, mildly, or not compromised):

    Neurologic status in expected range

    Dyspnea at rest and on exertion not present

    Restlessness, cyanosis, and fatigue not present

    PaO_2, $PaCO_2$, arterial pH, and O_2 saturation within normal limits

    End-tidal CO_2 in expected range

Other Examples

Patient will:

- Have pulmonary function within normal limits
- Describe plan for care at home
- Not use pursed-lip breathing
- Not experience shortness of breath or orthopnea

NIC Priority Interventions

Acid-Base Management: Promotion of acid-base balance and prevention of complications resulting from acid-base imbalance

Airway Management: Facilitation of patency of air passages

Nursing Activities

Assessments

- Assess lung sounds; respiratory rate, depth, and effort; and production of sputum as indicators of effective use of supportive equipment
- Monitor O_2 saturation with pulse oximeter
- Monitor blood gas results (eg, low PaO_2 and elevated $PaCO_2$ levels suggest respiratory deterioration)
- Monitor electrolyte levels

- Monitor mental status (eg, level of consciousness, restlessness, and confusion)
- Increase frequency of monitoring when patient appears somnolent
- Observe for cyanosis, especially of oral mucous membranes
- *(NIC) Airway Management:*
  Identify patient requiring actual/potential airway insertion
  Auscultate breath sounds, noting areas of decreased or absent ventilation and presence of adventitious sounds
  Monitor respiratory and oxygenation status, as appropriate

Patient/Family Teaching

- Explain proper use of supportive equipment (oxygen, suction, spirometer, IPPB)
- Instruct patient in breathing and relaxation techniques
- Explain to patient and family the reasons for low-flow oxygen and other treatments
- Inform patient and family that smoking is prohibited
- Instruct patient and family in plan for care at home, eg, medications, activity, supportive equipment, reportable signs and symptoms, and community resources
- *(NIC) Airway Management:*
  Instruct how to cough effectively
  Teach patient how to use prescribed inhalers, as appropriate

Collaborative Activities

- Consult with physician regarding future need for arterial blood gas (ABG) test and use of supportive equipment as indicated by a change in the patient's condition
- Report changes in correlated assessment data (eg, patient sensorium, breath sounds, respiratory pattern, ABGs, sputum, effect of medications)
- Administer prescribed medications (eg, sodium bicarbonate) to maintain acid-base balance
- Prepare patient for mechanical ventilation, if necessary
- *(NIC) Airway Management:*
  Administer humidified air or oxygen, as appropriate
  Administer bronchodilators, as appropriate
  Administer aerosol treatments, as appropriate
  Administer ultrasonic nebulizer treatments, as appropriate
  Administer humidified air or oxygen

Other

- Inform patient before beginning intended procedures, to lower anxiety and increase sense of control
- Reassure patient during periods of respiratory distress and/or anxiety
- Provide frequent oral hygiene
- Institute measures to reduce oxygen consumption (eg, control fever and pain, reduce anxiety)
- Institute plan of care for a patient on a ventilator, which may include:

  Ensuring adequate oxygen delivery by reporting abnormal ABGs, having ambu bag attached to oxygen source at bedside, and hyperoxygenating prior to suctioning

  Ensuring effective breathing pattern by assessing for synchronization and possible need for sedation

  Maintaining patent airway by suctioning patient and keeping an endotracheal (ET) tube or replacement at bedside

  Monitoring for complications (eg, pneumothorax, unilateral aeration)

  Verifying correct placement of ET tube

- *(NIC) Airway Management:*

  Position to maximize ventilation potential

  Position to alleviate dyspnea

  Insert oral or nasopharyngeal airway, as appropriate

  Remove secretions by encouraging coughing or suctioning

  Encourage slow, deep breathing; turning; and coughing

  Assist with incentive spirometer, as appropriate

  Perform chest physical therapy, as appropriate

Grieving, Anticipatory
(9.2.1.2) (1980, 1996)

Definition: Intellectual and emotional responses and behaviors by which individuals, families, and communities work through the process of modifying self-concept based on the perception of potential loss

Defining Characteristics

Subjective

Anger

Denial of potential loss
Denial of the significance of the loss
Expression of distress at potential loss
Guilt
Objective
Alteration in eating habits, sleep patterns, dream patterns
Altered activity level
Altered communication patterns
Altered libido
Bargaining
Difficulty taking on new or different roles
Potential loss of significant object
Resolution of grief prior to the reality of loss
Sorrow

Related Factors

To be developed

Other Related Factors (non-NANDA)
Impending death of self
Potential loss of body parts or functions
Potential loss of significant person, animal, or possession
Potential loss of social role

Suggestions for Use

Anticipatory grieving may be a normal, not necessarily maladaptive, response. If it requires no intervention, do not include it in the
patient care plan. *Anticipatory grieving* occurs *before* the loss. It
shares some defining characteristics with *Dysfunctional grieving*;
however, the following symptoms of *Dysfunctional grieving* would
rule out a diagnosis of *Anticipatory grieving*:

Exaggerated and prolonged feelings of guilt
Interference with life functioning
Prolonged anger or hostility
Suicidal thoughts

Suggested Alternative Diagnoses

Coping: individual, ineffective
Grieving, dysfunctional
Sorrow, chronic

NOC Suggested Outcomes

Coping: Actions to manage stressors that tax an individual's resources

Grief Resolution: Adjustment to actual or impending loss

Psychosocial Adjustment: Life Change: Psychosocial adaptation of an individual to a life change

Goals/Evaluation Criteria

Examples Using NOC Language

- Patient successfully resolves *Anticipatory grieving*, as demonstrated by successful Coping, Grief Resolution, and Psychosocial Adjustment: Life Change
- Patient demonstrates **Coping**, as evidenced by the following indicators (specify 1–5: never, rarely, sometimes, often, or consistently demonstrated):

    Identifies and uses effective coping patterns

    Seeks information concerning illness and treatment

    Uses available social supports

    Seeks professional help, as appropriate

    Reports decrease in physical symptoms of stress and in negative feelings

Other Examples

Patient/family will:

- Demonstrate ability to make mutual decisions regarding anticipated loss
- Express thoughts, feelings, and spiritual beliefs about loss
- Verbalize fears/concerns about potential loss
- Participate in grief work
- Not be preoccupied with loss
- Not experience somatic distress
- Express feelings of productivity, usefulness, empowerment, and optimism

NIC Priority Interventions

Grief Work Facilitation: Assistance with the resolution of a significant loss

Grief Work Facilitation: Perinatal Death: Assistance with the resolution of a perinatal loss

Nursing Activities

Assessments

- Assess past experience of patient/family with loss, existing support systems, and current grief work
- Determine cause and length of time since diagnosis of fetal/infant death
- *(NIC) Grief Work Facilitation:* Identify the loss

Patient/Family Teaching

- Teach characteristics of normal and abnormal grieving
- Discuss differences in individual patterns of grieving (eg, male vs. female)
- Help child to clarify misconceptions about death, dying, or loss
- *(NIC) Grief Work Facilitation:* Instruct in phases of the grieving process, as appropriate

Collaborative Activities

- Refer to appropriate resources, such as support groups, legal assistance, financial assistance, social services, chaplain, grief counselor, genetic counselor
- *(NIC) Grief Work Facilitation:* Identify sources of community support

Other

- Assist patient/family to verbalize fears/concerns of potential loss, including impact on the family unit
- Help patient/family to share mutual fears, plans, concerns, and hopes with each other
- For perinatal loss, encourage parents to hold infant while/after the baby dies, as appropriate
- *(NIC) Grief Work Facilitation:*

   Assist the patient to identify the nature of the attachment to the lost object or person

   Encourage expression of feelings about the loss

   Encourage identification of greatest fears concerning the loss

   Include significant others in discussions and decisions, as appropriate

   Use clear words, such as "dead" or "died," rather than euphemisms

   Encourage patient to implement cultural, religious, and social customs associated with the loss

   Encourage expression of feelings in ways comfortable to the child, such as writing, drawing, or playing

Grieving, Dysfunctional
(9.2.1.1) (1980, 1996)

Definition: Extended, unsuccessful use of intellectual and emotional responses by which individuals, families, [and] communities attempt to work through the process of modifying self-concept based upon the perception of loss

Defining Characteristics

Subjective
Alteration in dream patterns
Alteration in libido
Anger
Denial of loss
Expression of guilt
Expression of unresolved issues
Sadness

Objective
Alteration in activity level
Alteration in eating habits
Alteration in sleep patterns
Crying
Developmental regression
Difficulty in expressing loss
Idealization of lost object
Interference with life functioning
Labile affect
Onset or exacerbation of somatic or psychosomatic responses
Prolonged interference with life functioning
Reliving past experiences with little or no reduction (diminishment) of intensity of the grief
Repetitive use of ineffectual behaviors associated with attempts to reinvest in relationships

Related Factors

Actual or perceived object loss (object loss is used in the broadest sense). Objects may include people, possessions, a job, status, home, ideals, and parts and processes of the body.
[Chronic illness]
[Terminal illness]

Suggestions for Use

Most of the defining characteristics may also be present in the normal or anticipatory grief process. Grieving is dysfunctional only if it is prolonged (perhaps for more than a year after the loss) or if the symptoms are unusually numerous or severe. *Chronic sorrow* describes the patient's feelings, whereas grieving describes behaviors used in trying to cope with the loss. See "Suggestions for Use" for "Grieving, Anticipatory" on p. 175.

Suggested Alternative Diagnoses

Adjustment, impaired
Coping: individual, ineffective
Grieving, anticipatory
Sorrow, chronic
Thought processes, altered

NOC Suggested Outcomes

Coping: Actions to manage stressors that tax an individual's resources

Grief Resolution: Adjustment to actual or impending loss

Psychosocial Adjustment: Life Change: Psychosocial adaptation of an individual to a life change

Goals/Evaluation Criteria

Examples Using NOC Language

- Patient will satisfactorily resolve *Dysfunctional grieving,* as demonstrated by successful Coping, Grief Resolution, and Psychosocial Adjustment: Life Change
- See "Goals/Evaluation Criteria" for "Grieving, Anticipatory" on p. 176, for indicators for **Coping,** and for "Other Examples"

Other Examples

Patient will:
- Report adequate intake of food and fluids
- Report adequate social support
- Verbalize grief
- Verbalize meaning of loss

NIC Priority Interventions

Grief Work Facilitation: Assistance with the resolution of a significant loss

Grief Work Facilitation: Perinatal Death: Assistance with the resolution of a perinatal loss

Nursing Activities

See "Nursing Activities" for "Grieving, Anticipatory" on p. 177

Assessments

- Assess and document the presence and source of patient's grief

Patient/Family Teaching

- Provide patient/family with information about hospital and community resources, such as self-help groups

Collaborative Activities

- Initiate a patient care conference to review patient/family needs related to their stage of the grieving process and to establish a plan of care
- Seek support among peers and others to provide patient care as needed
- *(NIC) Grief Work Facilitation: Perinatal Death:* Notify laboratory or funeral home, as appropriate, for disposition of body

Other

- Acknowledge patient's and family's grief reactions while continuing necessary care activities
- Discuss with patient/family the impact of the loss on the family unit and its functioning
- Avoid confrontation of denial and, at the same time, do not reinforce denial
- Balance any misperceptions with reality
- Encourage independence in performance of self-care, assisting patient only as necessary
- Establish a schedule for contact with patient
- Establish a trusting relationship with patient and family
- Help patient/family to participate actively in decision-making process
- Provide a safe, secure, and private environment to facilitate patient/family grieving process
- Recognize and reinforce the strength of each family member
- *(NIC) Grief Work Facilitation: Perinatal Death:*
  Assist in keeping infant alive until parents arrive
  Baptize the infant, as appropriate
  Discuss plans that have been made (eg, burial, funeral, and infant name)

Describe mementos that will be obtained, including footprints, handprints, pictures, caps, gowns, blankets, diapers, and blood pressure cuffs, as appropriate

Prepare infant for viewing by bathing and dressing, including parents in activities as appropriate

Encourage family members to view and hold infant for as long as desired

Focus on normal features of infant, while sensitively discussing anomalies

Transfer infant to morgue or prepare body to be transported by family to funeral home

Growth, Risk for Altered
(6.6.2) (1998)

Definition: At risk for growth above the 97th percentile or below the 3rd percentile for age, crossing two percentile channels; disproportionate growth

Risk Factors

Prenatal

Congenital/genetic disorders

Infection

Maternal nutrition

Multiple gestation

Substance use/abuse

Teratogen exposure

Individual

Anorexia

Caregiver and/or individual maladaptive feeding behaviors

Chronic illness

Infection

Insatiable appetite

Malnutrition

Organic and inorganic factors

Prematurity

Substance abuse

Environmental

Deprivation

Lead poisoning

Natural disasters
Poverty
Teratogens
Violence
Caregiver
Abuse
Mental illness
Mental retardation
Severe learning disability

Suggestions for Use

There are many conditions, including other nursing diagnoses, that create risk for altered growth, for example, *Ineffective breast-feeding*. The diagnosis of *Risk for altered growth related to Ineffective breastfeeding* suggests goals focused on weight gain/loss but gives little guidance for nursing activities to correct the breast-feeding problem; whereas a diagnosis of *Ineffective breastfeeding related to maternal anxiety/ambivalence* provides direction for nursing activities to correct the breastfeeding problem and, indirectly, to correct the *Risk for altered growth*. When possible, use the more specific diagnoses rather than the more general diagnosis *Risk for altered growth*.

Because growth is routinely assessed in nursing care of children, a diagnostic statement is usually not required for that application—such assessment is usually included in pediatric standards of care. Likewise, this label is not appropriate for a child with failure to thrive. That condition may be described better by one of the family functioning diagnoses or by a diagnosis of *Altered nutrition: less than body requirements*.

Suggested Alternative Diagnoses

Breastfeeding, ineffective
Family coping: ineffective, disabling
Growth and development, altered
Individual coping, ineffective
Infant feeding pattern, ineffective
Nutrition: less than body requirements, altered
Parenting, altered
Self-care deficit: feeding

NOC Suggested Outcomes

To be developed

Goals/Evaluation Criteria

NOTE: This text can provide only examples of growth norms. Refer to pediatrics or child development texts for complete discussion of growth.

• The child will achieve expected growth norms (eg, weight, head circumference, bone age, mean body mass), that is: not above the 97th percentile or below the 3rd percentile for age

NIC Priority Interventions

To be developed

Nursing Activities

NOTE: Because this nursing diagnosis is so broad, not every possible nursing activity can be listed here. Refer to age-specific sections in growth and development texts for full lists of activities.

Assessments

• Assess the caretakers' knowledge, resources, support system, coping skills, and level of commitment to develop a plan of care for eliminating risk factors
• Conduct a thorough health assessment (eg, child's history, temperament, culture, family environment, developmental screening) to determine risk factors
• Monitor parent/child interactions and communication
• Assess adequacy of nutritional intake (eg, calories, nutrients)
• Monitor trends in weight loss or gain
• Take skinfold measurements
• Determine food preferences

Patient/Family Teaching

• Teach caregivers about normal growth patterns
• Teach patient/family about nutritional needs

Collaborative Activities

• Act as case manager to insure comprehensive care by coordinating medical, school, rehabilitation, and social services efforts
• Refer to nutritionist for diet teaching and planning

Other

• Assist caretakers to develop a plan of care. (For possible care plans/interventions, refer to "Nursing Activities" for the "Suggested Alternative Diagnoses" presented on p. 182.)
• Establish a therapeutic and trusting relationship with caretakers

Growth and Development, Altered
(6.6) (1986)

Definition: The state in which an individual demonstrates deviations in norms from his/her age group

Defining Characteristics

Objective

Altered physical growth

Decreased responses

Delay or difficulty in performing skills (eg, motor, social, or expressive) typical of age group

Flat affect

Inability to perform self-care or self-control activities appropriate for age

Listlessness

Related Factors

Effects of physical disability

Environmental and stimulation deficiencies

Inadequate caretaking

Inconsistent responsiveness

Indifference

Multiple caretakers

Prescribed dependence

Separation from significant others

Other Possible Related Factors (non-NANDA)

Abuse

Changes in family system

Congenital anomaly

Fetal distress during or after birth/delivery

Inadequate bonding

Inadequate prenatal care

Loss

Maternal acute/chronic disease

Neonatal disease

Poverty

Prematurity

Serious illness/injury

Traumatic separation
Unhealthy maternal lifestyle during pregnancy

Suggestions for Use

Use of this label is not recommended. It is too broad to suggest nursing actions. There are many nursing diagnoses that could be considered "alterations in growth and development" or that could be caused by altered growth and development (eg, *Self-care deficit, Urinary incontinence, Impaired verbal communication*, and *Altered parenting*). When possible, use the more specific labels. If the problem is potential rather than actual, use *Risk for altered growth* and/or *Risk for altered development*.

Because growth and development are routinely assessed in nursing care of children, a diagnostic statement is usually not required for that application—such assessment is usually included in pediatric standards of care. This label is not appropriate for a mentally impaired child (eg, *Altered growth and development related to Down syndrome*). Instead, diagnose the specific functional task that the child is unable to perform (eg, *Feeding self-care deficit*). Likewise, this label is probably not appropriate for a child with failure to thrive. That condition may be described better by one of the family functioning diagnoses or by a diagnosis of *Altered nutrition: less than body requirements. Altered growth and development* is most appropriately used for a child who is having difficulty achieving age-specific developmental tasks and growth norms.

Suggested Alternative Diagnoses

Bowel incontinence
Breastfeeding, ineffective
Communication, impaired verbal
Coping: family, ineffective, compromised
Coping: family, ineffective, disabling
Coping: individual, ineffective
Incontinence, urinary
Infant feeding pattern, ineffective
Nutrition: less than body requirements, altered
Parenting, altered
Self-care deficit (specify)

NOC Suggested Outcomes

Child Development: 2 months...Adolescence: Milestones of physical, cognitive, and psychosocial progression by 2 months (4 months, 2 years, and so on) of age. **NOTE:** NOC lists a separate outcome for each age group

Growth: A normal increase in body size and weight

Physical Aging Status: Physical changes that commonly occur with adult aging

Physical Maturation: Female: Normal physical changes in the female that occur with the transition from childhood to adulthood

Physical Maturation: Male: Normal physical changes in the male that occur with the transition from childhood to adulthood

Goals/Evaluation Criteria

Examples Using NOC Language

- Normal progression of **Physical Aging Status**, as evidenced by the following indicators (specify 1–5: extreme, substantial, moderate, mild, or no deviation from expected range):

    Mean body mass, bone density, basal metabolic rate, skin elasticity, and muscle strength

    Cardiac output, vital capacity, and blood pressure

    Hearing, visual, olfactory, and taste acuity

Other Examples

This section can only provide examples. Refer to *Nursing Outcomes Classification (NOC)* manual or pediatrics text for complete list of indicators for each age group: 2, 4, 6, and 12 months; 2, 3, 4, and 5 years; middle childhood; and adolescence.

- The child will achieve expected growth norms (eg, weight, head circumference, bone age, mean body mass), that is, not above the 97th percentile or below the 3rd percentile for age
- The child will achieve milestones of physical, cognitive, and psychosocial progression by (specify age of achievement), with no delay from expected range
- Examples of indicators of normal child development for a 6-month-old child are as follows: Rolls over, sits with support, grasps and mouths objects
- Physical maturation will progress normally (eg, for females: growth spurt between 9.5 and 14.5 years of age, breast develop-

ment, and onset of menstruation; for males: growth spurt between 10.5 and 16 years of age, voice change, penis enlargement, increased muscle mass)
- The patient will achieve the highest level of wellness, independence, and growth and development possible given patient's illness/disability status

NIC Priority Interventions

Developmental Enhancement: Facilitating or teaching parents/caregivers to facilitate the optimal gross motor, fine motor, language, cognitive, social, and emotional growth of preschool and school-aged children

Nutritional Monitoring: Collection and analysis of patient data to prevent or minimize malnourishment

Nutrition Therapy: Administration of food and fluids to support metabolic processes of a patient who is malnourished or at high risk for becoming malnourished

Self-Responsibility Facilitation: Encouraging a patient to assume more responsibility for own behavior

Nursing Activities

NOTE: Because this nursing diagnosis is so broad and nonspecific, not every possible nursing activity can be listed here. Refer to the *Nursing Interventions Classification (NIC)* manual and to age-specific sections in growth and development texts for full lists of activities for NIC priority interventions.

Assessments

- Assess the caretakers' knowledge, resources, support systems, coping skills, and level of commitment to develop a plan of care
- Conduct a thorough health assessment (eg, child's history, temperament, culture, family environment, developmental screening) to determine functional level
- Identify potential related physical problems (eg, dehydration, falls, upper respiratory infection, skin breakdown), and initiate plans to prevent them
- Monitor parent/child interactions and communication
- Assess adequacy of nutritional intake (eg, calories, nutrients)
- Monitor trends in weight loss or gain
- Take skinfold measurements
- Determine food preferences

- *(NIC) Self-Responsibility Facilitation:* Monitor level of responsibility that patient assumes

Patient/Family Teaching

- *(NIC) Developmental Enhancement:*

  Teach caregivers about normal developmental milestones and associated behaviors

  Demonstrate activities that promote development to caregivers

Collaborative Activities

- Act as case manager to ensure comprehensive care by coordinating medical, nutritional, school, rehabilitation, and social services
- *(NIC) Developmental Enhancement:* Refer caregivers to support group, as appropriate

Other

- Assist caretakers to develop a plan of care. (For possible care plans/interventions, refer to "Family Coping: Ineffective, Compromised," on pp. 96–98, and "Family Coping: Ineffective, Disabling," on pp. 100–101.)
- Assist patient in achieving next level of growth and development through appropriate mastery of tasks specific to his/her level
- Create an environment where ADLs can be performed with maximum independence
- Establish a therapeutic and trusting relationship with caretakers
- Help the family develop a strategy to integrate the patient as an accepted member of the family and community
- *(NIC) Developmental Enhancement:*

  Provide activities that encourage interaction among children

  Encourage child to express self through positive rewards or feedback for attempts

  Offer age-appropriate toys or materials

  Be consistent and structured with behavior management/modification strategies
- *(NIC) Self-Responsibility Facilitation:*

  Encourage patient to take as much responsibility for own self-care as possible

  Encourage parents to clearly communicate and follow through on expectations for responsible behavior in child, as appropriate

Health Maintenance, Altered
(6.4.2) (1982)

Definition: Inability to identify, manage, and/or seek out help to maintain health

Defining Characteristics

Subjective
Expressed interest in improving health behaviors

Objective
Demonstrated lack of adaptive behaviors to internal/external environmental changes
Demonstrated lack of knowledge regarding basic health practices
History of lack of health-seeking behavior
Reported or observed lack of equipment, financial, and/or other resources
Reported or observed impairment of personal support system
Reported or observed inability to take responsibility for meeting basic health practices in any or all functional pattern areas

Other Defining Characteristics (non-NANDA)
History of untreated, chronic symptoms of disease process
Limited use of health care agencies and personnel
Limited use of preventive health measures
Need to adhere to cultural/religious beliefs

Related Factors

Disabling spiritual distress
Dysfunctional grieving
Ineffective family coping
Ineffective individual coping
Lack of ability to make deliberate and thoughtful judgments
Lack of material resources
Lack of or significant alteration in communication skills (eg, written, verbal, and/or gestural)
Perceptual/cognitive impairment (complete/partial lack of gross- and/or fine-motor skills)
Unachieved developmental tasks

Other Related Factors (non-NANDA)
Cultural beliefs
Lack of social supports

Motor impairment
Religious beliefs

Suggestions for Use

Use this diagnosis for patients who *wish* to change an unhealthy lifestyle or who *lack knowledge* of their disease or condition. Do not use it to describe patients who are not motivated to change or learn. *Health-seeking behaviors* is a wellness diagnosis to be used for clients with a generally healthy lifestyle who are seeking to attain a higher level of wellness (eg, a client who wishes information about blood pressure screening).

Suggested Alternative Diagnoses

Adjustment, impaired
Coping: individual, ineffective
Denial, ineffective
Health-seeking behaviors
Knowledge deficit
Management of therapeutic regimen: family/individual, ineffective
Noncompliance (specify)

NOC Suggested Outcomes

Health Beliefs: Perceived Resources: Personal conviction that one has adequate means to carry out a health behavior

Health-Promoting Behavior: Actions to sustain or increase wellness

Health-Seeking Behavior: Actions to promote optimal wellness, recovery, and rehabilitation

Knowledge: Health Behaviors: Extent of understanding conveyed about the promotion and protection of health

Knowledge: Health Resources: Extent of understanding conveyed about health care resources

Knowledge: Treatment Regimen: Extent of understanding conveyed about a specific treatment regimen

Participation: Health Care Decisions: Personal involvement in selecting and evaluating health care options

Psychosocial Adjustment: Life Change: Psychosocial adaptation of an individual to a life change

Risk Detection: Actions taken to identify personal health threats

Social Support: Perceived availability and actual provision of reliable assistance from other persons

Treatment Behavior: Illness or Injury: Personal actions to palliate or eliminate pathology

Goals/Evaluation Criteria

Examples Using NOC Language

- Will demonstrate **Participation: Health Care Decisions**, as evidenced by the following indicators (specify 1–5: never, rarely, sometimes, often, or consistently demonstrated):

    Demonstrates self-direction in decision making

    Seeks information

    Identifies barriers and available supports for achieving desired outcomes

    Seeks services to meet desired outcomes

Other Examples

Patient will:

- Develop and follow strategies to maximize health
- Acknowledge adverse effects of health beliefs
- Demonstrate awareness that healthy behavior requires some effort, and confidence in ability to manage it
- Follow recommended treatment regimens
- Identify potential health risks created by lifestyle
- Verbalize and demonstrate knowledge of preventive health measures (eg, performs self-examinations, participates in health screenings)

NIC Priority Interventions

Health System Guidance: Facilitating a patient's location and use of appropriate health services

Support System Enhancement: Facilitating support to patient by family, friends, and community

Nursing Activities

Assessments

- Identify beliefs and knowledge deficits that interfere with health maintenance
- Assess availability and adequacy of support system

Patient/Family Teaching

- *(NIC) Health System Guidance:*

    Explain the immediate health care system, how it works, and what the patient/family can expect

    Give written instructions for purpose and location of health care activities, as appropriate

Inform the patient the meaning of signing a consent form

Inform patient of the cost, time, alternatives, and risks involved in a specific test or procedure

Provide patient with copy of Patient's Bill of Rights

Collaborative Activities

- Consult with social services to plan for health maintenance needs on discharge
- *(NIC) Health System Guidance:*

  Inform patient of appropriate community resources and contact persons

  Advise use of second opinion

  Coordinate referrals to relevant health care providers, as appropriate

  Coordinate/schedule time needed by each service to deliver care, as appropriate

  Assist individual to complete forms for assistance, such as housing and financial aid, as needed

Other

- Encourage discussion of preventive health measures specific to patient needs, such as dietary changes, cessation of smoking, stress reduction, and implementation of exercise program
- *(NIC) Health System Guidance:* Encourage the patient/family to ask questions about services and charges

Health-Seeking Behaviors (specify)
(5.4) (1988)

Definition: A state in which a patient in stable health* is actively seeking ways to alter personal health habits and/or the environment in order to move toward a higher level of health

Defining Characteristics

Subjective

Expression of concern about current environmental conditions on health status

---

*Stable health status is defined as age-appropriate, illness-prevention measures achieved; client reports good or excellent health; and signs and symptoms of disease, if present, are controlled.

Expressed desire for increased control of health practice
Expressed desire to seek a higher level of wellness
Stated unfamiliarity with wellness community resources
Objective
Demonstrated or observed lack of knowledge of health-promotion
  behaviors
Observed desire for increased control of health practice
Observed desire to seek a higher level of wellness
Observed unfamiliarity with wellness community resources

Related Factors

Specific to patient (to be developed)

Suggestions for Use

Use this label for well patients who wish information about disease prevention or health promotion. For patients with an unhealthy lifestyle, consider *Altered health maintenance*.

Suggested Alternative Diagnoses

Breastfeeding, effective
Family coping: potential for growth
Health maintenance, altered

NOC Suggested Outcomes

Adherence Behavior: Self-initiated action taken to promote wellness, recovery, and rehabilitation
Health Beliefs: Personal convictions that influence health behaviors
Health Orientation: Personal view of health and health behaviors as priorities
Health-Promoting Behavior: Actions to sustain or increase wellness

Goals/Evaluation Criteria

Examples Using NOC Language

• Demonstrates **Adherence Behavior**, as evidenced by the following indicators (specify 1–5: never, rarely, sometimes, often, or consistently demonstrated):
  Seeks health-related information from a variety of sources
  Describes strategies to eliminate unhealthy behavior
  Reports using strategies to maximize health
  Performs self-screening and self-monitoring
  Uses health services congruent with need

Other Examples

Patient will:

- Recognize and act on the need to alter personal health habits
- Have a sense of personal responsibility for making healthy choices
- Strive to balance exercise, work, leisure, and rest
- Maintain a healthy diet
- Avoid risky behaviors (eg, driving without seat-belt)
- Express the desire to seek a higher level of wellness

NIC Priority Interventions

Health Education: Development and provision of instruction and learning experiences to facilitate voluntary adaptation of behavior conducive to health in individuals, families, groups, or communities

Self-Modification Assistance: Reinforcement of self-directed change initiated by the patient to achieve personally important goals

Nursing Activities

Assessments

- Assess patient's motivation to change
- *(NIC) Health Education:*

  Determine personal context and sociocultural history of individual, family, or community health behavior

  Determine current health knowledge and lifestyle behaviors of individual, family, or target group

Patient/Family Teaching

- *(NIC) Health Education:*

  Target high-risk groups and age ranges that would benefit most from health education

  Prioritize identified learner needs based on client preference, skills of nurse, resources available, and likelihood of successful goal attainment

  Avoid use of fear or scare techniques as strategy to motivate people to change health or lifestyle behaviors

  Teach strategies that can be used to resist unhealthful behavior or risk taking, rather than give advice to avoid or change behavior

Use group presentations to provide support and lessen threat to learners experiencing similar problems or concerns, as appropriate

Collaborative Activities

- Consult with community services as a primary step toward health promotion for patient/family. Involve patient/family in consultation

Other

- Discuss with patient/family personal health habits and determine which behaviors may be changed to achieve optimal health (eg, through diet, smoking cessation, stress reduction, exercise program)
- Assist patient to recognize potential barriers to changing behaviors
- Stress the importance of self-monitoring when attempting behavior change
- Assist patient to identify extrinsic and intrinsic rewards that can serve as motivators for behavior change
- Help the patient to recognize small successes
- *(NIC) Health Education:* Plan long-term follow-up to reinforce health behavior or lifestyle adaptations

Home Maintenance Management, Impaired (6.4.1.1) (1980)

Definition: Inability to independently maintain a safe, growth-promoting immediate environment

Defining Characteristics

Subjective

Household members describe outstanding debts or financial crises

Household members express difficulty in maintaining their home in a comfortable fashion

Household [members] request assistance with home maintenance

Objective
Accumulation of dirt, food wastes, or hygienic wastes
Disorderly surroundings
Inappropriate household temperature
Lack of necessary equipment or aids
Offensive odors
Overtaxed (eg, exhausted, anxious) family members
Presence of vermin or rodents
Repeated hygienic disorders, infestations, or infections
Unwashed or unavailable cooking equipment, clothes, linen

Related Factors

Impaired cognitive or emotional functioning
Inadequate support system
Individual/family member disease or injury
Insufficient family organization or planning
Insufficient finances
Lack of knowledge
Lack of role modeling
Unfamiliarity with neighborhood resources

Other Defining Characteristics (non-NANDA)
Developmental disability
Home environment obstacles

Suggestions for Use

This diagnosis emphasizes inability to manage the home environment (eg, laundry, cleaning, and cooking. If the difficulty is with managing medications or treatments, use *Ineffective management of therapeutic regimen.* If it is primarily a difficulty in managing self-care, such as bathing and dressing, use *Self-care deficit* (specify). Differentiate also between this label and *Caregiver role strain.*

Suggested Alternative Diagnoses

Caregiver role strain
Coping: family, ineffective, compromised
Injury, risk for (trauma, falls)
Management of therapeutic regimen: family/individual, ineffective
Self-care deficit (specify)

NOC Suggested Outcomes

Parenting: Provision of an environment that promotes optimum growth and development of dependent children

Parenting: Social Safety: Parental actions to avoid social relationships that might cause harm or injury

Role Performance: Congruence of an individual's role behavior with role expectations

Self-Care: Instrumental Activities of Daily Living (IADLs): Ability to perform activities needed to function in the home or community

Goals/Evaluation Criteria

Examples Using NOC Language

- *Impaired home maintenance management* will be eliminated or moderated, as demonstrated by Parenting, Parenting: Social Safety, Role Performance, and Self-Care: Instrumental Activities of Daily Living

- **Role Performance** will be demonstrated, as evidenced by the following indicators (specify 1–5: not, slightly, moderately, substantially, or totally adequate):

    Ability to meet role expectations

    Performance of family role behaviors

Other Examples

Patient/family/household member will:

- Follow specific plan for home maintenance
- Identify options to overcome financial constraints
- Verbalize awareness of constraints on home situation due to illness of family member
- Verbalize knowledge of available resources
- Perform home maintenance tasks (eg, shopping, meal preparation, laundry, yard work, housework)
- Drive car (eg, for shopping)
- Remove environmental hazards from the home
- Provide for the physical needs of dependents in the home
- Provide supervision for children (eg, of playmates, day-care workers)

NIC Priority Interventions

Home Maintenance Assistance: Helping the patient/family to maintain the home as a clean, safe, and pleasant place to live

Nursing Activities

Assessments

- *(NIC) Home Maintenance Assistance:* Determine patient's home maintenance requirements

Patient/Family Teaching

- Provide written material regarding home maintenance
- *(NIC) Home Maintenance Assistance:* Provide information on how to make home environment safe and clean

Collaborative Activities

- Assess and document need for postdischarge follow-through with public health nurse
- Contact discharge planner/social worker to establish realistic plan for home maintenance
- *(NIC) Home Maintenance Assistance:*
  Provide information on respite care, as needed
  Offer homemaker services, as appropriate

Other

- Accept and support without judgment the realities of the home situation
- Help patient/family/household member identify obstacles/hazards in home that may impede home maintenance
- Help patient/family/household member identify strengths in family unit, as well as support systems that will assist in home maintenance
- Initiate discussion with patient/family about health status of all family members, as illness of other family members may affect home maintenance management
- *(NIC) Home Maintenance Assistance:*
  Involve patient/family in deciding home maintenance requirements
  Suggest necessary structural alterations to make home accessible
  Suggest services for pest control, as needed
  Suggest services for home repair, as needed
  Discuss cost of needed maintenance and available resources

Hopelessness
(7.3.1) (1986)

Definition: A subjective state in which an individual sees no alternatives or personal choices available and cannot mobilize energy on own behalf

Defining Characteristics

Subjective
Verbal cues (eg, despondent content, "I can't," sighing)

Objective
Closing eyes
Decreased appetite
Decreased affect
Decreased response to stimuli
Decreased verbalization
Increased/decreased sleep
Lack of initiative
Lack of involvement in care/passively allowing care
Passivity
Shrugging in response to speaker
Turning away from speaker
Avoiding eye contact (non-NANDA)

Related Factors

Abandonment
Failing or deteriorating physical condition
Long-term stress
Lost belief in transcendent values/God
Prolonged activity restrictions creating isolation
Lack of social supports (non-NANDA)

Suggestions for Use

Differentiate between this label and *Powerlessness. Hopelessness* implies that the person believes there *is* no solution to his/her problem ("no way out"). In *Powerlessness*, the person may know of a solution to the problem but believes it is beyond his/her control to achieve the solution. Long-term feelings of *Powerlessness* may lead to *Hopelessness*. Although both diagnoses share some defining characteristics, the following are specific only to *Powerlessness:* irritability, resentment, anger, guilt, and fear of alienation from caregivers. For some patients, *Hopelessness* may be a risk factor for suicide.

Suggested Alternative Diagnoses

Anxiety, death
Coping: individual, ineffective
Failure to thrive, adult
Grieving, dysfunctional (may be an etiology of Hopelessness)
Powerlessness
Spiritual distress, actual/risk
Violence: self-directed, risk for

NOC Suggested Outcomes

Decision Making: Ability to choose between two or more alternatives

Hope: Presence of internal state of optimism that is personally satisfying and life supporting

Mood Equilibrium: Appropriate adjustment of prevailing emotional tone in response to circumstances

Nutritional Status: Food and Fluid Intake: Amount of food and fluid taken into the body over a 24-hour period

Quality of Life: An individual's expressed satisfaction with current life circumstances

Sleep: Extent and pattern of sleep for mental and physical rejuvenation

Goals/Evaluation Criteria

Examples Using NOC Language

- *Hopelessness* will be eliminated, as evidenced by consistent Decision Making, presence of Hope, Mood Equilibrium, adequate Nutritional Status: Food and Fluid Intake, adequate Sleep, and expressed satisfaction with Quality of Life
- **Decision Making** will be demonstrated, as evidenced by the following indicators (specify 1–5: never, rarely, sometimes, often, or consistently demonstrated): Weighs and chooses among alternatives
- **Hope** will be exhibited, as evidenced by the following indicators (specify 1–5: none, limited, moderate, substantial, or extensive):
  Expression of faith, will to live, reasons to live, meaning in life, optimism, and belief in self and others
  Demonstration of a zest for life

Other Examples

Patient will:

- Identify personal strengths
- Initiate behaviors that may reduce feelings of hopelessness
- Report extent and pattern of sleep adequate to produce mental and physical rejuvenation
- Demonstrate appropriate mood and affect
- Maintain appropriate hygiene and grooming
- Ingest sufficient food and fluids to maintain stable weight
- Demonstrate interest in social and personal relationships
- Show interest in or satisfaction with achieving life goals

NIC Priority Interventions

Hope Instillation: Facilitation of the development of a positive outlook in a given situation

Nursing Activities

Assessments

- Assess and document potential for suicide
- Monitor affect and decision-making ability
- Monitor nutrition: intake and body weight
- Assess spiritual needs
- Determine adequacy of relationships and other social supports

Patient/Family Teaching

- Provide information on community resources, such as community agencies, social agencies, self-improvement classes, stress-reduction classes, counseling
- *(NIC) Hope Instillation:* Teach reality recognition by surveying the situation and making contingency plans

Collaborative Activities

- Obtain psychiatric consultation
- *(NIC) Hope Instillation:* Provide patient/family opportunity to be involved with support groups

Other

- Encourage active participation in group activities to provide opportunity for social supports and problem solving
- Explore with patient factors that contribute to feelings of hopelessness

- Provide positive reinforcement for behaviors that demonstrate initiative, such as eye contact, self-disclosure, reduction in amount of sleep time, self-care, increased appetite
- Schedule time with patient to provide opportunity to explore alternative coping measures
- *(NIC) Hope Instillation:*

    Assist patient/family to identify areas of hope in life

    Demonstrate hope by recognizing the patient's intrinsic worth and viewing the patient's illness as only one facet of the individual

    Help the patient expand spiritual self

    Employ guided life review and/or reminiscence, as appropriate

    Avoid masking the truth

    Involve the patient actively in own care

    Encourage therapeutic relationships with significant others

Hyperthermia
(1.2.2.3) (1986)

Definition: A state in which an individual's body temperature is elevated above his/her normal range

Defining Characteristics

Subjective

Nausea

Objective

Flushed skin

Increase in body temperature above normal range

Increased respiratory rate

Seizures/convulsions

[Skin] warm to touch

Tachycardia

Related Factors

Dehydration

Illness or trauma

Inability or decreased ability to perspire

Inappropriate clothing

Increased metabolic rate

Medication/anesthesia

[Prolonged] exposure to hot environment
Vigorous activity

Suggestions for Use

Nursing activities, such as removal of clothing or a cool sponge bath, are effective for mild *Hyperthermia*. However, severe *Hyperthermia* is a life-threatening condition requiring both medical and nursing intervention. An elevated temperature may not be a problem, but merely a symptom of a disease process/infection, and it is treated by a medication such as acetaminophen or aspirin. Most hyperthermias require no independent nursing treatment.

Suggested Alternative Diagnoses

Body temperature, risk for altered
Hyperthermia, risk for
Thermoregulation, ineffective

NOC Suggested Outcomes

Thermoregulation: Balance among heat production, heat gain, and heat loss
Thermoregulation: Neonate: Balance among heat production, heat gain, and heat loss during the neonatal period

Goals/Evaluation Criteria

Examples Using NOC Language

- Patient will demonstrate **Thermoregulation**, as evidenced by the following indicators (specify 1–5: extremely, substantially, moderately, mildly, or not compromised):
    Skin temperature in expected range
    Body temperature within normal limits
    Pulse and respiratory rates in expected range
    Skin color changes not present
    Drowsiness and irritability not present

Other Examples

Patient/family will:
- Demonstrate proper method of taking temperature
- Describe measures to prevent/minimize increase in body temperature
- Report early signs and symptoms of hyperthermia
  Infants will:
- Experience no respiratory distress, restlessness, or lethargy
- Use heat-dissipation posture

NIC Priority Interventions

Fever Treatment: Management of a patient with hyperpyrexia caused by nonenvironmental factors

Malignant Hyperthermia Precautions: Prevention or reduction of hypermetabolic response to pharmacologic agents used during surgery

Temperature Regulation: Attaining and/or maintaining body temperature within a normal range

Temperature Regulation: Intraoperative: Attaining and/or maintaining desired intraopertive body temperature

Vital Signs Monitoring: Collection and analysis of cardiovascular, respiratory, and body temperature data to determine and prevent complications

Nursing Activities

Also see "Nursing Activities" for "Body Temperature, Risk for Altered," on pp. 36–37

Assessments

- Monitor for seizure activity
- Monitor hydration (eg, skin turgor, moist mucous membranes)
- Monitor blood pressure, pulse, and respirations
- *For surgery patients:*

  Obtain personal and family history of malignant hyperthermia, deaths from anesthesia, or postoperative fever

  Monitor for signs of malignant hyperthermia (eg, fever, tachypnea, arrhythmias, blood pressure changes, mottled skin, rigidity, profuse sweating)

- *(NIC) Temperature Regulation:*

  Monitor temperature at least every 2 hours, as appropriate

  Institute a continuous core temperature monitoring device, as appropriate

  Monitor skin color and temperature

Patient/Family Teaching

- Instruct patient/family in measures for prevention and early recognition of hyperthermia (eg, heatstroke and heat exhaustion)
- *(NIC) Temperature Regulation:* Teach indications of heat exhaustion and appropriate emergency treatment, as appropriate

Collaborative Activities

- *(NIC) Temperature Regulation:*

  Administer antipyretic medication, as appropriate

Use cooling mattress and tepid baths to adjust altered body temperature, as appropriate

Other

- Remove excess clothing and cover patient with only a sheet
- Apply cool washcloths (or ice bag covered with a cloth) to axilla, groin, forehead, and nape of neck
- Encourage intake of oral fluids
- Use a circulating fan in patient's room
- Use a cooling blanket
- *For malignant hyperthermia:*
    Perform emergency care according to protocol
    Keep emergency equipment in operative areas according to protocol

Hypothermia
(1.2.2.2) (1986, 1988)

Definition: The state in which an individual's body temperature is reduced below normal range

Defining Characteristics

Objective
Cool skin
Cyanotic nail beds
Hypertension
Pallor
Piloerection
Reduction in body temperature below normal range
Shivering
Slow capillary refill
Cardiac dysrhythmias (non-NANDA)

Related Factors

Aging
Consumption of alcohol
Damage to hypothalamus
Decreased basal metabolic rate
Evaporation from skin in cool environment
Illness or trauma
Inability or decreased ability to shiver

Inactivity
Inadequate clothing
Medications causing vasodilation
[Prolonged] exposure to cool or cold environment

Other Related Factors (non-NANDA)
Hypothyroidism
Immaturity of newborn's temperature regulatory system
Loss of subcutaneous fat/malnutrition
Low birth weight

Suggestions for Use

Because severe *Hypothermia* (rectal temperature below 35°C or 95°F) may cause complications such as impaired myocardial or respiratory function, such low readings should be reported to the physician. Mild *Hypothermia* (95–97°F or 35–36°C) should respond to nursing interventions.

Suggested Alternative Diagnoses

Body temperature, risk for altered
Hypothermia, risk for
Infant behavior, disorganized, risk for
Thermoregulation, ineffective

NOC Suggested Outcomes

Thermoregulation: Balance among heat production, heat gain, and heat loss
Thermoregulation: Neonate: Balance among heat production, heat gain, and heat loss during the neonatal period

Goals/Evaluation Criteria

Also see "Goals/Evaluation Criteria" for "Hyperthermia," p. 203 and for "Risk for Altered Body Temperature," p. 35

Examples Using NOC Language

- Demonstrates **Thermoregulation**, as evidenced by the following indicators (specify 1–5: extremely, substantially, moderately, mildly, or not compromised):
    Presence of goose bumps and shivering when cold
    Reported thermal comfort

Other Examples
Patient/family will:
- Describe measures to prevent/minimize decrease in body temperature
- Report early signs and symptoms of hypothermia
- Maintain patient body temperature of at least 97°F (36°C)
Infant will:
- Use heat-retaining posture
- Have blood glucose within normal limits
- Not be lethargic

NIC Priority Interventions

Hypothermia Treatment: Rewarming and surveillance of a patient whose core body temperature is below 35°C

Temperature Regulation: Attaining and/or maintaining body temperature within a normal range

Temperature Regulation: Intraoperative: Attaining and/or maintaining desired intraopertive body temperature

Vital Signs Monitoring: Collection and analysis of cardiovascular, respiratory, and body temperature data to determine and prevent complications

Nursing Activities

Also see "Nursing Activities" for "Risk for Altered Body Temperature," pp. 36–37.

Assessments
- Record baseline vital signs
- Place patient on cardiac monitor
- Use a low-range thermometer, if necessary, to obtain accurate temperature
- Assess for symptoms of hypothermia (eg, skin color changes, shivering, fatigue, weakness, apathy, slurred speech)
- Assess for medical conditions that contribute to hypothermia (eg, diabetes, myxedema)
- *(NIC) Temperature Regulation:*
  Institute a continuous core temperature monitoring device, as appropriate
  Monitor temperature at least every 2 h, as appropriate
  Monitor newborn's temperature until stabilized

Patient/Family Teaching

- *(NIC) Temperature Regulation:*

  Teach patient, particularly elderly patients, actions to prevent hypothermia from cold exposure

  Teach indications of hypothermia and appropriate emergency treatment, as appropriate

Collaborative Activities

- For severe hypothermia, assist with core-warming techniques (eg, hemodialysis, peritoneal dialysis, colonic irrigation)

Other

- Provide warmth, dry clothing, heated blankets, mechanical heating devices, adjusted room temperature, hot-water bottles, submersion in warm water, and warm oral fluids, as tolerated
- Do not give intramuscular (IM) or subcutaneous medications to hypothermic patient

  For intraoperative patient:
- Regulate room temperature to maintain patient's warmth
- Cover patient's head and exposed body parts
- Warm blood before administering
- Cover patient with warm blanket for transport after surgery
- *(NIC) Temperature Regulation:*

  Wrap infant immediately after birth to prevent heat loss

  Apply stockinette cap to prevent heat loss of newborn

  Place newborn in isolette or under warmer, as needed

Incontinence, Bowel
(1.3.1.3) (1975, 1998)

Definition: Change in normal bowel habits characterized by involuntary passage of stool

Defining Characteristics

Subjective

Inability to recognize urge to defecate

Recognizes rectal fullness but reports inability to expel formed stool

Self-report of inability to feel rectal fullness

Objective

Constant dribbling of soft stool

Fecal odor

Fecal staining of clothing and/or bedding

Inability to delay defecation

Inattention to urge to defecate

Red perianal skin

Urgency

Related Factors

Abnormally high abdominal or intestinal pressure

Chronic diarrhea

Colorectal lesions

Dietary habits

Environmental factors (eg, inaccessible bathroom)

General decline in muscle tone

Immobility

Impaction

Impaired cognition

Impaired reservoir capacity

Incomplete emptying of bowel

Laxative abuse

Loss of rectal sphincter control

Lower motor nerve damage

Medications

Rectal sphincter abnormality

Self-care deficit—toileting

Stress

Upper motor nerve damage

Suggestions for Use

(1) Differentiate between this label and *Diarrhea*. (2) *Self-care deficit: toileting* may be the cause of *Bowel incontinence*. However, there seems to be no advantage to writing a diagnosis of *Bowel incontinence related to Self-care deficit: toileting*. A diagnosis such as *Toileting self-care deficit related to inability to ambulate to toilet or commode* provides more specific information about the self-care deficit and thus more guidance for nursing interventions to alleviate the problem.

Suggested Alternative Diagnoses

Diarrhea

Management of therapeutic regimen: individual, ineffective

Self-care deficit: toileting

NOC Suggested Outcomes

Bowel Continence. Control of passage of stool from the bowel

Bowel Elimination: Ability of the gastrointestinal tract to form and evacuate stool effectively

Goals/Evaluation Criteria

Examples Using NOC Language

- Patient will exhibit **Bowel Continence**, as evidenced by the following indicators (specify 1–5: never, rarely, sometimes, often, or consistently demonstrated):

    Maintains control of passage of stool

    Consistently identifies urge to defecate

    Consistently responds to urge in timely manner

    Manages bowel appliance independently

    Reaches toilet facility independently before defecating

Other Examples

Patient will:

- Have progressively fewer incontinent episodes
- Be free of skin irritation to perianal area

NIC Priority Interventions

Bowel Incontinence Care: Promotion of bowel continence and maintenance of perianal skin integrity

Bowel Incontinence Care: Encopresis: Promotion of bowel continence in children

Bowel Training: Assisting the patient to train the bowel to evacuate at specific intervals

Nursing Activities

Assessments

- Assess condition of perianal skin after each episode of incontinence
- Document frequency of incontinent episodes
- Assess for symptoms of encopresis
- Obtain toilet training history of child, including duration of encopresis and treatment efforts

- *(NIC) Bowel Incontinence Care:*
  Determine physical or psychologic cause of fecal incontinence
  Monitor diet and fluid requirements
  Monitor for adequate bowel evacuation
  Determine goals of bowel management program with patient/ family

Patient/Family Teaching

- Instruct patient/family about physiology of normal defecation
- For encopresis: Caution parents not to create feelings of anxiety, guilt, or inadequacy about toileting; teach parents ways to reward desired toileting behaviors
- *(NIC) Bowel Incontinence Care:*
  Instruct patient/family to record fecal output, as appropriate
  Discuss procedures and expected outcomes with patient
  Explain etiology of problem and rationale for actions

Collaborative Activities

- Obtain order from physician to institute bowel-training program (Program may include bulk-forming laxative; rectal suppository q day; digital stimulation; and scheduled use of bedpan, commode, or bathroom.)
- Refer for family therapy (eg, for incontinence with emotional etiology)

Other

- Provide care in an accepting, nonjudgmental manner
- Provide bedpan or assist to commode q _____
- Provide privacy for defecation
- Establish a regular time for defecation
- Provide foods high in bulk and ample fluids
- Reinforce that the goal of therapy is to help the child with encopresis learn new bowel habits while avoiding excessive involvement of the parent with daily aspects of bowel function and diet
- *(NIC) Bowel Incontinence Care:*
  Wash perianal area with soap and water and dry it thoroughly after each stool
  Use powder and creams on perianal area with caution
  Keep bed and clothing clean
  Implement bowel-training program, as appropriate
  Place on incontinent pads, as needed
  Provide protective pants, as needed

Incontinence, Urinary, Functional
(1.3.2.1.4) (1986, 1998)

Definition: Inability of usually continent person to reach toilet in time to avoid unintentional loss of urine

Defining Characteristics

Able to completely empty bladder
Amount of time required to reach toilet exceeds length of time between sensing urge and uncontrolled voiding
Loss of urine before reaching toilet
May only be incontinent in early morning
Senses need to void

Related Factors

Altered environmental factors
Impaired cognition
Impaired vision
Neuromuscular limitations
Psychologic factors
Weakened supporting pelvic structures

Suggestions for Use

None

Suggested Alternative Diagnoses

Incontinence, urinary, reflex
Incontinence, urinary, stress
Incontinence, urinary, total
Incontinence, urinary, urge
Self-care deficit: toileting
Urinary elimination, altered
Urinary retention

NOC Suggested Outcomes

Urinary Continence: Control of the elimination of urine
Urinary Elimination: Ability of the urinary system to filter wastes, conserve solutes, and collect and discharge urine in a healthy pattern

Goals/Evaluation Criteria
Examples Using NOC Language
- Demonstrates **Urinary Continence**, as evidenced by the following indicators (specify 1–5: never, rarely, sometimes, often, or consistently demonstrated):

    Recognizes urge to void

    Adequate time to reach toilet between urge and evacuation of urine

    Underclothing dry during day

    Underclothing or bedding dry during night

    Able to toilet independently

    Predictable pattern to passage of urine

Other Examples
Patient will:
- Use adaptive equipment to help with clothing and transfers when incontinence is related to impaired mobility

NIC Priority Interventions
Urinary Habit Training: Establishing a predictable pattern of bladder emptying to prevent incontinence for persons with limited cognitive ability who have urge, stress, or functional incontinence

Urinary Incontinence Care: Assistance in promoting continence and maintaining perineal skin integrity

Nursing Activities
Assessments
- *(NIC) Urinary Incontinence Care:*

    Identify multifactorial causes of incontinence (eg, urinary output, voiding pattern, cognitive function, preexistent urinary problems, postvoid residual, and medications)

    Monitor urinary elimination, including frequency, consistency, odor, volume, and color

    Obtain urine for culture and sensitivity testing, as needed

Patient/Family Teaching
- Discuss with patient/family ways to modify environment to reduce number of wetness episodes. Consider the following strategies:

    Improving environmental lighting to enhance vision

    Installing raised toilet seat and hand rails

Providing bedside commode, bedpan, and handheld urinal
Removing loose rugs

- Instruct patient/family in prompted voiding routine (frequent reminders) based on patient's pattern of toileting, to decrease wetness episodes
- Instruct patient/family in skin care and hygiene routine to prevent skin breakdown
- Offer strategies for bladder management during activities away from home
- *(NIC) Urinary Incontinence Care:*
  Explain etiology of problem and rationale for actions
  Discuss procedures and expected outcomes with patient
  Instruct patient/family to record urinary output and pattern, as appropriate
  Instruct patient to drink a minimum of 1500 mL fluids a day

Collaborative Activities

- Consult with physical/occupational therapy for assistance with manual dexterity
- *(NIC) Urinary Incontinence Care:* Refer to urinary continence specialist, as appropriate

Other

- *(NIC) Urinary Habit Training:*
  Establish interval of initial toileting schedule, based on voiding pattern
  Toilet patient or remind patient to void at prescribed intervals
  Use power of suggestion (eg, running water or flushing toilet) to assist patient to void
  Avoid leaving patient on toilet for more than 5 minutes
  Reduce toileting interval by one-half hour if more than three incontinence episodes in 24 h
  Increase toileting interval by 1 hr if patient is unable to void at two or more scheduled toileting times
  Increase the toileting interval by 1 h if patient has no incontinence episodes for three days until optimal 4-h interval is achieved
- *(NIC) Urinary Incontinence Care:*
  Assist to develop/maintain a sense of hope
  Modify clothing and environment to provide easy access to toilet [eg, obtain clothing that is easily removed; substitute elastic waistbands and Velcro for zippers, buttons, snap devices, and hooks, whenever feasible.]

Provide protective garments, as needed

Cleanse genital skin area at regular intervals

Provide positive feedback for any decrease in episodes of incontinence

Schedule diuretic administration to have least impact on lifestyle

Incontinence, Urinary, Reflex
(1.3.2.1.2) (1986, 1998)

Definition: An involuntary loss of urine occurring at somewhat predictable intervals when a specific bladder volume is reached

Defining Characteristics

Subjective

Incomplete emptying with lesion above sacral micturition center

No sensation of bladder fullness

No sensation of urge to void

No sensation of voiding

Sensation to urinate without voluntary inhibition of bladder contraction

Sensations associated with full bladder, such as sweating, restlessness, and abdominal discomfort

Objective

Complete emptying with lesion above pontine micturition center

Predictable pattern of voiding

Unable to cognitively inhibit or initiate voiding

Related Factors

Neurological impairment above level of sacral micturition center or pontine micturition center

Tissue damage from radiation cystitis, inflammatory bladder conditions, or radical pelvic surgery

Suggestions for Use

None

Suggested Alternative Diagnoses

Incontinence, urinary, functional

Incontinence, urinary, stress

Incontinence, urinary, total

Incontinence, urinary, urge

Self-care deficit: toileting
Urinary elimination, altered
Urinary retention

NOC Suggested Outcomes

Urinary Continence: Control of the elimination of urine
Urinary Elimination: Ability of the urinary system to filter wastes, conserve solutes, and collect and discharge urine in a healthy pattern

Goals/Evaluation Criteria

Also see NOC examples for "Incontinence, Urinary, Functional" p. 213

Examples Using NOC Language

- Demonstrates **Urinary Continence**, as evidenced by the following indicators (specify 1–5: never, rarely, sometimes, often, or consistently demonstrated):
    Voids in appropriate receptacle
    Voids >150 mL each time
    Absence of urinary tract infection (<100,000 WBC)

Other Examples

Patient will:
- Be free of skin breakdown
- Demonstrate intermittent self-catheterization procedure

NIC Priority Interventions

Urinary Habit Training: Improving bladder function for those with urge incontinence by increasing the bladder's ability to hold urine and the patient's ability to suppress urination
Urinary Catheterization, Intermittent: Regular periodic use of a catheter to empty the bladder

Nursing Activities

Assessments

- Assess for ability to recognize urge to void
- Identify voiding pattern (either voiding after specified intake or voiding after a specified interval)
- Monitor technique of patient/caregivers who perform intermittent catheterization
- For patients undergoing intermittent catheterization, monitor

color, odor, and clarity of urine and perform frequent urinalysis to monitor for infection
- Determine patient's readiness and ability to perform intermittent self-catheterization
- *(NIC) Urinary Habit Training:* Keep a continence specification record for three days to establish voiding pattern

Patient/Family Teaching

- Teach patient/family reportable signs/symptoms of autonomic dysreflexia, such as severe hypertension, severe headache, diaphoresis above level of injury, tachycardia of sudden onset
- Teach patient/family/caregivers technique for clean intermittent catheterization
- Teach signs and symptoms of urinary tract infection (eg, fever, chills, flank pain, hematuria, change in consistency and odor of urine)

Collaborative Activities

- Refer to enterostomal therapy nurse for instruction in clean intermittent self-catheterization, as appropriate
- Administer antibacterial therapy, per medical order, at initiation of intermittent catheterization

Other

- Assist patient in maintaining adequate hygiene and skin care routine. Consider the following strategies:
  Applying moisture barrier ointment or skin sealant
  Keeping skin dry
  Using collection device for urine
- Consider condom catheter collection device with leg bag
- Remind the patient to try to hold urine until scheduled elimination time
- Maintain fluid intake of approximately 2000 mL/day
  For intermittent urinary catheterization:
- Provide quiet room and privacy for procedure
- Use clean or sterile technique (per protocol) for catheterization
- Determine catheterization schedule, based on assessment of voiding patterns
- If output of >300 mL is obtained (for adults), catheterize more frequently
- *(NIC) Urinary Habit Training:*
  Establish interval of initial toileting schedule, based on voiding pattern

Toilet patient or remind patient to void at prescribed intervals

Use power of suggestion (eg, running water or flushing toilet) to assist patient to void

Avoid leaving patient on toilet for more than 5 minutes

Reduce toileting interval by one-half hour if more than three incontinence episodes occur in 24 h

Increase toileting interval by 1 h if patient is unable to void at two or more scheduled toileting times

Increase the toileting interval by 1 hr if patient has no incontinence episodes for three days until optimal 4-h interval is achieved

Incontinence, Urinary, Stress
(1.3.2.1.1) (1986)

Definition: The state in which an individual experiences a loss of urine of less than 50 mL occurring with increased abdominal pressure

Defining Characteristics

Subjective
Reported dribbling with increased abdominal pressure
Urinary urgency

Objective
Observed dribbling with increased abdominal pressure
Urinary frequency (more often than every 2 hours)

Related Factors

Degenerative changes in pelvic muscles and structural supports associated with increased age
High intraabdominal pressure (eg, obesity, gravid uterus)
Incompetent bladder outlet
Overdistention between voidings
Weak pelvic muscles and structural supports

Suggestions for Use

None

Suggested Alternative Diagnoses

Incontinence, urinary, functional
Incontinence, urinary, reflex

Incontinence, urinary, total
Incontinence, urinary, urge
Self-care deficit: toileting
Urinary elimination, altered
Urinary retention

NOC Suggested Outcomes

Urinary Continence: Control of the elimination of urine
Urinary Elimination: Ability of the urinary system to filter wastes, conserve solutes, and collect and discharge urine in a healthy pattern

Goals/Evaluation Criteria

Also see NOC examples for "Incontinence, Urinary, Functional" p. 213

Examples Using NOC Language

- Demonstrates **Urinary Continence**, as evidenced by the following indicators (specify 1–5: never, rarely, sometimes, often, or consistently demonstrated): No urine leakage with increased abdominal pressure (eg, sneezing, laughing, lifting)

Other Examples

Patient will:
- Describe a plan for treating the stress incontinence
- Maintain a voiding frequency of more than q2h

NIC Priority Interventions

Pelvic Floor Exercise: Strengthening the pubococcygeal muscles through voluntary, repetitive contraction to decrease stress or urge incontinence
Urinary Incontinence Care: Instituting a program to promote continence and to maintain perineal skin integrity

Nursing Activities

See "Nursing Activities" for " Incontinence, Urinary, Functional" pp. 213–215

Patient/Family Teaching

- Instruct patient in hygiene and skin care measures
- Teach self-administration of oral or topical estrogens to ameliorate symptoms

- Teach techniques that strengthen the sphincter and structural supports of the bladder (eg, pelvic muscle exercises, urine stop-and-start exercises)
- Inform patient that it may require several weeks of exercising to obtain improvement

Collaborative Activities

- Consult with physician regarding surgical or medical management of incontinent episodes

Other

- Assist patient to select appropriate garment/pad for short-term incontinence management
- Give positive feedback for doing pelvic floor exercises
- *(NIC) Urinary Incontinence Care:* Limit ingestion of bladder irritants (eg, cola, coffee, tea, and chocolate)

Incontinence, Urinary, Total
(1.3.2.1.5) (1986)

Definition: The state in which an individual experiences a continuous and unpredictable loss of urine

Defining Characteristics

Subjective
Unawareness of incontinence
Objective
Constant flow of urine occurs at unpredictable times without distention or uninhibited bladder contractions/spasms
Lack of perineal or bladder-filling awareness
Nocturia
Unsuccessful incontinence refractory treatments

Related Factors

Anatomic (fistula)
Independent contraction of detrusor reflex due to surgery
Neurologic dysfunction causing triggering of micturition at unpredictable times
Neuropathy preventing transmission of reflex indicating bladder fullness
Trauma or disease affecting spinal cord nerves

Suggestions for Use

None

Suggested Alternative Diagnoses

Incontinence, urinary, functional
Incontinence, urinary, reflex
Incontinence, urinary, stress
Incontinence, urinary, urge
Self-care deficit: toileting
Urinary elimination, altered
Urinary retention

NOC Suggested Outcomes

Urinary Continence: Control of the elimination of urine
Urinary Elimination: Ability of the urinary system to filter wastes, conserve solutes, and collect and discharge urine in a healthy pattern

Goals/Evaluation Criteria

Also see NOC examples for "Incontinence, Urinary, Functional" p. 213

Examples Using NOC Language

• Demonstrates **Urinary Continence**, as evidenced by the following indicators (specify 1–5: never, rarely, sometimes, often, or consistently demonstrated):

Responds in timely manner to urge

Absence of urinary tract infection (<100,000 WBC)

Other Examples

Patient/family will:

• Maintain adequate skin integrity
• Describe a plan of care for indwelling (ie, foley) catheter at home

NIC Priority Interventions

Urinary Incontinence Care: Institution of a program to promote continence and to maintain perineal skin integrity

Nursing Activities

See "Nursing Activities" for "Incontinence, Urinary, Functional" on pp. 213–215

Assessments

- Assess patient for presence of fistula (ie, urethral, vaginal, rectovaginal)
- Assess patient for skin breakdown and maintenance of adequate hygiene and skin care routine

Patient/Family Teaching

- Instruct patient/family in use of indwelling catheter management at home
- Instruct patient/family to report signs/symptoms of urinary tract infection (eg, fever, chills, flank pain, hematuria, change in consistency and odor of urine)

Collaborative Activities

- Consult physician about use of indwelling catheter

Other

For skin care, consider the following measures:

- Ensure skin is adequately dried
- Apply moisture barrier, ointment, or skin sealant
- *NIC Urinary Incontinence Care:* Limit fluids for 2 to 3 hours before bedtime, as appropriate

Incontinence, Urinary, Urge
(1.3.2.1.3) (1986)

Definition: The state in which an individual experiences involuntary passage of urine occurring soon after a strong sense of urgency to void

Defining Characteristics

Subjective

Bladder contraction/spasm

Objective

Frequency (voiding more often than every 2 hours)

Inability to reach toilet in time

Nocturia (urination more than two times per night)

Urinary urgency

Voiding in small amounts (less than 100 mL) or in large amounts (more than 500 mL)

Related Factors

Alcohol

Caffeine

Decreased bladder capacity (eg, history of pelvic inflammatory disease, abdominal surgery, indwelling urinary catheter)

Increased fluid intake

Increased urine concentration

Irritation of bladder stretch receptors, causing spasm (eg, bladder infection)

Overdistention of bladder

Suggestions for Use

None

Suggested Alternative Diagnoses

Incontinence, urinary, functional

Incontinence, urinary, reflex

Incontinence, urinary, stress

Incontinence, urinary, total

Self-care deficit: toileting

Urinary elimination, altered

Urinary retention

NOC Suggested Outcomes

Urinary Continence: Control of the elimination of urine

Urinary Elimination: Ability of the urinary system to filter wastes, conserve solutes, and collect and discharge urine in a healthy pattern

Goals/Evaluation Criteria

Also see NOC examples for "Incontinence, Urinary, Functional" p. 213

Examples Using NOC Language

• Demonstrates **Urinary Continence**, as evidenced by the following indicators (specify 1–5: never, rarely, sometimes, often, or consistently demonstrated):

  Responds in timely manner to urge

  Free of medications that interfere with urinary control

  Maintains environment barrier-free to independent toileting

  Urine passes without urgency

Other Examples

Patient will:
- Describe bladder management program to restore satisfactory urinary elimination pattern
- Have less frequent incontinent episodes

NIC Priority Interventions

Urinary Habit Training: Establishing a predictable pattern of bladder emptying to prevent incontinence for persons with limited cognitive ability who have urge, stress, or functional incontinence

Urinary Incontinence Care: Institution of a program to promote continence and to maintain perineal skin integrity

Nursing Activities

See "Nursing Activities" for "Incontinence, Urinary, Functional" p. 213–215

Patient/Family Teaching

- Instruct patient regarding techniques that will increase bladder capacity, such as initiating pelvic floor raising when feeling the urge to void and using a bladder-training schedule that lengthens the time between voids
- *(NIC) Urinary Incontinence Care:*
  Explain etiology of problem and rationale for actions
  Discuss procedures and expected outcomes with patient

Collaborative Activities

- Consult with physical/occupational therapist for assistance with manual dexterity
- Consult with physician regarding (1) antispasmodic/anticholinergic medications and (2) medical management (eg, electrostimulation therapy, investigation of underlying irritative or inflammatory bladder disorders, and surgical therapy)

Other

- Assist patient to void prior to sleep and encourage nighttime voids to reduce urgency
- Provide bedpan, bedside commode, and urinal nearby to encourage frequent voiding episodes

Incontinence, Urinary, Urge, Risk for
(1.3.2.1.6) (1998)

Definition: Risk for involuntary loss of urine associated with a sudden, strong sensation of urinary urgency

Risk Factors

Detrusor hyperreflexia from cystitis, urethritis, tumors, renal calculi, central nervous system disorders above pontine micturition center

Effects of medications, caffeine, or alcohol

Ineffective toileting habits

Involuntary sphincter relaxation

Small bladder capacity

Suggestions for Use

None

Suggested Alternative Diagnoses

Incontinence, urinary, urge

NOC Suggested Outcomes

To be developed

Goals/Evaluation Criteria

See "Goals/Evaluation Criteria" for "Incontinence, Urinary, Urge" pp. 223–224

NIC Priority Interventions

To be developed

Nursing Activities

Assessments

- Assess for risk factors (see "Risk Factors" above)
- Evaluate environment for barriers to timely toileting
- Assess patient's self-care abilities and mobility
- *(NIC) Urinary Incontinence Care:* Monitor urinary elimination, including frequency, consistency, odor, volume, and color

Patient/Family Teaching

- Instruct patient regarding techniques that will increase bladder capacity, such as initiating pelvic floor raising when feeling the urge to void and using a bladder-training schedule that lengthens the time between voids

- Discuss with patient/family ways to modify environment to remove obstacles and improve self-care ability. Consider the following strategies:

    Improving environmental lighting to enhance vision

    Installing a raised toilet seat and hand rails

    Providing a bedside commode, bedpan, and handheld urinal

    Using assistive devices (eg, wheelchairs, canes, walkers, and nonskid walking shoes)

Collaborative Activities

- Consult with a physical/occupational therapist for assistance with manual dexterity

Other

- Obtain clothing that is easily removed
- Substitute elastic waistbands and Velcro for zippers, buttons, snap devices, and hooks, whenever feasible
- Assist patient to void prior to sleep and encourage nighttime voids to reduce urgency
- Discourage use of bladder irritants, such as caffeine, alcohol, citrus juices, carbonated drinks, cigarette smoke, and certain spicy foods

Infant Behavior, Disorganized
(6.8.2) (1994, 1998)

Definition: Disintegrated physiological and neurobehavioral responses to the environment

Defining Characteristics

Regulatory Problems
Inability to inhibit
Irritability

State-Organization System
Active-awake (fussy, worried gaze)
Diffuse/unclear sleep
Irritable or panicky crying
Quiet-awake (staring, gaze aversion)
State oscillation

Attention-Interaction System

Abnormal response to sensory stimuli (eg, difficult to soothe, inability to sustain alert status

Motor system

Altered primitive reflexes

Finger splay, fisting, or hands to face

Hyperextension of arms and legs

Increased, decreased, or limp tone

Jittery, jerky, uncoordinated movement

Tremors, startles, twitches

Physiologic

"Time-out" signals (eg, gaze, grasp, hiccup, cough, sneeze, sigh, slack jaw, open mouth, tongue thrust)

Bradycardia, tachycardia, or arrhythmias

Bradypnea, tachypnea, apnea

Feeding intolerances (aspiration or emesis)

Oximeter desaturation

Pale, cyanotic, mottled, or flushed color

Related Factors

Prenatal

Congenital or genetic disorders

Teratogenic exposure

Postnatal

Feeding intolerance

Invasive/painful procedures

Malnutrition

Oral/motor problems

Pain

Prematurity

Individual

Gestational age

Illness

Immature neurologic system

Postconceptual age

Environmental

Physical environment inappropriateness

Sensory deprivation

Sensory inappropriateness

Sensory overstimulation

Caregiver
Cue knowledge deficit
Cue misreading
Environmental stimulation contribution

Suggestions for Use

This diagnosis is most useful for infants, especially premature infants, in neonatal intensive care units. Immature neurologic development and increased or noxious environmental stimuli create a situation in which the infant must use energy for adaptation rather than for growth and development.

Suggested Alternative Diagnoses

Disorganized infant behavior, risk for
Growth and development, altered
Organized infant behavior, potential for enhanced
Thermoregulation, ineffective

NOC Suggested Outcomes

Child Development: 2 Months, 4 Months, 6 Months, and 12 Months: Milestones of physical, cognitive, and psychosocial progression by 2 months, 4 months, 6 months, and 12 months of age. [**NOTE:** NOC lists these separately for each age group.]

Muscle Function: Adequacy of muscle contraction needed for movement

Neurologic Status: Extent to which the peripheral and central nervous systems receive, process, and respond to internal and external stimuli

Sleep: Extent and pattern of sleep for mental and physical rejuvenation

Thermoregulation: Balance among heat production, heat gain, and heat loss

Thermoregulation, Neonate: Balance among heat production, heat gain, and heat loss during the neonatal period

Goals/Evaluation Criteria

Examples Using NOC Language

- **Neurologic Status** is normal, as evidenced by the following indicators (specify 1–5: extremely, substantially, moderately, mildly, or not compromised):

Neurologic Status: consciousness, central motor control, cranial sensory/motor function, spinal sensory/motor function, and autonomic function

Breathing pattern

Rest-sleep pattern

Seizure activity not present

- **Thermoregulation** is not compromised, as evidenced by the following indicators (specify 1–5: extremely, substantially, moderately, mildly, or not compromised):

Skin temperature in expected range

Body temperature within normal limits

Skin color changes not present

Pulse and respiratory rates in expected range

Muscle twitching not present

Other Examples

Infant will:

- Exhibit organized neurobehavioral functioning in all systems
- Not be restless or lethargic
- Utilize nonshivering thermogenesis
- Demonstrate no delay from expected range of development: 2 months (eg, displays some head control in upright position), 4 months (eg, controls head well), 6 months (eg, sits with support), and 12 months (eg, has precise pincer grasp). **NOTE:** Refer to a child development or pediatrics text for a comprehensive list of developmental milestones for each age.
- Exhibit adequate muscle function (eg, tone and contraction of muscle; control, steadiness, and speed of muscle movement)
Parent/Caregiver will:
- Recognize infant behavioral cues that communicate stress
- Modify the environment in response to infant's behaviors
- Demonstrate appropriate handling techniques to enhance normal development

NIC Priority Interventions

Environmental Management: Manipulation of the patient's surroundings for therapeutic benefit

Positioning: Moving the patient or a body part to provide comfort, reduce the risk of skin breakdown, promote skin integrity, and/or promote healing

Nursing Activities

Assessments

- Determine whether infant is achieving developmental milestones
- Monitor for signs of stress and maladaptation
- Identify infant's self-regulatory behaviors (eg, sucking, hand-to-mouth movements)
- Observe for causative external environmental factors (eg, lights, handling, noise)
- Assess for causative internal factors, such as pain and hunger
- Monitor sleep pattern

Patient/Family Teaching

- Teach parents about infant's needs and abilities
- Demonstrate gentle handling of the baby
- Model appropriate response to infant's behavioral cues
- Instruct parents on normal growth and development

Other

- Use sheepskin, water bed, or other protective mattress/pad for infants who do not tolerate frequent position changes
- Encourage parents to hold infant and participate in care to the extent possible
- Provide a consistent caregiver
- Observe for signs of pain and intervene aggressively to treat pain and/or remove painful stimuli (eg, medicate with analgesics before painful procedures)
- Space interventions/handling to allow infant to have uninterrupted sleep for 3 or 4 hours at a time
- Position infant in correct body alignment
- Provide boundaries (eg, swaddle, hold close) during all treatments/activities
- *(NIC) Environmental Management:*

    Avoid unnecessary exposure, drafts, overheating, or chilling.

    Control or prevent undesirable or excessive noise, when possible

    Reduce environmental stimuli, as appropriate [eg, speak in a soft tone at the bedside; limit conversation; open and close incubator slowly and quietly; do not tap on incubator; place rolled blankets near infant's head to absorb sound; cover incubator or warmer during sleep periods]

Infant Behavior, Disorganized, Risk for
(6.8.1) (1994)

Definition: Risk for alteration in integration and modulation of the physiologic and behavioral systems of functioning (ie, autonomic, motor, state, organizational, self-regulatory, and attention-interaction systems)

Risk Factors

Environmental overstimulation
Invasive/painful procedures
Lack of containment/boundaries
Oral/motor problems
Pain
Prematurity

Suggestions for Use

This diagnosis is most useful for infants, especially premature infants, in neonatal intensive care units. Immature neurologic development and increased or noxious environmental stimuli create the risk for a situation in which the infant must use energy for adaptation rather than for growth and development.

Suggested Alternative Diagnoses

Disorganized infant behavior
Development, risk for altered
Growth, risk for altered
Growth and development, altered
Organized infant behavior, potential for enhanced
Thermoregulation, ineffective

NOC Suggested Outcomes

Child Development: 2 Months, 4 Months, 6 Months, and 12 Months: Milestones of physical, cognitive, and psychosocial progression by 2 months, 4 months, 6 months, and 12 months of age. [**NOTE:** NOC lists a separate outcome for each age group.]
Comfort Level: Feelings of physical and psychologic ease
Neurologic Status: Extent to which the peripheral and central nervous systems receive, process, and respond to internal and external stimuli

Pain Level: Amount of reported or demonstrated pain

Sleep: Extent and pattern of sleep for mental and physical rejuvenation

Goals/Evaluation Criteria

Examples Using NOC Language

For **Thermoregulation** and **Neurological Status** indicators, refer to "Goals/Evaluation Criteria" for "Disorganized Infant Behavior," pp. 228–229

- Demonstrates **Pain Level**, as evidenced by the following indicators (specify 1–5: severe, substantial, moderate, slight, or none):

    Oral or facial expressions of pain

    Protective body positions

    Restlessness or muscle tension

    Change in heart rate or blood pressure

Other Examples

Refer to "Goals/Evaluation Criteria" for "Infant Behavior, Disorganized," pp. 228–229

Infant will:

- Receive sufficient and restful sleep

NIC Priority Interventions

Environmental Management: Manipulation of the patient's surroundings for therapeutic benefit

Newborn Monitoring: Measurement and interpretation of physiologic status of the neonate the first 24 hours after delivery

Nursing Activities

Refer to "Nursing Activities" for " Infant Behavior, Disorganized," p. 230

The following assessments should be performed the first 24 hours after delivery.

- *(NIC) Newborn Monitoring:*

    Temperature, until stabilized

    Respiratory rate and breathing pattern

    For respiratory distress, hypoglycemia, and anomalies, if mother has diabetes

    Newborn's color

    For signs of hyperbilirubinemia

    Infant's ability to suck

    Newborn's first feeding

Newborn's weight
Newborn's first voiding and bowel movement
Umbilical cord
Male newborn's response to circumcision

Infant Behavior: Organized, Potential for Enhanced (6.8.3) (1994)

Definition: A pattern of modulation of the physiologic and behavioral systems of functioning of an infant (ie, autonomic, motor, state, organizational, self-regulatory, and attentional-interactional systems) that is satisfactory but that can be improved, resulting in higher levels of integration in response to environmental stimuli

Defining Characteristics

Objective
Definite sleep-wake states
Response to visual/auditory stimuli
Stable physiologic measures
Use of some self-regulatory behaviors

Related Factors

Pain
Prematurity

Suggestions for Use

Because this is a wellness diagnosis, related factors are not needed in the diagnostic statement.

Suggested Alternative Diagnoses

Family coping: potential for growth
Infant behavior, disorganized, risk for

NOC Suggested Outcomes

Child Development: 2 Months, 4 Months, 6 Months, and 12 Months: Milestones of physical, cognitive, and psychosocial progression by 2 months, 4 months, 6 months, and 12 months of age. [**NOTE:** NOC lists a separate outcome for each age group.]

Neurological Status: Extent to which the peripheral and central nervous systems receive, process, and respond to internal and external stimuli

Sleep: Extent and pattern of sleep for mental and physical rejuvenation

Thermoregulation: Balance among heat production, heat gain, and heat loss

Thermoregulation: Neonate: Balance among heat production, heat gain, and heat loss during the neonatal period

Goals/Evaluation Criteria
Examples Using NOC Language

For **Neurological Status** indicators, see "Examples Using NOC Language" for "Infant Behavior, Disorganized," on pp. 228–229

- Demonstrates no delay from expected range of **Child Development** (2, 4, 6, and 12 months). [**NOTE:** Refer to pediatrics or child development text or *Nursing Outcomes Classification (NOC)* manual for specific examples of normal growth and development in each age group.]
- Demonstrates **Thermoregulation**, as evidenced by the following indicators (specify 1–5: extremely, substantially, moderately, mildly, or not compromised):
    Body temperature within normal limits
    Respiratory distress [not present]
    Restlessness or lethargy [not present]
    Skin color changes
    Nonshivering thermogenesis
    Use of heat-retention or heat-dissipation posture
    Weaning from crib to Isolette
    Blood glucose within normal limits

Other Examples
Infant will:
- Exhibit normal neurobehavioral functioning in all systems
- Demonstrate no maladaptive or abnormal compensatory behaviors
- Have normal pattern, amount, and quality of sleep
- Be wakeful at appropriate times

NIC Priority Interventions

Environmental Management: Attachment Process: Manipulation of the patient's surroundings to facilitate the development of the parent-infant relationship

Sleep Enhancement: Facilitation of regular sleep-wake cycles

Nursing Activities

Assessments

- Monitor infant's pattern and amount of sleep
- Assess ability to regulate all physical and behavioral systems (eg, cardiac, respiratory, sleep-wake states, reciprocal interactions, self-regulatory)

Patient/Family Teaching

- Teach family measures to promote sleep (eg, comforting behaviors, lifestyle changes, consistent schedules)
- Review the developmental needs of infants (eg, stimulation, sleep requirements)
- Help parents to identify the infant's signs of overstimulation and stress
- Role model and teach parents to provide age-appropriate auditory, visual, tactile, vestibular, and gustatory stimulation daily. Some examples are the following:

  Auditory: Classical music; high-pitched, melodic speaking
  Visual: Face-to-face positioning with eye contact; mobiles and toys in black, white, and red contrasting colors
  Tactile: Skin-to-skin contact; massage; firm, gentle touch
  Vestibular: Rocking
  Gustatory: Pacifier, sucking fingers (nonnutritive sucking)

- Explain that developmental stimulation should occur when infant is alert
- Teach parents to provide developmental stimulation frequently and for short periods rather than long periods
- Role model and teach parents to use gentle touch; a soft, melodic tone of voice; and mutual gazing
- Teach parents to respond to all of the infant's vocalizations

Collaborative Activities

- Schedule medications and treatments to support infant's sleep pattern
- *(NIC) Environmental Management: Attachment Process:* Develop policies that permit presence of significant others as much as desired

Other

- Adjust environment (eg, light, noise, temperature, mattress, and bed) to promote sleep

- Maintain infant's usual bedtime routines, (eg, rocking, pacifier)
- Use massage, positioning, and touch to relax infant and promote sleep
- Schedule treatments to minimize interference with infant's sleep (allow cycle of at least 90 minutes)
- Support the infant's self-regulatory behaviors (eg, hand-to-mouth movements, sucking on fingers, limb flexion) for coping with environmental stimuli
- *(NIC) Environmental Management: Attachment Process:*
  Limit number of people in delivery room
  Place infant bassinet at head of mother's bed
  Maintain warm body temperature of newborn
  Provide comfortable chair for father/significant other
  Provide sufficiently long tubing to allow freedom of movement, as appropriate
  Maintain consistency of staff assignment over time
  Maintain low level of stimuli in patient and family environment
  Explain options and then let family choose hospital environment and visitation plan that best meets their needs
  Permit father/significant other to sleep in room with mother
  Reduce interruptions by hospital personnel

Infant Feeding Pattern, Ineffective
(6.5.1.4) (1992)

Definition: A state in which an infant demonstrates an impaired ability to suck or coordinate the suck-swallow response

Defining Characteristics

Objective
Inability to coordinate sucking, swallowing, and breathing
Inability to initiate or sustain an effective suck

Related Factors

Anatomical abnormalities
Neurologic impairment/delay
Oral hypersensitivity
Prematurity
Prolonged NPO

Suggestions for Use

This label describes a baby with sucking or swallowing difficulties. It focuses on the nutritional needs of the infant. The goal of nursing activities is to prevent weight loss or promote weight gain. Use the defining characteristics in Table 3 on p. 42 to discriminate among this label and the suggested alternative diagnoses.

Suggested Alternative Diagnoses

Breastfeeding, ineffective
Breastfeeding, interrupted
Growth, risk for altered
Nutrition: less than body requirements, altered

NOC Suggested Outcomes

Breastfeeding Establishment: Infant: Proper attachment of an infant to and sucking from the mother's breast for nourishment during the first 2–3 weeks

Breastfeeding Maintenance: Continued nourishment of an infant through breastfeeding

Muscle Function: Adequacy of muscle contraction needed for movement

Nutritional Status: Food and Fluid Intake: Amount of food and fluid taken into the body over a 24-hour period

Goals/Evaluation Criteria

Examples Using NOC Language

- Demonstrates **Breastfeeding Establishment: Infant**, as evidenced by the following indicators (specify 1–5: not, slightly, moderately, substantially, or totally adequate):
  Proper alignment and latch-on response
  Proper areolar grasp and compression
  Correct suck and tongue placement
  Audible swallow
  Six or more urinations per day (after infant 2–3 days of age)
- Demonstrates **Breastfeeding Maintenance**, as evidenced by the following indicators (specify 1–5: not, slightly, moderately, substantially, or totally adequate):
  Infant's growth and development is in normal range
  Mother's freedom from breast tenderness

Other Examples

- Infant coordinates suck and swallow with respirations while maintaining heart rate and color
- Oral food and fluid intake are adequate

NIC Priority Interventions

Enteral Tube Feeding: Delivering nutrients and water through an intestinal tube

Lactation Counseling: Use of an interactive helping process to assist in maintenance of successful breastfeeding

Nonnutritive Sucking: Provision of sucking opportunities for infant who is gavage fed or who can receive nothing by mouth

Tube Care: Umbilical Line: Management of a newborn with an umbilical catheter

Nursing Activities

Assessments

- Assess infant's readiness for nipple feeding:

    Coordination of sucking, swallowing, and breathing (34 weeks)

    Presence of gag reflex (32 weeks)

    Presence of mature sucking reflex (32–34 weeks)

    Presence of rooting reflex (28–36 weeks)

- Assess daily whether the infant is ready to advance. Consider a feeding flow sheet to facilitate assessment; document infant's state, oxygen needs, preferred nipple, position, formula type/temperature, amount of feeding taken in first 10 minutes, total feeding, total feeding time, daily weight, and stool pattern

- At each feeding, assess infant's nipple feeding skills by evaluating if infant:

    Actively initiates swallow in coordination with suck

    Actively sucks liquid from bottle

    Completes feeding in acceptable time

    Coordinates sucking, swallowing, and breathing

    Loses minimal liquid from mouth

- At each feeding, assess respiratory function and behavioral state and monitor infant for problems such as regurgitation, abdominal distention, and increased residuals

- If infant must be tube fed:

    Monitor for proper placement of the tube (eg, check for gastric residual or follow appropriate protocol)

    Monitor for presence of bowel sounds

- *(NIC) Lactation Counseling:*
  Determine knowledge base about breastfeeding
  Determine mother's desire and motivation to breastfeed
  Evaluate mother's understanding of infant's feeding cues (eg, rooting, sucking, and alertness)
  Monitor maternal skill with latching infant to the nipple

Patient/Family Teaching

- Teach the following to increase success with nipple feeding:
  Avoid techniques that interrupt infant's learning by allowing passive flow of liquid without infant's active participation (eg, jiggling bottle, moving nipple up and down, moving nipple in and out of infant's mouth, moving infant's jaw up and down)
  Burp the infant frequently
  Choose the most appropriate nipple (consider size, shape, firmness, size of hole)
  Consider varying formula (eg, by thickness, taste, temperature)
  Calming the infant prior to feeding; during feeding, remove nipple at first sign of respiratory or state changes
  Feed the premature infant when fully alert and eager
  Overfill bottle above amount of scheduled feeding to make sucking easier and to minimize sucking of air
  Position the infant in a semiupright position with head slightly forward and chin tilting down
  Provide consistent caregivers to better read infant's cues and facilitate infant learning; involve mother at earliest opportunity
  Remain relaxed and patient during feeding, allow brief rest periods, pace the infant to complete feeding in appropriate time (too quickly may compromise safety, too slowly may increase fatigue and calorie expenditure)
  Use facilitation techniques (eg, prior to feeding, increase oral sensitivity by stroking the infant's lips, cheeks, and tongue; during feeding, place your fingers on each cheek and under the jaw midway between the chin and throat to provide inward and forward support of the cheeks and tongue)
- If infant must be tube fed, inform parents on importance of meeting infant sucking needs
- *(NIC) Lactation Counseling:*
  Demonstrate suck training, as appropriate
  Instruct about infant stool and urination patterns, as appropriate
  Instruct on signs of problems to report to health care practitioner

Collaborative Activities

- Establish support network to ensure that mother has help with day-to-day lactation/breastfeeding problems as they occur
- Refer to a lactation specialist or breastfeeding support group, as needed
- Refer to a physical or occupational therapist any infant who is not progressing with feeding or has structural or oral motor defects
- If infant cannot maintain oral nutrition, provide enteral tube feedings, according to protocol
- Consult with physician/nutritionist regarding type and strength of enteral feeding

Other

- Arrange for home visit within 72 hours of discharge
- Determine most appropriate feeding method (eg, nipple feeding; intermittent gavage; continuous feeding with nasogastric (NG) tube, jejunal tube, or gastrostomy)
- If infant must be tube fed:
    Elevate head of the bed or hold infant during feedings
    Offer pacifier to infant during feeding
    Talk to infant during feeding
    Perform daily skin care around feeding device. Keep feeding site dry.
    Change feeding containers and tubing every 24 hours.

Infection, Risk for
(1.2.1.1) (1986)

Definition: The state in which an individual is at increased risk for being invaded by pathogenic organisms

Risk Factors

Chronic disease
Immunosuppression
Inadequate acquired immunity
Inadequate primary defenses (eg, broken skin, traumatized tissue, decrease in ciliary action, stasis of body fluids, change in pH secretions, altered peristalsis)
Inadequate secondary defenses (eg, decreased hemoglobin, leukopenia, suppressed inflammatory response)

Insufficient knowledge to avoid exposure to pathogens
Invasive procedures
Malnutrition
Pharmaceutical agents
Rupture of amniotic membranes
Tissue destruction and increased environmental exposure
Trauma

Suggestions for Use

Do not use this label routinely for patients with surgical incisions. For the common surgical population, maintaining routine standards of care will prevent incision infection. Likewise, do not use *Risk for infection* routinely for patients who have an indwelling catheter. Aseptic technique is expected. Everyone is, in a sense, at risk for infection. Therefore, use this nursing diagnosis only for those patients who are at higher than "usual" risk—for example, those with nutritional deficits or compromised immune systems. For patients with actual infection, use a collaborative problem (eg, Potential Complication: Sepsis).

Suggested Alternative Diagnoses

Injury, risk for
Nutrition: less than body requirements, altered
Protection, altered
Skin integrity, impaired

NOC Suggested Outcomes

Immune Status: Adequacy of natural and acquired appropriately targeted resistance to internal and external antigens
Knowledge: Infection Control: Extent of understanding conveyed about prevention and control of infection
Risk Control: Actions to eliminate or reduce actual, personal, and modifiable health threats
Risk Detection: Actions taken to identify personal health threats
Goals/Evaluation Criteria

Examples Using NOC Language

- Risk factors for infection will be eliminated as evidenced by adequacy of patient's Immune Status, substantial Knowledge: Infection Control, and consistently demonstrated Risk Detection and Risk Control behaviors

- Patient will demonstrate **Risk Control**, as evidenced by the following indicators (specify 1–5: never, rarely, sometimes, often, or consistently demonstrated):

  Obtains appropriate immunizations

  Monitors environmental and personal behavior risk factors

  Avoids exposure to health threats

  Modifies lifestyle to reduce risk

Other Examples

Patient/family will:
- Be free of signs and symptoms of infection
- Demonstrate adequate personal hygiene
- Indicate gastrointestinal, respiratory, genitourinary, and immune status within normal limits
- Describe factors contributing to infection transmission
- Report signs and symptoms of infection and follow screening and monitoring procedures

NIC Priority Interventions

Immunization/Vaccination Administration: Provision of immunizations for prevention of communicable disease

Infection Control: Minimizing the acquisition and transmission of infectious agents

Infection Protection: Prevention and early detection of infection in a patient at risk

Nursing Activities

Assessments

- Monitor for signs/symptoms of infection (eg, temperature, pulse rate, drainage, appearance of wound, secretions, appearance of urine, skin temperature, skin lesions, fatigue, malaise)
- Assess for factors that increase vulnerability to infection (eg, advanced age, immunocompromise, malnutrition)
- Monitor laboratory values (eg, CBC, absolute granulocyte count, differential results, cultures, serum protein, and albumin)
- Observe performance of personal hygiene practices to protect against infection

Patient/Family Teaching

- Explain to patient/family why illness and/or therapy increases the risk for infection
- Instruct in performance of personal hygiene practices to protect against infection
- Teach parents recommended immunization schedule for diphtheria, tetanus, pertussis, polio, measles, mumps, and rubella)
- Explain rationale/benefits for and side effects of immunizations
- Provide patient/family a method for keeping a record of immunizations (eg, form, diary)
- Teach safe methods of food handling/preparation/storage
- *(NIC) Infection Control:*

  Instruct patient on appropriate hand-washing techniques

  Instruct visitors to wash hands on entering and leaving the patient's room

  Teach patient and family about signs and symptoms of infection and when to report them to the health care provider

Collaborative Activities

- Refer patient/family to social services and/or community resources to assist in managing home, hygiene, and nutrition
- Follow agency protocol for reporting suspected infections and/or positive cultures
- Refer to social services for help in paying for immunizations (eg, insurance coverage and health department clinics)
- *(NIC) Infection Control:* Administer antibiotic therapy, as appropriate

Other

- Help patient/family identify factors in their environment, lifestyle, or health practices that increase risk of infection
- Protect patient from cross-contamination by not assigning same nurse to another patient with an infection and not rooming patient with an infected patient
- *(NIC) Infection Control:*

  Clean the environment appropriately after each patient use

  Maintain isolation techniques, as appropriate

  Institute universal precautions

  Limit the number of visitors, as appropriate

Injury, Risk for
(1.6.1) (1978)

Definition: A state in which the individual is at risk of injury as a result of environmental conditions interacting with the individual's adaptive and defensive resources.

Risk Factors

Internal

Abnormal blood profile (eg, leukocytosis or leukopenia)
Altered clotting factors
Biochemical/regulatory function (eg, sensory dysfunction)
Decreased hemoglobin
Developmental age (physiological, psychosocial)
Effector dysfunction
Immune/autoimmune disorder
Integrative dysfunction
Malnutrition
Physical (eg, broken skin, altered mobility)
Psychologic (affective orientation)
Sickle cells
Thalassemia
Thrombocytopenia
Tissue hypoxia

External

Biological
Immunization level of community
Microorganisms

Chemical
Drugs (eg, pharmaceutical agents, alcohol, caffeine, nicotine, preservatives, cosmetics, and dyes)
Nutrients (eg, vitamins, food types)
Poisons
Pollutants

Physical
Design, structure, and arrangement of community, building, or equipment
Mode of transport or transportation
People/provider (nosocomial agents; staffing patterns; cognitive, affective, and psychomotor patterns)

Suggestions for Use

This is a broad label that includes internal risk factors such as altered clotting factors and decreased hemoglobin. It is important to identify only those patients who are at unusually high risk for this problem. Everyone has at least some risk for accidents and injury, but the label should be used only for those who require nursing intervention to prevent injury. **NOTE:** It may be useful to use the label *Sensory/perceptual alterations* as an etiology for *Risk for injury.*

This label consists of seven subcategories that describe *injury* more specifically: *Latex allergy response; Risk for latex allergy response;* and *Risk for suffocation, poisoning, trauma, aspiration, and disuse syndrome.* When possible, use these more specific labels instead of *Risk for injury* because they provide clearer direction for nursing care. They need no further specification except for *Risk for trauma,* which includes wounds, burns, and fractures, as well as many other risk factors.

Some nurses use the label *Risk for injury* to describe the potential for such conditions as malignant hyperthermia. It is also sometimes used as a general description for the potential for fetal distress that exists during labor. Those conditions are more usefully described as collaborative problems; however, for nurses who do not use collaborative problems, this text includes goals and nursing interventions for those situations.

Suggested Alternative Diagnoses

Aspiration, risk for
Home maintenance management, impaired
Infection, risk for
Latex allergy response
Latex allergy response, risk for
Poisoning, risk for
Protection, altered
Sensory/perceptual alterations (visual, auditory, kinesthetic, gustatory, tactile, olfactory)
Suffocation, risk for
Thought processes, altered
Trauma, risk for
Violence: self-directed, risk for

NOC Suggested Outcomes

Parenting: Social Safety: Parental actions to avoid social relationships that might cause harm or injury

Risk Control: Actions to eliminate or reduce actual, personal, and modifiable health threats

Safety Behavior: Fall Prevention: Individual or caregiver actions to minimize risk factors that might precipitate falls

Goals/Evaluation Criteria

Examples Using NOC Language

- *Risk for injury* will be decreased, as evidenced by Parenting: Social Safety and Safety Behavior: Fall Prevention.
- **Risk Control** will be demonstrated, as evidenced by the following indicators (specify 1–5: never, rarely, sometimes, often, or consistently demonstrated):

   Monitors environmental and personal behavior risk factors
   Develops and follows selected risk control strategies
   Modifies lifestyle to reduce risk

Other Examples

   Patient/family will:

- Provide a safe environment (eg, eliminate clutter and spills, place handrails, and use rubber shower mats and grab bars)
- Identify risks that increase susceptibility to injury
- Avoid physical injury

   Parents will:

- Recognize risk of and monitor for abuse
- Screen playmates, caregivers, and other social contacts
- Recognize signs of gang membership and other high-risk social behaviors

NIC Priority Interventions

Electronic Fetal Monitoring: Intrapartum: Electronic evaluation of fetal heart-rate response to uterine contractions during intrapartal care

Fall Prevention: Instituting special precautions with patient at risk for injury from falling

Labor Induction: Initiation or augmentation of labor by mechanical or pharmacological methods

Latex Precautions: Reducing the risk of a systemic reaction to latex. [**NOTE:** Although this is listed as a priority intervention, no nursing activities will be listed for it. If the patient requires Latex Precautions, use a diagnosis of *Risk for* or actual *Latex allergy response* rather than *Risk for injury*.]

Malignant Hyperthermia Precautions: Prevention or reduction of a hypermetabolic response to pharmacologic agents used during surgery. [**NOTE:** Although NIC lists this as a priority intervention, no nursing activities are provided for it here. If the patient requires Malignant Hyperthermia Precautions, use a nursing diagnosis of *Risk for hyperthermia* instead of *Risk for injury.*]

Nursing Activities

Because this diagnostic label is so broad, nursing activities vary greatly depending on the problem etiology. It is not possible to anticipate every possible nursing activity that might be used for this diagnosis.

Assessments

- Identify factors that affect safety needs, eg: changes in mental status, degree of intoxication, fatigue, maturational age, medications, and motor and/or sensory deficit (eg, with gait, balance)
- Identify environmental factors that create risk for falls (eg, slippery floors, throw rugs, open stairways, windows, swimming pools)
- Check patient for presence of constrictive clothing, cuts, burns, or bruises
- *(NIC) Electronic Fetal Monitoring: Intrapartum:*
  Institute electronic fetal monitoring during intrapartal care, according to agency protocols
  Review obstetrical history for pertinent information that may influence induction, such as gestational age and length of prior labor and such contraindications as complete placenta previa, classical uterine incision, and pelvic structural deformities

Patient/Family Teaching

- Instruct patient/family in techniques to prevent injury at home. Specify techniques.
- Instruct patient to use caution in use of heat-therapy devices
- Provide educational materials related to strategies and measures to prevent injury
- Provide information on environmental hazards and characteristics (eg, stairs, windows, cupboard locks, swimming pools, streets, gates)

- *(NIC) Electronic Fetal Monitoring: Intrapartum:*

    Instruct woman and support person(s) about the reason for electronic monitoring, as well as information to be obtained

    Discuss appearance of rhythm strip with mother and support person

Collaborative Activities

- Refer to educational classes in the community
- *(NIC) Electronic Fetal Monitoring: Intrapartum:*

    Keep physician informed of pertinent changes in the fetal heart rate, interventions for nonreassuring patterns, subsequent fetal response, labor progress, and maternal response to labor

    Assist with procedures to induce labor, if indicated, according to agency protocols and procedures

Other

For adults:

- Reorient patient to reality and immediate environment when necessary
- Assist patient with ambulation, as needed
- Provide assistive devices for walking (eg, cane, walker)
- Use heating devices with caution to prevent burns in patients with sensory deficit
- Use an alarm to alert caretaker when patient is getting out of bed or leaving room
- If necessary, use physical restraints to limit risk of falling
- Place bell or call light with in reach of dependent patient at all times
- Instruct patient to call for assistance with movement, as appropriate
- Remove environmental hazards (eg, provide adequate lighting)
- Make no unnecessary changes in physical environment (eg, furniture placement)
- Ensure that patient wears proper shoes (eg, nonskid soles, secure fasteners)

    For children:

- Raise side rails when not present at bedside
- For children old enough to climb over bed rails, use a crib with a net or "bubble top"
- *(NIC) Electronic Fetal Monitoring: Intrapartum:* Calibrate equipment, as appropriate, for internal monitoring with a spiral electrode and/or intrauterine pressure catheter

Knowledge Deficit (specify)
(8.1.1) (1980)

Definition: Absence or deficiency of cognitive information related to specific topic

Defining Characteristics

Subjective
Verbalization of the problem
Objective
Inaccurate follow-through of instruction
Inaccurate performance on tests
Inappropriate or exaggerated behaviors (eg, hysteria, hostility, agitation, or apathy)

Related Factors

Cognitive limitation
Information misinterpretation
Lack of exposure
Lack of interest in learning
Lack of recall
Unfamiliarity with information resources

Suggestions for Use

Knowledge deficit is not recommended as a problem label for the following reasons:

- *Knowledge deficit* is not truly a human response. "Response" suggests a behavior or action; *Knowledge deficit* is simply a state of being.
- *Knowledge deficit* does not necessarily describe a health state.
- *Knowledge deficit* does not necessarily describe a *problem*. Nursing diagnoses should reflect altered functioning; but *Knowledge deficit* simply means the person lacks some knowledge, not that her/his functioning is changed as a result of that lack of knowledge.

Knowledge deficit can contribute to a number of problem responses, including *Anxiety, Altered parenting, Self-care deficit,* or *Ineffective coping.* Therefore, it may be used effectively as the etiology of a nursing diagnosis (eg, *Risk for injury (trauma) related to lack of knowledge of proper application of seat belts when pregnant* or *Anxiety related to lack of knowledge of procedures involved in bone marrow aspiration*).

If *Knowledge deficit* is used as the problem part of a nursing diagnosis, one goal must be "Patient will acquire knowledge about...." This causes the nurse to focus on giving information rather than focusing on the behaviors caused by the patient's lack of knowledge, reinforcing the belief that giving information will change behavior and solve problems. On the other hand, when *Knowledge deficit* is used as an etiology, it focuses attention on behaviors that indicate self-doubt, decisional conflict, anxiety, and so on. Note the difference in nursing care suggested by the following diagnostic statements:

Knowledge deficit (bone marrow aspiration) related to lack of prior experience

Anxiety related to knowledge deficit (bone marrow aspiration)

Patient teaching is an important intervention for most patients and for all nursing diagnoses (eg, *Constipation, Ineffective breast-feeding*). Therefore, it is not necessary, or even desirable, to have a *Knowledge deficit* diagnosis on every patient's care plan. Nurses should include teaching as one of the nursing interventions for all the other diagnoses that they make.

Some patients, such as a newly diagnosed diabetic, require a great deal of teaching in order to acquire necessary self-care skills. Such *special* teaching plans should be a part of the routine care on standardized care plans for these patients and should not require an individualized nursing diagnosis. However, if the agency does not have a standardized plan or protocol, it will be necessary to write an individualized teaching plan. Even then, *Knowledge deficit* should be used as the etiology of a response, for example, *Risk for altered health maintenance (diabetes management) related to knowledge deficit (medication, diet, exercise, and skin care) secondary to new diagnosis.*

If used at all, *Knowledge deficit* should describe conditions in which the patient needs new or additional knowledge. It should not be used for problems involving the patient's *ability* to learn (eg, *Knowledge deficit related to severe anxiety about outcome of surgery*). Rakel and Bulechek (1990) propose a diagnosis of *Situational learning disability: Impaired ability to learn* or *Situational learning disability: Lack of motivation to learn* for such conditions. However, these are not yet NANDA labels.

At least two studies have shown that *Knowledge deficit* is one of the diagnoses most frequently used (misused) by nurses (Gordon

1985; Lambert and Jones 1989). This may be due in part to premature diagnosing: it is easy to recognize a knowledge deficit, label it as a problem, and not look beyond that to the *human response* to the lack of knowledge. Misuse of this diagnosis also occurs because of the mistaken belief that information giving effectively changes human behavior.

Suggested Alternative Diagnoses

Adjustment, impaired
Individual coping, ineffective
Denial, ineffective
Health maintenance, altered
Home maintenance management, impaired
Management of therapeutic regimen: community/family/individual, ineffective
Noncompliance (specify)

NOC Suggested Outcomes

Knowledge: [specify]: Extent of understanding conveyed about, [eg,] Breastfeeding.

[**NOTE:** NOC has 14 Knowledge outcomes: Breastfeeding, Child Safety, Diet, Disease Process, Energy Conservation, Health Behaviors, Health Resources, Infection Control, Medication, Personal Safety, Prescribed Activity, Substance Use Control, Treatment Procedure(s), and Treatment Regimen. Conceivably, any subject or outcome could be placed after the NOC "Knowledge:" outcome.]

Goals/Evaluation Criteria

Examples Using NOC Language

- Demonstrates **Knowledge: Diet**, as evidenced by the following indicators (specify 1–5: none, limited, moderate, substantial, or extensive):

    Description of recommended diet
    Explanation of rationale for recommended diet
    Selection of foods recommended in diet
    Development of strategies to change dietary habits
    Performance of self-monitoring activities

Other Examples

Patient/family will:
- Identify need for additional information regarding prescribed treatment (eg, diet information about)

• Demonstrate ability to _____ (specify skill or behavior)

NIC Priority Interventions

Health System Guidance: Facilitating a patient's location and use of appropriate health services

Teaching, Disease Process: Assisting the patient to understand information related to a specific disease process

Teaching, Individual: Planning, implementing, and evaluating a teaching program designed to address a patient's particular needs

Teaching, Infant Care: Instructs the patient on nurturing and physical care needed during the first year of life

Teaching, Preoperative: Assisting a patient to understand and mentally prepare for surgery and the postoperative recovery period

Teaching, Prescribed Activity/Exercise: Preparing a patient to achieve and/or maintain a prescribed level of activity

Teaching, Prescribed Diet: Preparing a patient to correctly follow a prescribed diet

Teaching, Prescribed Medication: Preparing a patient to safely take prescribed medications and monitor their effects

Teaching, Procedure/Treatment: Preparing a patient to understand and mentally prepare for a prescribed procedure or treatment

Teaching, Psychomotor Skill: Preparing a patient to perform a psychomotor skill

Teaching, Safe Sex: Providing instruction concerning sexual protection during sexual activity

Teaching, Sexuality: Assisting individuals to understand physical and psychosocial dimensions of sexual growth and development

Nursing Activities

NOTE: Because *Knowledge deficit* is such a broad label, this text provides only general activities. Refer to the *Nursing Interventions Classification (NIC)* manual for nursing activities associated with a specific intervention, such as Teaching Safe Sex or Teaching Psychomotor Skill.

Assessments

• Check for accurate feedback to ensure that patient understands prescribed treatment and other relevant information

- *(NIC) Teaching: Individual:*

  Determine patient's learning needs

  Appraise the patient's current level of knowledge and understanding of content [eg, knowledge of prescribed procedure/treatment]

  Determine the patient's ability to learn specific information (eg, developmental level, physiologic status, orientation, pain, fatigue, unfulfilled basic needs, emotional state, and adaptation to illness)

  Determine the patient's motivation to learn specific information (ie, health beliefs, past noncompliance, bad experiences with health care/learning, and conflicting goals)

  Appraise the patient's learning style

Patient/Family Teaching

- Provide teaching at patient's level of understanding, repeating information as necessary
- Use multiple teaching approaches, return demonstrations, and verbal and written feedback.
- *(NIC) Teaching: Individual:*

  Establish rapport

  Establish teacher credibility, as appropriate

  Set mutual, realistic learning goals with the patient

  Provide an environment conducive to learning

  Select appropriate teaching methods/strategies

  Select appropriate educational materials

  Reinforce behavior, as appropriate

  Provide time for the patient to ask questions and discuss concerns

  Document on the permanent medical record the content presented, the written materials provided, and the patient's understanding of the information or patient behaviors that indicate learning

  Include the family/significant others, as appropriate

Collaborative Activities

- Provide information on community resources that will help the patient maintain his/her treatment regimen
- Develop a coordinated multidisciplinary teaching plan. Specify plan.
- Plan with patient and physician adjustment in treatment to facilitate patient's ability to follow prescribed treatment

Other
- Interact with patient in a nonjudgmental manner to facilitate learning

Latex Allergy Response
(1.6.1.6) (1998)

Definition: An allergic response to natural latex rubber products

Defining Characteristics

Type I Reactions: Immediate. Abdominal pain; contact urticaria to generalized symptoms; edema of sclera or eyelids; edema of the lips, tongue, uvula, and/or throat; erythema of the eyes; facial edema; facial erythema; facial itching; flushing; general discomfort; generalized edema; hypotension, syncope, cardiac arrest; immediate, <1 hour, reactions to latex proteins (can be life threatening); increasing complaint of total body warmth; itching of the eyes; nasal congestion; nasal erythema; nasal itching; nausea; oral itching; respiratory arrest; restlessness; rhinorrhea; shortness of breath, tightness in chest; tearing of the eyes; wheezing, bronchospasm

Type IV Reactions: Delayed onset (hours), eczema, irritation, reaction to additives causes discomfort (eg, thirams, carbamates), redness

Irritant Reactions: Blisters, chapped or cracked skin, erythema

Related Factors

No immune mechanism response

Suggestions for Use

For situations that frequently cause sensitization allergy to latex, see "Risk Factors" for "Latex Allergy Response, Risk for" on pp. 256–257. For both diagnoses, nursing care would focus on avoiding exposure to latex. When an actual allergic reaction occurs, the dermatitis must be treated medically and the nursing diagnoses of *Impaired skin integrity* and *Risk for infection* may be used.

Suggested Alternative Diagnoses

Body image disturbance
Infection, risk for
Latex allergy response, risk for

Skin integrity, impaired

NOC Suggested Outcomes

To be developed

Goals/Evaluation Criteria

The patient will:
- Regain skin integrity, as evidenced by good hydration; reduced inflammation, scaling, and flaking; decreased inflammation; and verbalizations of reduced itching
- Experience restful sleep
- Not experience respiratory complications (eg, asthma)
- Exhibit a positive self-concept, as evidenced by expressed feelings of self-worth and satisfaction with interpersonal interactions
- Not experience recurrence of the allergic response to latex

NIC Priority Interventions

Not yet published. The following seems logical:

Latex Precautions: Reducing the risk of a systemic reaction to latex

Nursing Activities

Assessments

- Identify source(s) of latex to which the patient was (or might be) exposed
- Assess skin for signs of healing (eg, decreased redness, flaking and scaling)
- Assess comfort level
- Assess sleep/rest pattern
- Observe for signs of *Body image disturbance* or *Social isolation*
- Observe for development of asthmatic response (eg, wheezing, dyspnea)
- *(NIC) Latex Precautions:*
  Monitor latex-free environment
  Monitor patient for signs and symptoms of a systemic reaction

Patient/Family Teaching

- Explain the relationship between skin dryness, the symptom of itching, and the prescribed therapy (ie, hydration)
- Explain that scratching will only produce more itching
- Suggest that the client wear loose-fitting, open-weave, cotton clothing and avoid rough or tightly woven fabrics
- Explain that keeping the home and work environments at a con-

stant temperature (68°F to 75°F) and humidity (about 50 percent) will help decrease itching
- Advise against self-treating with leftover medication at home
- Explain that the skin lesions are not contagious (unless they are infected)
- Teach to bathe daily for 15 to 20 minutes and apply emollient or prescribed medication within 4 minutes after the bath
- Teach to use warm, not hot, water for bathing
- *(NIC) Latex Precautions:*
  Instruct patient and family about latex content in products and substitution with nonlatex products, as appropriate; wearing a medical alert tag; and notifying care providers
  Instruct patient and family about signs of a reaction
  Instruct patient and family about emergency treatment
  Instruct visitors about latex-free environment

Collaborative Activities
- *(NIC) Latex Precautions:* Report information to physician, pharmacist, and other care providers, as indicated

Other
- Encourage client to maintain existing social activities
- Provide alternatives for supplies/ equipment containing latex (eg, condoms, balloons, gloves, urinary/intravenous catheters)
- *(NIC) Latex Precautions:*
  Place allergy band on patient
  Post sign indicating latex precautions
  Survey environment and remove latex products

Latex Allergy Response, Risk for
(1.6.1.7) (1998)

Definition: At risk for allergic response to natural latex rubber products

Risk Factors
Allergies to bananas, avocados, tropical fruits, kiwis, and chestnuts
Allergies to poinsettia plants
Conditions needing continuous or intermittent catheterization
History of allergies and asthma

History of reactions to latex (eg, balloons, condoms, gloves)

Multiple surgical procedures, especially from infancy (eg, spina bifida)

Professions with daily exposure to latex (eg, medicine, nursing, dentistry)

Suggestions for Use

This label may be more useful than actual *Latex allergy response*. See "Suggestions for Use"on page 254.

Suggested Alternative Diagnoses

Body image disturbance

Infection, risk for

Skin integrity, impaired

NOC Suggested Outcomes

To be developed

Goals/Evaluation Criteria

The patient will:

• Not experience allergic reaction to latex (eg, no skin lesions or symptoms)

• Identify and avoid environmental sources of latex

NIC Priority Interventions

NIC priority interventions have not yet been published. However, the following seems to be a logical choice:

Latex Precautions: Reducing the risk of a systemic reaction to latex

Nursing Activities

Also see "Nursing Activities" for "Latex Allergy Response," on pp. 255–256

Assessments

• Identify source(s) of latex to which the patient is (or may be) exposed—both at work and at home

• Assess patient/family knowledge of sources of latex

• Assess knowledge of sensitization and allergic reactions

• *(NIC) Latex Precautions:*

Question patient or appropriate other about history of neural tube defect (eg, spina bifida) or congenital urological condition (eg, exstrophy of the bladder)

Question patient or appropriate other about history of systemic reactions to natural rubber latex (eg, facial or scleral edema, tearing eyes, urticaria, rhinitis, and wheezing)

Patient/Family Teaching

- Teach information about sensitization and allergic reactions, as needed
- Advise against self-treating if allergic reaction is suspected
- *(NIC) Latex Precautions:* Instruct patient and family about risk factors for developing a latex allergy

Collaborative Activities

- Help develop agency and organizational policies to decrease worker exposure to latex products
- *(NIC) Latex Precautions:* Refer patient to allergist for allergy testing, as appropriate

Other

- For clients with risk factors (eg, allergy to bananas, history of asthma), provide alternatives (or sources for alternatives) for supplies/equipment containing latex (eg, condoms, balloons, gloves, urinary catheters, intravenous catheters)

Loneliness, Risk for
(3.1.3) (1994)

Definition: A subjective state in which an individual is at risk of experiencing vague dysphoria

Risk Factors

Affectional deprivation [eg, death of a spouse]
Cathectic deprivation [eg, no one to talk to]
Physical isolation [eg, isolation because of infectious disease]
Social isolation [eg, shunning by peer group]

Suggestions for Use

Discriminate between this diagnosis and *Social isolation*. *Social isolation* is objective (perceived by others); *Loneliness* is subjective (an inner feeling state). *Social isolation* may be the risk factor or etiology of *Loneliness*. *Loneliness* better describes the feeling response brought about solitude that is not desired by the person.

For *Loneliness* that is brought about by physical disability or disfigurement, see *Body image disturbance*.

Suggested Alternative Diagnoses

Body image disturbance
Grieving, dysfunctional
Relocation stress syndrome
Social interaction, impaired
Social isolation

NOC Suggested Outcomes

Grief Resolution: Adjustment to actual or impending loss
Social Interaction Skills: An individual's use of effective interaction behaviors
Social Involvement: Frequency of an individual's social interactions with persons, groups, or organizations
Social Support: Perceived availability and actual provision of reliable assistance from other persons

Goals/Evaluation Criteria

Examples Using NOC Language

- Demonstrates resolution of *Loneliness*, as evidenced by Grief Resolution, Social Interaction Skills, and Social Support
- Demonstrates **Social Involvement**, as evidenced by the following indicators (specify 1–5: none, limited, moderate, substantial, or extensive):
    Interaction with close friends, neighbors, family members, and/or members of work group(s)
    Participation as a member of a church, club, or volunteer group
    Participation in leisure activities

Other Examples

Patient will:
- Use time alone in a positive way when socialization is not possible
- Identify reasons for feelings of loneliness
- Describe a plan for increasing meaningful relationships
- Use effective interpersonal communication skills (eg: self-disclosure, cooperation, sensitivity, assertiveness, consideration, genuineness, trust, and compromise). Specify skills most relevant to patient

- Verbalize adequacy of social supports (eg, assistance provided by others)
- Indicate willingness to ask others for help
- Effectively accomplish grief work (eg, express feelings, verbalize acceptance of loss)

NIC Priority Interventions

Family Integrity Promotion: Promotion of family cohesion and unity

Socialization Enhancement: Facilitation of another person's ability to interact with others

Visitation Facilitation: Promoting beneficial visits by family and friends

Nursing Activities

Assessments

- Assess the patient's perceived and actual support systems
- Determine risk factors for loneliness (eg, lack of energy needed for social interaction, poor communication skills)
- Compare client's desire for visitation/social interaction to actual visitation/social interaction
- Monitor patient's response to visits from family and friends
- *(NIC) Family Integrity Promotion*
  Determine typical family relationships
  Monitor current family relationships

Patient/Family Teaching

- Teach social skills, as needed (eg, role model self-disclosure)
- Teach patient to monitor own behaviors that contribute to social isolation

Collaborative Activities

- Refer patient to group or program for increased understanding and practice of communication and interaction skills
- *(NIC) Family Integrity Promotion:*
  Refer family to support group of other families dealing with similar problems
  Refer for family therapy, as indicated

Other

- Encourage patient to talk about feelings of loneliness
- Assist patient to discover new interests
- Role-play communication skills and techniques with patient
- Help patient identify strengths and limitations in communicating

- Give positive feedback when patient uses effective social interaction skills
- Help patient to recognize available social supports
- Encourage patient to reach out to others who have similar interests
- Facilitate family visitation
- *(NIC) Family Integrity Promotion:*
  Assist family to maintain positive relationships
  Provide for care of patient by family members, as appropriate
  Encourage patient to develop closeness in one existing relationship

Management of Therapeutic Regimen: Community, Ineffective (5.2.3) (1994)

Definition: A pattern of regulating and integrating into community processes programs for treatment of illness and the sequelae of illness that are unsatisfactory for meeting health-related goals

Defining Characteristics

Deficits in people and programs to be accountable for illness care of aggregates

Deficits in advocates for aggregates

Deficits in community activities for secondary and tertiary prevention

Illness symptoms above the norm expected for the number and type of population

Number of health care resources are insufficient for the incidence or prevalence of illness(es)

Unavailable health care resources for illness care

Unexpected acceleration of illness(es)

Related Factors

To be developed by NANDA

Related Factors (Non-NANDA)

Lack of community programs for disease prevention, smoking cessation, alcohol abuse, and so forth

Complex population needs

Ineffective communication among subgroups and community

Failure of society to value the community and subgroups
Failure of community/subgroups to value self
Government policies

Also see "Defining Characteristics" for "Management of Therapeutic Regimen: Community, Ineffective," p. 261

Suggestions for Use

This diagnosis is appropriate for a community in which one or more groups are underserved—perhaps because of insufficient resources, ineffective management of available resources, exposure to risk factors such as toxic chemicals, and so forth. This diagnosis is more narrowly focused on health care delivery than is *Ineffective community coping*, which describes the general adaptation and problem-solving processes of the community.

Suggested Alternative Diagnoses

Community coping, ineffective

NOC Suggested Outcomes

Not yet developed

Goals/Evaluation Criteria

The community will:
- Identify needed resources
- Budget resources for illness prevention and care
- Identify factors affecting the community's ability to meet health care needs of specific aggregates
- Obtain advocates who are accountable for health care of specific aggregates
- Develop plans for prevention and treatment of illnesses
- Experience a trend in illness symptoms toward the norm for that illness

NIC Priority Interventions

Environmental Management: Community: Monitoring and influencing of the physical, social, cultural, economic, and political conditions that affect the health of groups and communities

Health Policy Monitoring: Surveillance and influence of government and organization regulations, rules, and standards that affect nursing systems and practices to ensure quality care of patients

Nursing Activities

Assessments

- *(NIC) Environmental Management: Community:*
  Initiate screening for health risks from the environment
  Monitor status of known health risks
- *(NIC) Health Policy Monitoring:* Assess implications and requirements of proposed policies and standards for quality patient care

Teaching

- *(NIC) Environmental Management: Community:* Conduct educational programs for targeted risk groups
- *(NIC) Health Policy Monitoring:* Acquaint policy makers with implications of current and proposed policies and standards for patient welfare

Collaborative Activities

- *(NIC) Environmental Management: Community:*
  Participate in multidisciplinary teams to identify threats to safety in the community
  Collaborate in the development of community action programs
  Coordinate services to at-risk groups and communities
  Work with environmental groups to secure appropriate governmental regulations

Other

- *(NIC) Health Policy Monitoring:*
  Review proposed policies and standards in organizational, professional, and governmental literature and in the popular media
  Promote governmental policy to reduce specified risks
  Identify and resolve discrepancies between health policies and standards and current nursing practice
  Lobby policy makers to make changes in health policies and standards to benefit patients
  Testify in organization, profession, and public forums to influence the formulation of health policies and standards that benefit patients
  Assist consumers of health care to be informed of current and proposed changes in health policies and standards and the implications for health outcomes
- *(NIC) Environmental Management: Community:* Encourage neighborhoods to become active participants in community safety

Management of Therapeutic Regimen: Families, Ineffective (5.2.2) (1994)

Definition: A pattern of regulating and integrating into family processes a program for treatment of illness and the sequelae of illness that are unsatisfactory for meeting specific health goals

Defining Characteristics

Subjective

Verbalized desire to manage the treatment of illnesses and prevention of the sequelae

Verbalized difficulty with regulation/integration of one or more effects or prevention of complications

Verbalizes that family did not take action to reduce risk factors for progression of illness and sequelae

Objective

Acceleration [expected or unexpected] of illness symptoms of a family member

Inappropriate family activities for meeting the goals of a treatment or prevention program

Lack of attention to illness and its sequelae

Related Factors

Complexity of health care system

Complexity of therapeutic regimen

Decisional conflicts

Economic difficulties

Excessive demands made on individual or family

Family conflict

Suggestions for Use

Use this diagnosis for families who are motivated to follow a therapeutic regimen but who are having difficulty doing so. It is not appropriate for families who are not interested in adhering to the treatment program. This diagnosis is more narrowly focused than *Altered family processes* or *Ineffective family coping*, both of which include problems other than managing the patien's family's treatment program. It is difficult to differentiate this label from *Ineffective individual management of therapeutic regimen* because individuals typically are a part of a family.

Suggested Alternative Diagnoses

Coping: family, ineffective, disabling
Family processes, altered
Health maintenance, altered
Management of therapeutic regimen: individual, ineffective

NOC Suggested Outcomes

Not yet developed

Goals/Evaluation Criteria

The family will:

- Indicate a desire to manage the therapeutic regimen/program
- Identify factors interfering with adhering to the therapeutic regimen
- Adjust usual activities as needed to incorporate the treatment programs of family members (eg, diet, school activities)
- Experience a decrease in illness symptoms among family members

NIC Priority Interventions

Family Involvement: Facilitating family participation in the emotional and physical care of the patient

Family Mobilization: Utilization of family strengths to influence patient's health in a positive direction

Family Process Maintenance: Minimization of family process disruption effects

Nursing Activities

Also see "Nursing Activities" for "Management of Therapeutic Regimen: Individual, Ineffective" on pp. 271–272

Assessments

- Assess present status of family coping and processes
- Assess family members' levels of understanding of illness, complications, and recommended treatments
- Assess family members' readiness to learn
- Identify family cultural influences and health beliefs
- (*NIC*) *Family Involvement:*

   Identify family members' capabilities for involvement in care of patient

   Determine physical, emotional, and educational resources of primary caregiver

   Monitor family structure and roles

Identify individual family members' understanding and beliefs about the situation

Determine level of patient dependency on family, as appropriate for age or illness

Identify and respect family's coping mechanisms

Patient/Family Teaching

- Teach family time management/organization skills
- Provide caregivers with skills needed for patient's therapy
- Teach strategies for maintaining or restoring patient's health
- Teach strategies for care of a dying patient
- *(NIC) Family Involvement:* Facilitate family understanding of the medical aspects of illness

Collaborative Activities

- Help family to identify community health care resources
- Refer family to family support groups

Other

- Involve family in discussion of strengths and resources
- Assist patient/family to establish realistic goals
- Assist family members to plan and implement patient therapies and lifestyle changes
- Support maintenance of family routines and rituals in hospital (eg, private meals together, family discussions)
- Discuss family's plans for child care when parents must be absent
- Plan patient home care activities to decrease disruption of family routine
- *(NIC) Family Involvement:*

  Encourage care by family members during hospitalization, when appropriate

  Encourage family members to keep or maintain family relationships, as appropriate

  Assist primary caregiver to acquire needed care delivery supplies

  Support primary caregiver in the use of relief services opportunities

Management of Therapeutic Regimen: Individual, Effective (5.2.4) (1994)

Definition: A pattern of regulating and integrating into daily living a program for treatment of illness and its sequelae that are satisfactory for meeting specific health goals

Defining Characteristics

Subjective

Verbalized desire to manage the treatment of illness and prevention of sequelae

Verbalized intent to reduce risk factors for progression of illness and sequelae

Objective

Appropriate choices of daily activities for meeting the goals of a treatment or prevention program

Illness symptoms are within a normal range of expectation

Suggestions for Use

This diagnosis does not need to include related factors because it is a wellness diagnosis.

Suggested Alternative Diagnoses

None

NOC Suggested Outcomes

Adherence Behavior: Self-initiated action taken to promote wellness, recovery, and rehabilitation

Compliance Behavior: Actions taken on the basis of professional advice to promote wellness, recovery, and rehabilitation

Knowledge: Treatment Regimen: Extent of understanding conveyed about a specific treatment regimen

Participation: Health Care Decisions: Personal involvement in selecting and evaluating health care options

Risk Control: Actions to eliminate or reduce actual, personal, and modifiable health threats

Symptom Control Behavior: Personal actions to minimize perceived adverse changes in physical and emotional functioning

Goals/Evaluation Criteria

Examples Using NOC Language

- Demonstrates **Adherence Behavior**, as evidenced by the following indicators (specify 1–5: never, rarely, sometimes, often, or consistently demonstrated):

   Uses health-related information from a variety of sources to develop health strategies

   Provides rationale for adopting a regimen

   Describes rationale for deviating from a recommended regimen

   Performs self-monitoring

- Demonstrates **Participation: Health Care Decisions**, as evidenced by the following indicator (specify 1–5: never, rarely, sometimes, often, or consistently demonstrated): Evaluates satisfaction with health care outcomes

- Demonstrates **Risk Control**, as evidenced by the following indicators (specify 1–5: never, rarely, sometimes, often, or consistently demonstrated):

   Monitors environmental and personal behavior risk factors

   Participates in screening for associated health problems and identified risks

Other Examples

Patient will:

- Describe and follow prescribed health regimens (eg, diet, exercise)
- Change/modify health regimen as directed by health provider
- Report symptom control

NIC Priority Interventions

Anticipatory Guidance: Preparation of patient for an anticipated developmental and/or situational crisis

Health System Guidance: Facilitating a patient's location and use of appropriate health services

Nursing Activities

Assessments

- Assess patient's knowledge of health promotion and disease prevention
- Identify patient's usual methods of coping and problem solving

Patient/Family Teaching

- Help patient to plan for the future by providing information on the usual course of the patient's illness

- Teach stress management techniques
- *(NIC) Health System Guidance:*

  Explain the immediate health care system, how it works, and what the patient/family can expect

  Inform the patient of accreditation and State Health Department requirements for judging the quality of a facility

  Give written instructions for purpose and location of health care activities, as appropriate

  Inform patient how to access emergency services by telephone and vehicle, as appropriate

Collaborative Activities

- Offer information on community resources specific to health goals of the patient (eg, support groups)
- *(NIC) Health System Guidance:* Identify and facilitate communication among health care providers and patient/family, as appropriate

Other

- Help patient to identify and prepare for upcoming developmental milestones, role changes, or situational crises
- Help patient to identify situational obstacles that interfere with adherence to therapeutic regimen
- Plan to visit patient at strategic developmental/situational times
- *(NIC) Health System Guidance:* Encourage the patient/family to ask questions about services and charges

Management of Therapeutic Regimen: Individual, Ineffective (5.2.1) (1992)

Definition: A pattern of regulating and integrating into daily living a program for treatment of illness and the sequelae of illness that is unsatisfactory for meeting specific health goals

Defining Characteristics

Subjective

Choices of daily living ineffective for meeting the goals of a treatment or prevention program

[Statements that patient/family] did not take action to include treatment regimens in daily routines

[Statements that patient/family] did not take action to reduce risk factors for progression of illness and sequelae

Verbalized desire to manage the treatment of illness and prevention of sequelae

Verbalized difficulty with regulation/integration of one or more prescribed regimens for treatment of illness and its effects or prevention of complications

Objective

Acceleration [expected or unexpected] of illness symptoms

Related Factors

Complexity of health care system

Complexity of therapeutic regimen

Decisional conflicts

Family conflict

Family patterns of health care

Inadequate number and types of cues to action

Knowledge deficits

Mistrust of regimen and/or health care personnel

Perceived barriers

Perceived benefits

Perceived seriousness

Perceived susceptibility

Powerlessness

Social support deficits

Suggestions for Use

Use this diagnosis for patients who wish to follow a therapeutic regimen and are motivated to do so but are having difficulty with it. For example, the diagnosis is appropriate for a patient who is trying to lose weight and has the necessary information but finds it difficult to adhere to a low-calorie diet because her business requires her to eat out frequently. It is not appropriate for an obese patient who is not interested in dieting or losing weight.

Suggested Alternative Diagnoses

Adjustment, impaired

Denial, ineffective

Health maintenance, altered

Noncompliance (specify)

NOC Suggested Outcomes

Knowledge: Treatment Regimen: Extent of understanding conveyed about a specific treatment regimen

Participation: Health Care Decisions: Personal involvement in selecting and evaluating health care options

Treatment Behavior: Illness or Injury: Personal actions to palliate or eliminate pathology

Goals/Evaluation Criteria

Refer to "Goals/Evaluation Criteria" for "Management of Therapeutic Regimen, Individual, Effective" p. 268

Other Examples

Patient will:

- Develop and follow plan to achieve therapeutic regimen
- Identify obstacles that interfere with adherence to the therapeutic regimen
- Avoid risk-taking behaviors
- Recognize and report symptoms of change in disease status
- Use therapeutic equipment/devices correctly

NIC Priority Interventions

Behavior Modification: Promotion of a behavior change

Self-Modification Assistance: Reinforcement of self-directed change initiated by the patient to achieve personally important goals

Nursing Activities

Assessments

- Assess patient's level of understanding of illness, complications, and recommended treatments to determine knowledge deficit
- Interview patient/family to determine "problem areas" in integrating treatment regimen into lifestyle
- *(NIC) Self-Modification Assistance:*
  Appraise the patient's reasons for wanting to change
  Appraise the patient's present knowledge and skill level in relationship to the desired change
  Appraise the patient's social and physical environment for extent of support of desired behaviors

Patient/Family Teaching

- Identify essential treatments
- Offer information on community resources specific to health goals of patient (eg, support groups)

- Assist patient to identify situational obstacles that interfere with adherence to therapeutic regimen
- Provide information on illness, complications, and recommended treatments
- *(NIC) Self-Modification Assistance:* Instruct the patient on how to move from continuous reinforcement to intermittent reinforcement

Collaborative Activities

- Collaborate with other health care providers to determine how to modify therapeutic regimen without jeopardizing patient's health

Other

- Assist patient to develop realistic plan to achieve adherence to therapeutic regimen. Plan should include the following:
    Identification of modifications/adaptations in ADLs
    Identification of support systems to achieve therapeutic goals
    Identification of actions patient/family are willing to take (eg, dietary changes, exercise modification, sleep pattern changes, medication and treatment schedules, sexual activity modifications, role changes)
- Provide coaching and support to motivate patient's continued adherence to therapy
- *(NIC) Self-Modification Assistance:*
    Encourage the patient to examine personal values and beliefs and satisfaction with them
    Assist the patient in identifying a specific goal for change
    Assist the patient in identifying target behaviors that need to change to achieve the desired goal
    Explore with the patient potential barriers to change behavior
    Identify with the patient the most effective strategies for behavior changes
    Encourage the patient to identify appropriate, meaningful reinforcers/rewards
    Foster moving toward primary reliance on self-reinforcement versus family or nurse rewards
    Assist the patient in identifying the circumstances or situations in which the behavior occurs (eg, cues/triggers)
    Explain to the patient the importance of self-monitoring in attempting behavior change

Memory, Impaired
(8.3.1) (1994)

Definition: The state in which an individual experiences the inability to remember or recall bits of information or behavioral skills. Impaired memory may be attributed to pathophysiologic or situational causes that are either temporary or permanent.

Defining Characteristics

Forgets to perform a behavior at a scheduled time
Inability to determine if a behavior was performed
Inability to learn or retain new skills or information
Inability to perform a previously learned skill
Inability to recall factual information
Inability to recall recent or past events
Observed or reported experiences of forgetting

Related Factors

Acute or chronic hypoxia
Anemia
Decreased cardiac output
[Depression]
Excessive environmental disturbances
Fluid and electrolyte imbalance
Neurologic disturbances

Suggestions for Use

Use this diagnosis only if it is possible for the patient's memory to improve. If the impairment is permanent, consider using it as an etiology of another diagnosis—for example, *Self-care deficit* or *Risk for injury. Impaired memory* is also a defining characteristic for some other diagnoses, such as *Chronic confusion* and *Altered thought processes,* in which other symptoms are also present.

Suggested Alternative Diagnoses

Confusion, chronic
Environmental interpretation syndrome, impaired
Thought processes, altered
Tissue perfusion, altered (cerebral)

NOC Suggested Outcomes

Child Development: 12 months…Adolescence: Milestones of physical, cognitive, and psychosocial progression by 12 months (2 years, 3 years, etc.) of age. [**NOTE:** NOC lists a separate outcome and indicators for each age group.]

Cognitive Orientation: Ability to identify person, place, and time

Memory: Ability to cognitively retrieve and report previously stored information

Neurologic Status: Consciousness: Extent to which an individual arouses, orients, and attends to the environment

Goals/Evaluation Criteria

Examples Using NOC language

- Demonstrates unimpaired Memory and Child Development: 12 months…Adolescence
- Demonstrates **Cognitive Orientation**, as evidenced by the following indicators (specify 1–5: never, rarely, sometimes, often, or consistently demonstrated): Identifies significant other; current place; and correct day, month, year, and season
- Demonstrates **Neurologic Status: Consciousness**, as evidenced by the following indicators (specify 1–5: extremely, substantially, moderately, mildly, or not compromised):
    Opens eyes to external stimuli
    Obeys commands
    Attends to environmental stimuli

Other Examples

Patient will:
- Use techniques to help improve memory
- Accurately recall immediate, recent, and remote information
- Verbalize being better able to remember

NIC Priority Interventions

Memory Training: Facilitation of memory

Nursing Activities

Assessments

- Assess for depression, anxiety, and increased stressors that may be contributing to memory loss
- Assess neurologic function to determine whether patient has memory loss only or also has problems, such as dementia, which need to be referred for further treatment

- Assess extent and nature of memory loss (eg, immediate, recent, or remote events; gradual or sudden loss)
- Determine history and present pattern of alcohol use
- Determine which medications or street drugs the client is taking that might affect memory (eg, marijuana)
- *(NIC) Memory Training:* Monitor patient's behavior during therapy

Patient/Family Teaching

- Explain to the older patient that short-term memory loss frequently occurs with aging
- *(NIC) Memory Training:* Structure the teaching methods according to patient's organization of information

Collaborative Activities

- Refer patients with sudden memory loss to physician
- *(NIC) Memory Training:* Refer to occupational therapy, as appropriate

Other

- Label items (eg, the bathroom door, the sink, the refrigerator) to increase recall
- Do not rearrange furniture in the room or the patient's home
- Help the patient to relax in order to improve concentration
- *(NIC) Memory Training:*

  Discuss with patient/family any practical memory problems experienced

  Stimulate memory by repeating patient's last expressed thought, as appropriate

  Reminisce about past experiences with patient, as appropriate

  Implement appropriate memory techniques, such as visual imagery, mnemonic devices, memory games, memory cues, association techniques, making lists, using computers, or using name tags, or rehearsing information

  Assist in associated-learning tasks, such as practice learning and recalling verbal and pictorial information presented, as appropriate

  Provide for orientation training, such as patient rehearsing personal information and dates, as appropriate

  Provide opportunity for concentration, such as a game matching pairs of cards, as appropriate

  Provide opportunity to use memory for recent events, such as questioning patient about a recent outing

Provide for picture recognition memory, as appropriate

Encourage patient to participate in group memory training programs, as appropriate

Mobility: Bed, Impaired
(6.1.1.1.6) (1998)

Definition: Limitation of independent movement from one bed position to another [specify level]

Defining Characteristics

Impaired ability to do the following:

Move from supine to long-sitting or long-sitting to supine

Move from supine to prone or prone to supine

Move from supine to sitting or sitting to supine

Turn side to side

"Scoot" or reposition self in bed

Related Factors

To be developed

Suggestions for Use

(1) When the patient's bed mobility cannot be improved, this label should be used as a related or risk factor for other nursing diagnoses, such as *Risk for impaired skin integrity*.

(2) Specify level of mobility, the same as you would for *Impaired physical mobility* and *Impaired wheelchair mobility:*

Level 0: Is completely independent

Level 1: Requires use of equipment or device

Level 2: Requires help from another person for assistance, supervision, or teaching

Level 3: Requires help from another person and equipment/device

Level 4: Is dependent; does not participate in activity

(3) See "Suggestions for Use" for "Mobility: Physical, Impaired" on p. 279

Suggested Alternative Diagnoses

Disuse syndrome, risk for

Injury, risk for

Mobility: physical, impaired

Skin integrity, risk for impaired

NOC Suggested Outcomes

Because this is a new NANDA label, NOC has not yet published suggested outcomes for it. However, the following choices seem appropriate.

Joint Movement: Active: Range of motion of joints with self-initiated movement

Mobility Level: Ability to move purposefully

Goals/Evaluation Criteria

The patient will:

- Perform full range-of-motion of all joints
- Turn self in bed or state realistic level of assistance needed
- Demonstrate correct use of assistive devices (eg, trapeze)
- Request repositioning assistance, as needed

NIC Priority Interventions

To be developed

Nursing Activities

Assessments

- Perform ongoing assessment of patient's mobility level
- Assess level of consciousness
- Assess muscle strength and joint mobility (range of motion)
- Assess need for assistance from home health agency or other organization
- Assess need for durable medical equipment

Patient/Family Teaching

- Instruct in active/passive range-of-motion exercises to improve muscle strength and endurance
- Instruct in turning techniques and correct body alignment

Collaborative Activities

- Use occupational/physical therapists as resources in developing plan to maintain/increase bed mobility

Other

- Position call light/button within easy reach
- Provide assistive devices (eg, trapeze)
- Provide positive reinforcement during activities
- Implement pain control measures before beginning exercises or physical therapy
- Ensure care plan includes number of personnel needed to turn patient

Mobility: Physical, Impaired
(6.1.1.1) (1973, 1998)

Definition: A limitation in independent, purposeful physical movement of the body or of one or more extremities [specify level]:

Level 0: Is completely independent

Level 1: Requires use of equipment or device

Level 2: Requires help from another person for assistance, supervision, or teaching

Level 3: Requires help from another person and equipment/ device

Level 4: Is dependent; does not participate in activity

Defining Characteristics

Objective

Decreased reaction time

Difficulty turning

Engages in substitutions for movement (eg, increased attention to other's activity, controlling behavior, focus on pre-illness/disability activity)

Gait changes (eg, decreased walk, speed, difficulty initiating gait, small steps, shuffles feet, exaggerated lateral postural sway)

Limited ability to perform fine-motor skills

Limited ability to perform gross-motor skills

Limited range of motion

Movement-induced shortness of breath

Movement-induced tremor

Postural instability during performance of routine activities of daily living

Slowed movement

Uncoordinated or jerky movements

Related Factors

Altered cellular metabolism

Body mass index above 75th age-appropriate percentile

Cognitive impairment

Cultural beliefs regarding age-appropriate activity

Decreased muscle strength, control, and/or mass

Depressive mood state or anxiety

Developmental delay

Discomfort

Intolerance to activity/decreased strength and endurance

Joint stiffness or contractures
Lack of knowledge regarding value of physical activity
Lack of physical or social environmental supports
Limited cardiovascular endurance
Loss of integrity of bone structures
Medications
Musculoskeletal impairment
Neuromuscular impairment
Pain
Prescribed movement restrictions
Reluctant to initiate movement
Sedentary lifestyle or disuse or deconditioning
Selective or generalized malnutrition
Sensoriperceptual impairments

Suggestions for Use

Use *Impaired physical mobility* to describe individuals with limited ability for independent physical movement, such as decreased ability to move arms or legs or generalized muscle weakness, or when nursing interventions will focus on restoring mobility and function or preventing further deterioration. For example, an appropriate diagnosis would be *Impaired physical mobility related to ineffective management of Chronic pain secondary to rheumatoid arthritis.*

Do not use this label to describe temporary immobility that cannot be changed by the nurse (eg, traction, prescribed bedrest) or permanent paralysis. In these and many other instances, *Impaired physical mobility* can be used effectively as the etiology of a problem. An example of this would be *Impaired tissue integrity (decubitus ulcer) related to Impaired physical mobility +4.* When appropriate, use more specific labels, such as *Impaired bed mobility, Impaired transfer ability, Impaired wheelchair mobility,* or *Impaired walking.*

Suggested Alternative Diagnoses

Disuse syndrome, risk for
Injury, risk for
Mobility: bed, impaired
Mobility: wheelchair, impaired
Self-care deficit
Transfer ability, impaired
Walking, Impaired

NOC Suggested Outcomes

Ambulation: Walking: Ability to walk from place to place

Ambulation: Wheelchair: Ability to move from place to place in a wheelchair

Joint Movement: Active: Range of motion of joints with self-initiated movement

Mobility Level: Ability to move purposefully

Self-Care: Activities of Daily Living (ADLs): Ability to perform the most basic physical tasks and personal care activities

Transfer Performance: Ability to change body locations

Goals/Evaluation Criteria

Examples Using NOC Language

- Demonstrates **Mobility Level**, as evidenced by the following indicators (specify 1–5: is dependent [does not participate], requires assistive person and device, requires assistive person, is independent with assistive device, or is completely independent):

    Balance performance
    Body positioning performance
    Muscle and joint movement
    Transfer performance
    Ambulation: walking
    Ambulation: wheelchair

Other Examples

Patient will:

- Demonstrate correct use of assistive devices with supervision
- Request assistance with mobilization activities, as needed
- Perform activities of daily living independently with assistive devices (specify activity and device)
- Bear weight
- Walk with effective gait for _____ (specify distance)
- Transfer to and from chair/wheelchair
- Maneuver wheelchair effectively

NIC Priority Interventions

Exercise Therapy, Ambulation: Promotion and assistance with walking to maintain or restore autonomic and voluntary body functions during treatment and recovery from illness or injury

Exercise Therapy, Joint Mobility: Use of active or passive body movement to maintain or restore joint flexibility

Positioning: Moving the patient or a body part to provide comfort, reduce the risk of skin breakdown, promote skin integrity, and/or promote healing

Nursing Activities

Assessment is an ongoing process to determine the performance level of the patient's Impaired mobility

Level 1 Nursing Activities

- Assess need for home health assistance and need for durable medical equipment
- Teach patient about and monitor use of mobility devices (eg, cane, walker, crutches, or wheelchair)
- Instruct and assist him/her with transfer process (eg, bed to chair)
- Refer to physical therapist for an exercise program
- Provide positive reinforcement during activities
- Assist patient to use supportive, nonskid footwear for walking
- (NIC) Positioning:
  Instruct the patient how to use good posture and good body mechanics while performing any activity
  Monitor traction devices for proper setup

Level 2 Nursing Activities

- Assess patient's learning needs
- Assess need for assistance from home health agency and need for durable medical equipment
- Instruct and encourage patient in active/passive range-of-motion exercises to maintain or develop muscle strength and endurance
- Instruct and encourage patient to use a trapeze and/or weights to enhance and maintain strength of upper extremities.
- Teach techniques for safe transfer and ambulation.
- Instruct patient regarding weight-bearing status
- Instruct patient regarding correct body alignment
- Use occupational/physical therapist as a resource in developing a plan for maintaining/increasing mobility
- Provide positive reinforcement during activities
- Supervise all mobilization attempts and assist patient, as necessary
- Use a gait belt when assisting with transfer or ambulation

Levels 3 and 4 Nursing Activities

- Determine patient motivation level for maintaining or restoring mobility of joints and muscles

- Use occupational/physical therapist as resource in planning patient care activities
- Encourage patient/family to view limitations realistically
- Provide positive reinforcement during activities
- Administer analgesics before beginning exercises
- Develop a plan specifying the following:
  - Type of assistive device
  - Positioning of patient in bed/chair
  - Ways to transfer/turn patient
  - Number of personnel needed to mobilize patient
  - Necessary elimination equipment (eg, bedpan, urinal, fracture pan)
  - Schedule of activities
- *(NIC) Positioning:*
  - Monitor traction devices for proper setup
  - Place on an appropriate therapeutic mattress/bed
  - Position patient in proper body alignment
  - Place in the designated therapeutic position (eg, avoid placing the amputation stump in the flexion position; elevate the affected body part, as appropriate; immobilize or support the affected body part, as appropriate)
  - Turn the immobilized patient at least every 2 hours, according to a specific schedule
  - Place bed-positioning switch and call light within easy reach
  - Encourage active range-of-motion exercises

Mobility: Wheelchair, Impaired
(6.1.1.1.4) (1998)

Definition: Limitation of independent operation of wheelchair within environment [specify level]

Defining Characteristics

Impaired ability to operate manual or power wheelchair on an incline or decline

Impaired ability to operate manual or power wheelchair on even or uneven surface

Impaired ability to operate wheelchair on curbs

Related Factors

To be developed

Suggestions for Use

Specify levels of mobility, which are the same as the options for *Impaired physical mobility* and *Impaired bed mobility:*

Level 0: Is completely independent

Level 1: Requires use of equipment or device

Level 2: Requires help from another person for assistance, supervision, or teaching

Level 3: Requires help from another person and equipment/device

Level 4: Is dependent; does not participate in activity

See "Suggestions for Use" for "Mobility: Physical, impaired" on p. 279

Suggested Alternative Diagnoses

Injury, risk for

Mobility: physical, impaired

Skin integrity, risk for impaired

Transfer ability, impaired

NOC Suggested Outcomes

Because this is a new NANDA label, NOC has not yet published suggested outcomes for it. However, the following seem to be appropriate choices.

Ambulation: Wheelchair: Ability to move from place to place in a wheelchair

Joint Movement: Active: Range of motion of joints with self-initiated movement

Mobility Level: Ability to move purposefully

Goals/Evaluation Criteria

Examples Using NOC Language

For each indicator in this set of goals, specify the following parameters: Is dependent (does not participate), requires assistive person and device, requires assistive person, is independent with assistive device, or is completely independent.

• Patient will demonstrate **Ambulation: Wheelchair**, as evidenced by the following indicators:

   Transfers to and from wheelchair

   Propels wheelchair safely

   Maneuvers curbs, doorways, and ramps

• Demonstrates **Mobility Level**, as evidenced by the following indicators: Balance performance, muscle movement, joint movement, body positioning performance, and transfer performance

Other Examples

Patient will:

- Request assistance with mobilization activities, as needed
- Perform activities of daily living independently with/without assistive devices (specify activity and device)
- Demonstrate moderate active movement of all joints or specify affected joints

NIC Priority Interventions

Because this is a new NANDA label, NIC has not yet published priority interventions for it. However, the following choices seem appropriate.

Exercise Therapy: Joint Mobility: Use of active or passive body movement to maintain or restore joint flexibility

Positioning: Wheelchair: Placement of a patient in a properly selected wheelchair to enhance comfort, promote skin integrity, and foster independence

Nursing Activities

Assessments

- Assess patient's learning needs regarding use of wheelchair
- Assess need for assistance from home health agency and need for special modifications to wheelchair (eg, motor)
- Assess joint mobility and muscle strength
- Assess cognitive abilities
- Determine patient's motivation level for using wheelchair
- *(NIC) Positioning: Wheelchair:*

  Check patient's position in the wheelchair while patient sits on selected pad and wears proper footwear

  Monitor for patient's inability to maintain correct posture in wheelchair

Patient/Family Teaching

- *(NIC) Positioning: Wheelchair*

  Instruct patient on exercises to increase upper body strength, as appropriate

  Teach how to operate wheelchair, as appropriate

Collaborative Activities

- Collaborate with physical and occupational therapist, as needed

(eg, to be certain that wheelchair size and type is appropriate for patient)

Other

- Provide positive reinforcement during activities
- Supervise attempts to operate wheelchair on curbs and inclines
- Encourage patient/family to view limitations realistically
- *(NIC) Positioning: Wheelchair:*

  Check that foot rests have at least 2 inches of clearance from the floor

  Ensure that wheelchair allows at least 2 to 3 inches of clearance from the back of knee to front of sling seat

  Provide modifications or appliances to wheelchair to correct for patient problems or muscle weakness

Nausea
(9.1.2) (1998)

Definition: An unpleasant, wavelike sensation in the back of the throat, epigastrium, or throughout the abdomen that may or may not lead to vomiting

Defining Characteristics

Subjective

Reports "nausea" or "sick to stomach"

Objective

Accompanied by pallor, cold and clammy skin, increased salivation, tachycardia, gastric stasis, and diarrhea

Accompanied by swallowing movements affected by skeletal muscles

Usually precedes vomiting, but may be experienced after vomiting or when vomiting does not occur

Related Factors

Chemotherapy

Irritation to the gastrointestinal system

Postsurgical anesthesia

Stimulation of neuropharmacologic mechanisms

Suggestions for Use

This label is appropriate for short-term episodes of nausea/vomiting (eg, postoperatively). When *Nausea* is severe/prolonged and may compromise adequate nutrition, use *Risk for altered nutrition: less than body requirements related to Nausea.*

Suggested Alternative Diagnoses

Fluid volume deficit, risk for
Nutrition: less than body requirements, risk for altered

NOC Suggested Outcomes

Because this is a new NANDA label, NOC has not yet published suggested outcomes for it. However, the following may be appropriate:

Comfort Level: Feelings of physical and psychologic ease

Fluid Balance: Balance of water in the intracellular and extracellular compartments of the body

Nutritional Status: Food and Fluid Intake: Amount of food and fluid taken into the body over a 24-hour period

Goals/Evaluation Criteria

Examples Using NOC Language

- Demonstrates **Fluid Balance**, as evidenced by the following indicators (specify 1–5: extremely, substantially, moderately, mildly, or not compromised):

    24-hour intake and output balanced
    Body weight stable
    Sunken eyes not present
    Abnormal thirst not present
    Skin hydration not compromised
    Moist mucous membranes
    Serum electrolytes within normal limits (WNL)
    Urine specific gravity WNL

- Demonstrates **Nutritional Status: Food and Fluid Intake**, as evidenced by the following indicators (specify 1–5: not, slightly, moderately, substantially, or totally adequate):

    Oral food, tubefeeding, or TPN intake
    Oral or IV fluid intake

Other Examples

The patient will:

- Report relief from nausea
- Identify measures that decrease nausea

NIC Priority Interventions

Because this is a new NANDA label, NIC has not yet published priority interventions for it. However, the following may be appropriate:

Fluid Management: Promotion of fluid balance and prevention of complications resulting from abnormal or undesired fluid levels

Fluid Monitoring: Collection and analysis of patient data to regulate fluid balance

Nutritional Monitoring: Collection and analysis of patient data to prevent or minimize malnourishment

Nursing Activities

Assessment

- Monitor patient's subjective symptoms of nausea
- Monitor urine color, quantity, and specific gravity
- *(NIC) Nutritional Monitoring:*
  Monitor trends in weight loss and gain
  Monitor for dry, flaky skin with depigmentation
  Monitor skin turgor, as appropriate
  Monitor gums for swelling, sponginess, receding, and increased bleeding
  Monitor energy level, malaise, fatigue, and weakness
  Monitor caloric and nutrient intake
- *(NIC) Fluid Management:*
  Maintain accurate intake and output record
  Monitor food/fluid ingested and calculate daily caloric intake, as appropriate
  Monitor nutrition status
  Monitor hydration status (eg, moist mucous membranes, adequacy of pulses, and orthostatic blood pressure), as appropriate

Patient/Family Teaching

- Teach patient to use voluntary swallowing and/or deep breathing to suppress the vomiting reflex
- Teach to eat slowly
- Teach to restrict fluids 1 hour before, 1 hour after, and during meals
- Instruct to avoid the smell of food preparation at home (eg, let someone else prepare meals, stay out of the kitchen, go for a walk during meal preparation)

Collaborative Activities

- Administer prescribed antiemetics
- Consult with physician to provide adequate pain control with medications that do not cause nausea for the patient
- *(NIC) Fluid Management:* Administer IV therapy, as prescribed

Other

- Elevate head of bed or place in lateral position to prevent aspiration (for clients with decreased mobility)
- Keep client and bedding clean when vomiting occurs
- Remove odor-producing substances immediately (eg, bedpans, food)
- Do not schedule pain- or nausea-producing procedures near mealtimes
- Provide oral care after vomiting
- Apply cool, damp cloth to patient's wrists, neck, and forehead
- Offer cold foods and other foods with little odor
- *(NIC) Nutritional Monitoring:* Note significant changes in nutritional status and initiate treatments, as appropriate

Noncompliance (specify)
(5.2.1.1) (1973, 1998)

Definition: The extent to which a person's and/or caregiver's behavior coincides or fails to coincide with a health-promoting or therapeutic plan agreed upon by the person (and/or family, and/or community) and health care professional. In the presence of an agreed-upon, health-promoting or therapeutic plan, person's or caregiver's behavior may be fully, partially [adherent], or non-adherent and may lead to clinically effective, partially effective, or ineffective outcomes.

Defining Characteristics

Objective

Behavior indicative of failure to adhere (by direct observation or by statements of patient or significant others)

Evidence of development of complications

Evidence of exacerbation of symptoms

Failure to keep appointments

Failure to progress

Objective tests (eg, physiologic measures, detection of physiologic markers)

Related Factors

Health Care Plan

Complexity

Cost

Duration
Intensity
Significant others
Individual Factors
Cultural influences
Health beliefs
Individual's value system
Knowledge and skill relevant to the regimen behavior
Motivational forces
Personal and developmental abilities
Spiritual values
Health System
Access and convenience of care
Client-provider relationships
Communication and teaching skills of the provider
Credibility of provider
Financial flexibility of plan
Individual health coverage
Provider continuity and regular follow-up
Provider reimbursement of teaching and follow-up
Satisfaction with care
Network
Involvement of members in health plan
Perceived beliefs of significant others
Social value regarding plan

Suggestions for Use

Noncompliance describes failure to adhere to a therapeutic recommendation after having made an informed decision *to* do so and after expressing an intention to do so. If the patient is informed and *intends* to follow instructions, then nursing intervention can be directed at finding and removing the factors that keep him or her from doing so. For example, a patient may state, "My husband doesn't need to lose weight, and he loves fried food and pastries. He just won't eat the diet foods, and I really don't have time to cook one meal for myself and one for the rest of the family." This client would like to comply with her diet, but situational factors make it difficult. You could write a nursing diagnosis of *Noncompliance with low-calorie diet related to inconvenience of preparing special foods and lack of family support.* That diagnosis does suggest independent nursing interventions.

Noncompliance should *not* be used for a patient who makes an informed decision to not follow a therapeutic recommendation, for instance, when a patient decides to stop taking a medication with unpleasant side effects. Nursing intervention might then be directed at convincing the patient of the value of continuing with the therapy, but the nurse should balance this approach with respect for the patient's autonomy when he or she has truly made an informed decision. Remember that a decision to refuse therapy can be as rational as a decision to have therapy.

Noncompliance should not be used for patients who are unable to follow instructions (eg, weakness, cognitive disability) or who lack necessary information. If those factors are contributing to *Noncompliance*, then it is better to use the diagnosis *Altered health maintenance.*

Some nurses believe that *Noncompliance* is a negative label. When using this diagnosis, be sure to express the etiology in neutral, nonjudgmental terms. Geissler (1991) has suggested the term *nonadherence*, although it is not yet a NANDA label.

Suggested Alternative Diagnoses

Denial, ineffective
Health maintenance, altered
Management of therapeutic regimen: family/individual, ineffective

NOC Suggested Outcomes

Adherence Behavior: Self-initiated action taken to promote wellness, recovery, and rehabilitation
Compliance Behavior: Actions taken on the basis of professional advice to promote wellness, recovery, and rehabilitation
Pain Level: Amount of reported or demonstrated pain
Symptom Control Behavior: Personal actions to minimize perceived adverse changes in physical and emotional functioning
Treatment Behavior: Illness or Injury: Personal actions to palliate or eliminate pathology

Goals/Evaluation Criteria

Examples Using NOC Language

• *Noncompliance* will be decreased, as demonstrated by Compliance, Symptom Control, and Treatment Behavior: Illness or Injury
• **Adherence Behavior** will be demonstrated, as evidenced by the following indicators:

Reports using strategies to eliminate unhealthy behavior and maximize health

Describes rationale for deviating from a recommended regimen

Weighs risks/benefits of health behavior

Uses health services congruent with need

Other Examples

Patient will:

- Not abuse health care providers physically or verbally
- Use pain control measures
- Comply with prescribed medication and treatment regimens
- Keep appointments with health care providers
- Report significant treatment effects and side effects
- Report controlling illness symptoms

NIC Priority Interventions

Health System Guidance: Facilitating a patient's location and use of appropriate health services

Self-Modification Assistance: Reinforcement of self-directed change initiated by the patient to achieve personally important goals

Nursing Activities

Assessments

- Identify probable cause of patient's noncompliant behavior

Patient/Family Teaching

- Help patient/family to understand the need for following the prescribed treatment and the consequences of noncompliance
- *(NIC) Health System Guidance:*

  Inform patient of appropriate community resources and contact persons

  Give written instructions for purpose and location of health care activities, as appropriate

Collaborative Activities

- Consult with physician about possible alteration in medical regimen to encourage patient's compliance
- *(NIC) Health System Guidance:*

  Coordinate referrals to relevant health care providers, as appropriate

  Identify and facilitate communication among health care providers and patient/family, as appropriate.

Coordinate/schedule time needed by each service to deliver care, as appropriate

Provide follow-up contact with patient, as appropriate

Assist individual to complete forms for assistance, such as housing and financial aid, as needed

Other

- Encourage the patient to express feelings and concerns about hospitalization and relationship with health care providers
- Provide emotional support to family members to help them maintain a positive relationship with patient
- Give positive reinforcement for compliance to encourage ongoing positive behaviors
- Develop a written contract with the patient, and evaluate compliant behaviors on a continuing basis. Specify contract.
- *(NIC) Self-Modification Assistance:*

  Encourage the patient to examine personal values and beliefs and satisfaction with them

  Explore with the patient potential barriers to change behavior

  Identify with the patient the most effective strategies for behavior change

  Assist the patient in formulating a systematic plan for behavior change [including intrinsic and extrinsic rewards/reinforcers]

  Assist the patient in identifying even small successes

Nutrition: Less Than Body Requirements, Altered (1.1.2.2) (1975)

Definition: The state in which an individual is experiencing an intake of nutrients insufficient to meet metabolic needs

Defining Characteristics

The author recommends using this label only if one of the following cues is present:

Body weight 20 percent or more under ideal for height and frame

Food intake less than metabolic needs—either total calories or specific nutrients (non-NANDA)

Loss of weight with adequate food intake

Reported inadequate food intake less than the RDA (recommended daily allowance)

Subjective

Abdominal cramping

Abdominal pain with or without pathology

Perceived inability to ingest food

Reported altered taste sensation

Reported lack of food

Satiety immediately after ingesting food

Indigestion (non-NANDA)

Objective

Aversion to eating

Capillary fragility

Diarrhea and/or steatorrhea

Evidence of lack of food

Excessive loss of hair

Hyperactive bowel sounds

Lack of information, misinformation

Lack of interest in food

Misconceptions

Pale conjunctival and mucous membranes

Poor muscle tone

Refusal to eat (non-NANDA)

Sore, inflamed buccal cavity

Weakness of muscles required for swallowing or mastication

Related Factors

Inability to ingest or digest food or absorb nutrients due to biologic, psychologic, or economic factors, including the following:

Chemical dependence (specify)

Chronic illness (specify)

Difficulty in chewing or swallowing

Economic factors

Food intolerance

High metabolic needs

Inadequate sucking reflex in the infant

Lack of basic nutritional knowledge

Limited access to food

Loss of appetite

Nausea/vomiting

Parental neglect

Psychologic impairment (specify)

Suggestions for Use

Use this label for patients who are able to eat but unable to ingest, digest, or absorb nutrients to adequately meet metabolic needs. Inadequate ingestion might occur because of decreased appetite, nausea, poverty, or many other situations. Examples of patients unable to digest food or absorb particular nutrients are those with allergies, diarrhea, lactose intolerance, or poorly fitting dentures.

Do not use this label routinely for persons who are NPO or for those completely unable to ingest food for other reasons (eg, unconscious patients). Nurses cannot prescribe independent nursing interventions for a diagnosis such as *Altered nutrition: less than body requirements related to NPO.* They cannot give the missing nutrients, and they cannot change the NPO order. Additionally, the patient is often NPO for only a short time before and after surgery; thus, any lack of nutrients is temporary and resolves without nursing intervention. Long-term NPO status is a risk factor for other nursing diagnoses, such as *Risk for altered oral mucous membrane,* and for collaborative problems such as Potential Complication: Electrolyte imbalance.

The patient might have a total nutritional deficit or perhaps be deficient in only one nutrient. When the deficit is something other than total, it should be specified like the following example: *Altered nutrition: less than body requirements **for protein** related to lack of knowledge of nutritious foods and limited budget for food.*

Suggested Alternative Diagnoses

Breastfeeding, ineffective
Dentition, altered
Failure to thrive, adult
Infant feeding pattern, ineffective
Management of therapeutic regimen: individual, ineffective
Nausea
Self-care deficit: feeding
Swallowing, impaired

NOC Suggested Outcomes

Nutritional Status: Extent to which nutrients are available to meet metabolic needs

Nutritional Status: Food and Fluid Intake: Amount of food and fluid taken into the body over a 24-hour period

Nutritional Status: Nutrient Value: Adequacy of nutrients taken into the body

Goals/Evaluation Criteria
Examples Using NOC Language
- Demonstrates **Nutritional Status: Food, Fluid, and Nutrient Intake**, as evidenced by the following indicators (specify 1–5: not, slightly, moderately, substantially, or totally adequate):
    Oral food, tube feeding, or TPN intake
    Oral or IV fluid intake

Other Examples
Patient will:
- Maintain weight at ____Kg or gain ____Kg by ____(specify date)
- Describe components of nutritionally adequate diet
- Verbalize willingness to follow diet
- Tolerate prescribed diet
- Maintain body mass and weight WNL
- Have laboratory values (eg, transferrin, albumin, and electrolytes) WNL
- Report adequate energy levels

NIC Priority Interventions

Eating Disorders Management: Prevention and treatment of severe diet restriction and overexercising or bingeing and purging of food and fluids

Nutrition Management: Assistance with or provision of a balanced dietary intake of foods and fluids

Weight Gain Assistance: Facilitation of body weight gain

Nursing Activities
General Activities for all Altered Nutrition
Assessments
- Determine patient motivation for changing eating habits
- Monitor laboratory values, especially transferrin, albumin, and electrolytes
- *(NIC) Nutrition Management:*
    Ascertain patient's food preferences
    Determine patient's ability to meet nutritional needs
    Monitor recorded intake for nutritional content and calories
    Weigh patient at appropriate intervals

Patient/Family Teaching

- Teach a method for meal planning
- Teach patient/family foods that are nutritious, yet inexpensive
- *(NIC) Nutrition Management:* Provide appropriate information about nutritional needs and how to meet them

Collaborative Activities

- Confer with dietitian to establish protein requirements for patients with inadequate protein intake or protein losses (eg, patients with anorexia nervosa or glomerular disease/peritoneal dialysis)
- Confer with physician regarding need for appetite stimulant, supplemental feedings, nutritional tube feedings, or TPN so that adequate caloric intake is maintained
- Refer to physician to determine cause of altered nutrition
- Refer to appropriate community nutritional programs (eg, Meals on Wheels, food banks) if patient cannot buy or prepare adequate food
- *(NIC) Nutrition Management:* Determine—in collaboration with dietitian, as appropriate—number of calories and type of nutrients needed to meet nutrition requirements [especially for patients with high-energy needs, such as postoperative patients and those with burns, trauma, fever, and wounds].

Other

- Develop meal plan with patient to include schedule of meals, eating environment, patient likes/dislikes, food temperature
- Encourage family members to bring food of patient's preference from home
- Assist patient to write realistic weekly goals for exercise and food intake
- Encourage patient to display food and exercise goals in a prominent location and review them daily
- Offer largest meal during time of day when patient's appetite is greatest
- Create a pleasant environment for meals (eg, remove unsightly supplies/excretions)
- Avoid invasive procedures before meals
- Feed patient, as needed
- *(NIC) Nutrition Management:*
  Encourage patient to wear properly fitted dentures and/or acquire dental care

Provide patient with high-protein, high-calorie, nutritious finger
  foods and drinks that can be readily consumed, as appropriate
Teach patient how to keep a food diary, as needed

Difficulty in Chewing/Swallowing

Also refer to "Nursing Activities" under the preceding "General
Activities for all Altered Nutrition," on pp. 295–296, and to "Nursing Activities" for "Swallowing, Impaired" on pp. 467–468

Assessments

- Assess and document degree of chewing/swallowing difficulty

Collaborative Activities

- Request occupational therapy consultation

Other

- Reassure patient and provide calm atmosphere during meals
- Have suction catheters available at bedside and suction during
  meals, as needed
- Place patient in semi-Fowler or high-Fowler position to facilitate
  swallowing; have patient remain in this position for 30 minutes
  following meals to prevent aspiration
- Place food on unaffected side of mouth to facilitate swallowing
- When feeding patient, use syringe, if necessary, to facilitate
  swallowing
- *(NIC) Nutrition Management:* Encourage patient to wear properly fitted dentures and/or acquire dental care

Nausea/Vomiting

Also refer to "Nursing Activities" under "General Activities for
all Altered Nutrition," on pp. 295–296, and to "Nursing Activities"
for "Nausea," on pp. 287–288

Assessments

- Identify factors precipitating nausea and vomiting
- Document color, amount, and frequency of emesis

Patient/Family Teaching

- Instruct patient in slow, deep breathing and voluntary swallowing to decrease nausea and/or vomiting

Collaborative Activities

- Administer antiemetics and/or analgesics before eating or on
  prescribed schedule

Other

- Minimize factors that may precipitate nausea and vomiting. Specify factors.
- Offer cool, wet washcloth to be placed on forehead or back of neck
- Offer oral hygiene before meals
- Limit diet to ice chips and clear liquids when symptoms are severe; progress with diet, as appropriate

Loss of Appetite

Also refer to "Nursing Activities" under "General Activities for all Patients with Altered Nutrition," on pp. 295–296

Assessments

- Identify factors that may contribute to patient's loss of appetite (eg, medications, emotional concerns)

Other

- Give positive feedback to patient who shows increased appetite
- Provide foods in accordance with patient's personal, cultural, and religious preferences
- *(NIC) Nutrition Management:*

  Offer snacks (eg, frequent drinks and fresh fruits/fruit juice), as appropriate

  Provide a variety of high-calorie, nutritious foods from which to select

Eating Disorders

Also refer to "Nursing Activities" under "General Activities for all Patients with Altered Nutrition," on pp. 295–296

Assessments

- Monitor patient for behaviors associated with weight loss

Collaborative Activities

- Consult dietitian to determine daily caloric intake necessary to attain target weight
- Notify physician if patient refuses to eat
- Work with physician, nutritionist, and patient to set weight and intake goals

Other

- Establish a trusting, supportive relationship with patient
- Communicate expectations for appropriate intake of food/fluid and amount of exercise
- Confine patient's eating to scheduled meals and snacks
- Accompany patient to bathroom after meals/snacks to observe for self-induced vomiting
- Develop behavior modification program specific to patient's needs
- Provide positive reinforcement for weight gain and appropriate eating behaviors but do not focus interactions on food or eating
- Explore with patient and significant others personal issues (eg, body image) that contribute to eating behaviors
- Communicate that the patient is responsible for choices about eating and physical activity
- Discuss the benefits of healthy eating behaviors and the consequences of noncompliance

Nutrition: More Than Body Requirements, Altered (1.1.2.1) (1975)

Definition: The state in which an individual is experiencing an intake of nutrients that exceeds metabolic needs

Defining Characteristics

The author recommends using this diagnosis only if one or more of the following NANDA defining characteristics is present:

Triceps skinfold greater than 15 mm in men and 25 mm in women

Weight 20 percent over ideal for height and frame

Subjective

Reports of little or no exercise

Objective

Concentration of food intake at end of day

Dysfunctional eating pattern, pairing food with other activities

Eating in response to external cues, such as time of day or social situation

Eating in response to internal cues other than hunger (eg, anxiety, [anger, depression, boredom, stress, loneliness])

Sedentary activity level

<u>Other Possible Defining Characteristics (non-NANDA)</u>

Rapid transition across growth percentiles in infants or children

Reported or observed higher baseline weight at beginning of each pregnancy

Related Factors

Excessive intake in relation to metabolic need

<u>Other Possible Related Factors (non-NANDA)</u>

Chemical dependence

Concentrating food intake at end of day

Decreased metabolic requirements (eg, secondary to prescribed bed rest)

Dysfunctional eating patterns

Eating in response to external cues (eg, time of day or social situation)

Eating in response to internal cues other than hunger (eg, anxiety)

Ethnic/cultural norms

Increased appetite

Lack of basic nutritional knowledge

Lack of physical exercise

Medications that stimulate appetite

Use of food as reward or comfort measure

Obesity in one or both parents

Use of solid food as major food source before 5 months of age

Selecting foods that do not meet daily requirements

Substituting sweets for addiction

Suggestions for Use

This diagnosis is most appropriate for patients who are motivated to lose weight (eg, a woman who has gained weight after pregnancy). For patients who are overweight but not motivated to participate in a weight loss program, consider *Altered health maintenance* instead. Note that *Altered nutrition: more than body requirements* focuses attention on nutrition instead of on lifestyle changes necessary for weight loss (eg, exercise). Eating in response to stressors might be described better as *Ineffective individual coping*.

Although some of the nursing actions and one of the NIC interventions specify "eating disorders management" as an intervention for this diagnosis, the focus of nursing for a patient who is bingeing and purging is much more complex than excess calorie intake; this diagnosis has limited use in that situation.

Suggested Alternative Diagnoses

Coping: individual, ineffective
Health maintenance, altered
Management of therapeutic regimen: individual, ineffective
Nutrition: risk for more than body requirements, altered

NOC Suggested Outcomes

Nutritional Status: Food and Fluid Intake: Amount of food and fluid taken into the body over a 24-hour period
Nutritional Status: Nutrient Intake: Adequacy of nutrients taken into the body

Goals/Evaluation Criteria

Examples Using NOC Language

• Demonstrates **Nutritional Status: Food and Fluid Intake**, as evidenced by the following indicators (specify 1–5: not, slightly, moderately, substantially, or totally adequate): oral food and fluid intake [not excessive]

Other Examples

Patient will:

• Acknowledge weight problem
• Verbalize desire to lose weight
• Participate in a structured weight-loss program
• Participate in a regular exercise program
• Approach ideal weight _____ (specify)
• Refrain from binge eating
• Experience adequate, but not excessive, intake of calories, fats, carbohydrates, vitamins, minerals, iron, and calcium

NIC Priority Interventions

Eating Disorders Management: Prevention and treatment of severe diet restriction and overexercising or bingeing and purging of food and fluids
Nutrition Management: Assisting with or providing a balanced dietary intake of foods and fluids
Weight Reduction Assistance: Facilitating loss of weight and/or body fat

Nursing Activities

Assessments

- Monitor patient for behaviors associated with weight gain
- *(NIC) Weight Reduction Assistance:*
  Determine patient's desire and motivation to reduce weight or body fat
  Determine current eating patterns by having patients keep a diary of what, when, and where they eat
- *(NIC) Nutrition Management:* Weigh patient at appropriate intervals

Patient/Family Teaching

- *(NIC) Nutrition Management:*
  Provide appropriate information about nutritional needs and how to meet them
  Encourage patient to follow a diet of complex carbohydrates and protein, and avoid simple sugars, fast food, caffeine, soft drinks
- *(NIC) Weight Reduction Assistance:*
  Discuss with patient and family the influence of alcohol consumption on food ingestion
  Instruct on how to read labels when purchasing food, to control amount of fat and calorie density of food obtained
  Teach food selections, in restaurants and social gatherings, that are consistent with planned calorie and nutrient intake
  Instruct on how to calculate percentage of fat in food products

Collaborative Activities

- Confer with dietitian to implement weight-loss program that includes dietary management and energy expenditure
- *(NIC) Nutrition Management:* Determine—in collaboration with dietitian, as appropriate—number of calories and type of nutrients needed to meet nutrition requirements
- *(NIC) Weight Reduction Assistance:* Encourage attendance at support groups for weight loss (eg, [Take Off Pounds Sensibly (TOPS) Club] or Weight Watchers)

Other

- Develop a trusting, supportive relationship with patient
- Help patient to identify physical problems that may be related to obesity/eating disorder
- For patient with compulsive eating disorder, establish expectations for appropriate eating behaviors, intake of food/fluid, and amount of exercise

- Explore with patient personal issues that may contribute to overeating
- Communicate that the patient, alone, is responsible for choices about eating and physical activity
- Provide positive reinforcement for weight loss, maintenance of dietary regimen, improved eating behaviors, and exercise
- Focus on the patient's feelings about herself or himself, rather than on the obesity
- Discuss with patient emotions or high-risk situations that stimulate eating (eg, types of foods, social situations, interpersonal stresses, unmet personal expectations, eating in secret/private)
- *(NIC) Weight Reduction Assistance:*
  Set a weekly goal for weight loss
  Assist patient to identify motivation for eating and internal and external cues associated with eating
  Determine with the patient the amount of weight loss desired
  Assist with adjusting diet to lifestyle and activity level
  Set a realistic plan with the patient to include reduced food intake and increased energy expenditure. [Plan should specify frequency of meals and snacks and include include self-monitoring activities.]
  Encourage substitution of undesirable habits with favorable habits
  Plan an exercise program, taking into consideration the patient's limitations
  Encourage use of internal reward systems when goals are accomplished

Nutrition: More Than Body Requirements, Risk for Altered (1.1.2.3) (1980)

Definition: The state in which an individual is at risk of experiencing an intake of nutrients that exceeds metabolic needs

Risk Factors

Subjective

Increased appetite

Eating in response to internal cues other than hunger (eg, anxiety)

Reported use of solid food as major food source before 5 months of age

Objective

Obesity in one or both parents

Concentration of food intake at end of day

Dysfunctional eating patterns

Eating in response to external cues (eg, time of day or social situation)

Observed use of food as reward or comfort measure

Pairing food with other activities

Rapid transition across growth percentiles in infants or children

Reported or observed higher baseline weight at beginning of each pregnancy

Other Possible Risk Factors (non-NANDA)

Chemical dependence

Decreased metabolic requirements

Ethnic/cultural norms

Lack of basic nutritional knowledge

Lack of physical exercise

Suggestions for Use

See "Suggestions for Use" for "Nutrition: More Than Body Requirements, Altered" p. 300

Suggested Alternative Diagnoses

Coping: individual, ineffective

Health maintenance, altered

Management of therapeutic regimen: individual, ineffective

NOC Suggested Outcomes

Nutritional Status: Food and Fluid Intake: Amount of food and fluid taken into the body over a 24-hour period

Goals/Evaluation Criteria

Examples Using NOC Language

- Demonstrates **Nutritional Status: Food and Fluid Intake**, as evidenced by the following indicators (specify 1–5: not, slightly, moderately, substantially, or totally adequate): oral food and fluid intake not excessive

Other Examples

Patient will:

- Acknowledge presence of risk factors
- Participate in a regular exercise program

- Maintain ideal weight ____ (specify)
- Eat a balanced diet

NIC Priority Interventions

Nutrition Management: Assisting with or providing a balanced dietary intake of foods and fluids

Weight Management: Facilitating maintenance of optimal body weight and percent body fat

Nursing Activities

Assessments

- Monitor presence of risk factors for weight gain
- *(NIC) Weight Management:*
  Determine patient's ideal body weight
  Determine patient's ideal percent body fat
- *(NIC) Nutrition Management:* Weigh patient at appropriate intervals

Patient/Family Teaching

- Provide information regarding available community resources, such as dietary counseling, exercise programs, self-help groups
- *(NIC) Weight Management:*
  Discuss with the patient the relationship between food intake, exercise, weight gain, and weight loss
  Discuss with patient the medical conditions that may affect weight
  Discuss with patient the habits and customs and cultural and heredity factors that influence weight
  Discuss risks associated with being over- and underweight
  Assist in developing well-balanced meal plans consistent with level of energy expenditure

Other

- Develop a weight-management plan
- Develop a plan for management of eating to include the following:
  Frequency of meals and snacks
  Diet high in complex carbohydrates and protein
  Avoidance of simple sugars, fast food, caffeine, and soft drinks
  Recognition of high-risk situations (eg, types of foods, social situations, interpersonal stresses, unmet personal expectations, eating in secret/private)
- Provide frequent positive reinforcement for good nutrition and exercise

Oral Mucous Membrane, Altered
(1.6.2.1.1) (1982, 1998)

Definition: Disruptions of the lips and soft tissue of the oral cavity

Defining Characteristics

Subjective

Oral pain/discomfort
Self-report of bad taste
Self-report of difficulty eating or swallowing
Self-report of diminished or absent taste

Objective

Bleeding
Coated tongue
Desquamation
Difficult speech
Edema
Enlarged tonsils beyond what is developmentally appropriate
Fissures, cheilitis
Geographic tongue
Gingival hyperplasia
Gingival or mucosal pallor
Gingival recession, pockets deeper than 4 mm
Halitosis
Hyperemia
Macroplasia
Mucosal denudation
Oral lesions or ulcers
Presence of pathogens
Purulent drainage or exudates
Red or bluish masses (eg, hemangiomas)
Smooth, atrophic, sensitive tongue
Stomatitis
Vesicles, nodules, or papules
White patches/plaques, spongy patches, or white curdlike exudate
Xerostomia (dry mouth)

Other Defining Characteristics (non-NANDA)
Discomfort with hot or cold foods
Dry mouth
Dry, cracked lips
Lack of or decreased salivation

Related Factors

Aging-related loss of connective, adipose, or bony tissue
Barriers to oral self-care
Barriers to professional care
Chemotherapy
Chemical (eg, alcohol, tobacco, acidic foods, regular use of inhalers)
Cleft lip or palate
Decreased platelets
Dehydration
Depression
Diminished hormone levels (women)
Immunocompromised
Immunosuppression
Impaired salivation
Ineffective oral hygiene
Infection
Lack of or decreased salivation
Loss of supportive structures
Malnutrition or vitamin deficiency
Mechanical (eg, ill-fitting dentures, braces, tubes [endotracheal/ nasogastric])
Medication side effects
Mouth breathing
NPO for more than 24 hours
Pathologic conditions—oral cavity
Radiation therapy
Stress
Surgery in oral cavity
Trauma (eg, drugs, noxious agents)

Suggested Alternative Diagnoses

Dentition, altered
Tissue integrity, impaired

NOC Suggested Outcomes

Oral Health: Condition of the mouth, teeth, gums, and tongue
Tissue Integrity: Skin and Mucous Membranes: Structural intactness and normal physiologic function of skin and mucous membranes

Goals/Evaluation Criteria

Examples Using NOC Language

- Demonstrates **Oral Health**, as evidenced by the following indicators (specify 1–5: extremely, substantially, moderately, mildly, or not compromised):

  Cleanliness of mouth, teeth, gums, tongue, dentures, or dental appliances

  Moisture of oral mucosa and tongue

  Color of mucosa membranes [pink]

  Integrity of oral mucosa, tongue, gum[s], and [teeth]

  Breath free of halitosis

- Demonstrates **Tissue Integrity: Skin and Mucous Membranes**, as evidenced by the following indicators (specify 1–5: extremely, substantially, moderately, mildly, or not compromised):

  Tissue lesion free

  Sensation in expected range

Other Examples

Patient will:

- Ingest foods and fluids with increasing comfort
- Perform essential oral hygiene as prescribed/instructed

NIC Priority Interventions

Oral Health Restoration: Promotion of healing for a patient who has an oral mucosa or dental lesion

Nursing Activities

Assessments

- Identify irritating substances such as tobacco, alcohol, food, medications, extremes in food temperature, seasonings
- Assess patient's understanding of and ability to perform oral care
- *(NIC) Oral Health Restoration:*

  Determine the patient's perception of changes in taste, swallowing, quality of voice, and comfort

  Monitor patient every shift for dryness of the oral mucosa

  Monitor for signs and symptoms of glossitis and stomatitis

  Monitor for therapeutic effects of topical anesthetics, oral protective pastes, and topical or systemic analgesics, as appropriate

Patient/Family Teaching

- *(NIC) Oral Health Restoration:*
  Reinforce oral hygiene regimen as part of discharge teaching
  Instruct patient to avoid commercial mouthwashes
  Instruct patient to report signs of infection to physician immediately

Collaborative Activities

- Confer with physician regarding an order for antifungal mouthwash or oral topical anesthetic if fungal infection exists.
- *(NIC) Oral Health Restoration:*
  Consult physician if signs and symptoms of glossitis and stomatitis persist or worsen
  Apply topical anesthetics, oral protective pastes, and topical or systemic analgesics, as needed

Other

- Provide mouth care prior to meals and as needed
- Avoid use of sugared candies and gum
- Clean dentures after each meal
- *(NIC) Oral Health Restoration:*
  Plan small, frequent meals; select soft foods; and serve chilled or room-temperature foods
  Assist patient to select soft, bland, and nonacidic foods
  Increase mouth care to every 2 hours and twice at night if stomatitis is not controlled
  Use a soft toothbrush for removal of dental debris
  Encourage frequent rinsing of the mouth with any of the following: sodium bicarbonate solution, warm saline, or hydrogen peroxide solution
  Avoid use of lemon-glycerin swabs
  Discourage smoking and alcohol consumption
  Remove dentures in case of severe stomatitis

Pain
(9.1.1) (1978, 1996)

Definition: An unpleasant sensory and emotional experience arising from actual or potential tissue damage or described in terms of such damage (International Association for the Study of Pain); sudden or slow onset of any intensity from mild to severe with an anticipated or predictable end and a duration of less than 6 months

Defining Characteristics

Subjective

Verbal or coded report

Objective

Antalgic gestures

Antalgic position

Autonomic alteration in muscle tone (may span from listless to rigid)

Autonomic responses (eg, diaphoresis; blood pressure, respiration, or pulse changes; pupillary dilation)

Changes in appetite and eating

Distraction behavior (eg, pacing, seeking out other people and/or activities, repetitive activities)

Expressive behavior (eg, restlessness, moaning, crying, vigilance, irritability, sighing)

Facial mask [of pain]

Guarding or protective behavior

Narrowed focus (eg, altered time perception, impaired thought processes, reduced interaction with people and environment)

Observed evidence [of pain]

Self-focus

Sleep disturbance (eyes lack luster, "hecohe look," fixed or scattered movement, grimace)

Other Defining Characteristics (non-NANDA)

Communication of pain descriptors (eg, pain, discomfort, nausea, night sweats, muscle cramps, itching skin, numbness, tingling of extremities)

Grimacing

Limited attention span

Pacing

Pallor

Withdrawal

Related Factors

Injury agents (eg, biologic, chemical, physical, psychologic)

Suggestions for Use

Pain can be diagnosed on the patient's report alone because that is sometimes the only sign of *Pain*. None of the other defining characteristics taken alone would be sufficient to diagnose *Pain*.

The related factors indicate that a patient can suffer both physical and psychologic *Pain.* Qualifier words should be added to this diagnosis to indicate the severity, location, and nature of the pain. Two examples of appropriate diagnoses are as follows: *Severe, stabbing chest pain related to fractured ribs,* and *Mild frontal headache related to sinus congestion.*

It is important to differentiate between *Pain* and *Chronic pain* because the nursing focus is different for each. Acute pain (eg, postoperative incision pain) is usually a collaborative problem managed primarily by administering narcotic analgesics. There are a few independent nursing interventions for acute *Pain,* such as teaching the patient to splint the incision while moving, but these alone would not provide adequate pain relief. The nurse takes a more active role in teaching patients self-management of *Chronic pain.* When pain is acute or caused by a stressor not amenable to nursing intervention (eg, surgical incision), it may be an etiology rather than a problem. Two such examples of appropriate diagnoses are as follows: *Ineffective airway clearance related to weak cough secondary to Pain from chest incision* and *Sexual dysfunction related to partner's severe Chronic pain secondary to arthritis.*

In differentiating between *Pain* and *Chronic pain,* the comparison in Table 4 may be helpful.

Table 4

Defining Characteristics	Pain	Chronic Pain
Duration less than 6 months	X	
Duration longer than 6 months		X
Autonomic responses, such as pallor, increase in vital signs, and diaphoresis	X	
Personality changes		X
Weight Loss		X

Pain can also be the etiology (ie, related factor) for other nursing diagnoses, such as *Powerlessness related to inability to cope with Chronic pain* and *Self-care deficit: dressing/grooming, related to joint Pain with movement.*

Suggested Alternative Diagnosis

Pain, chronic

NOC Suggested Outcomes

Comfort Level: Feelings of physical and psychologic ease
Pain Control Behavior: Personal actions to control pain
Pain: Disruptive Effects: Observed or reported disruptive effects of pain on emotions and behavior
Pain Level: Amount of reported or demonstrated pain

Goals/Evaluation Criteria

Examples Using NOC Language

- Demonstrates **Pain: Disruptive Effects**, as evidenced by the following indicators (specify 1–5: severe, substantial, moderate, slight, or none):
    Impaired role performance or interpersonal relationships
    Compromised work, life enjoyment, or sense of control
    Impaired concentration
    Disrupted sleep
    Lack of appetite or difficulty eating
- Demonstrates **Pain Level**, as evidenced by the following indicators (specify 1–5: severe, substantial, moderate, slight, or none):
    Oral or facial expressions of pain
    Protective body positions
    Restlessness or muscle tension
    Change in respiratory rate, heart rate, or blood pressure

Other Examples

Patient will:

- Demonstrate individualized relaxation techniques that are effective for achieving comfort
- Maintain pain level at _____ or less (on scale of 0–10)
- Report physical and psychologic well-being
- Recognize causal factors and use measures to prevent pain
- Report pain to health care provider
- Use analgesic and nonanalgesic relief measures appropriately

NIC Priority Interventions

Analgesic Administration: Use of pharmacologic agents to reduce or eliminate pain
Conscious Sedation: Administration of sedatives, monitoring of the patient's response, and provision of necessary physiologic support during a diagnostic or therapeutic procedure

Pain Management: Alleviation of pain or a reduction in pain to a level of comfort that is acceptable to the patient

Patient-Controlled Analgesia (PCA) Assistance: Facilitating patient control of analgesic administration and regulation

Nursing Activities

Assessments

- Use self-report as first choice to obtain assessment information
- Ask patient to rate pain/discomfort on a scale of 0 to 10 (0 = no pain/discomfort, 10 = worst pain)
- Use pain flow sheet to monitor pain relief of analgesics and possible side effects
- Assess the impact of religion, culture, beliefs, and circumstances on patient's pain and responses
- In assessing patient's pain, use words that are consistent with patient's age and developmental level
- *(NIC) Pain Management:*

  Perform a comprehensive assessment of pain to include location, characteristics, onset/duration, frequency, quality, intensity or severity of pain, and precipitating factors

  Observe for nonverbal cues of discomfort, especially in those unable to communicate effectively

Patient/Family Teaching

- Include in discharge instructions the specific medication to be taken, frequency of administration, potential side effects, potential medication interactions, specific precautions when taking the medication (eg, physical activity limitations, dietary restrictions), and name of person to notify about unrelieved pain
- Instruct patient to inform nurse if pain relief is not achieved
- Inform patient of procedures that may increase pain and offer suggestions for coping
- Correct misconceptions about narcotic/opioid analgesics (eg, risks of addiction and overdose)
- *(NIC) Pain Management:*

  Provide information about the pain, such as causes of the pain, how long it will last, and anticipated discomforts from procedures

  Use pain-control measures before pain becomes severe

  Teach the use of nonpharmacologic techniques (eg, biofeedback, transcutaneous electrical nerve stimulation [TENS], hypnosis, relaxation, guided imagery, music therapy, distraction, play therapy, activity therapy, acupressure, hot/cold application, and massage) before, after, and if possible, during painful activities; before pain occurs or increases; and along with other pain-relief measures

Collaborative Activities

- Manage immediate postoperative pain with scheduled opiate (eg, q4 hours for 36 hours) or PCA
- *(NIC) Pain Management:* Notify physician if measures are unsuccessful or if current complaint is a significant change from patient's past experience of pain

Other

- Adjust frequency of dosage as indicated by pain assessment and side effects
- Help patient identify comfort measures that have worked in the past, such as distraction, relaxation, or application of heat/cold
- Attend to comfort needs and other activities to assist relaxation, including the following measures:

  Offer position change, back rubs, and relaxation

  Change bed linen, as necessary

  Provide care in an unhurried, supportive manner

  Involve patient in decisions regarding care activities
- Help patient focus on activities rather than on pain/discomfort by providing diversion through television, radio, tapes, and visitors
- Note that the elderly have increased sensitivity to analgesic effects of opiates, with higher peak effect and longer duration of pain relief
- Be alert to possible drug-drug and drug-disease interactions in the elderly, who often have multiple illnesses and take multiple medications
- Use a positive approach in order to optimize patient response to analgesics (eg, "This will help relieve your pain.")
- Explore feelings about fear of addiction. To reassure patient, ask, "If you didn't have this pain, would you still want to take this drug?"
- *(NIC) Pain Management:*

  Incorporate the family in the pain relief modality, if possible

  Control environmental factors that may influence the patient's response to discomfort (eg, room temperature, lighting, and noise)

  Ensure pretreatment analgesia and/or nonpharmacologic strategies before painful procedures.

Pain, Chronic
(9.1.1.1) (1986, 1996)

Definition: An unpleasant sensory and emotional experience arising from actual or potential tissue damage or described in terms of such damage (International Association for the Study of Pain); sudden or slow onset of any intensity from mild to severe, constant or recurring, without an anticipated or predictable end and a duration of greater than 6 months

Defining Characteristics

Verbal or coded report or observed evidence of the following:
Protective behavior
Guarding behavior
Facial mask
Irritability
Self-focusing
Restlessness
Depression

Subjective

Fatigue
Fear of reinjury

Objective

Atrophy of involved muscle group
Altered ability to continue previous activities
Anorexia
Changes in sleep pattern
Reduced interaction with people
Sympathetic mediated responses (eg, temperature, cold, changes of body position, hypersensitivity)
Weight changes

Related Factors

Chronic physical-psychosocial disability (eg, metastatic cancer, neurologic injury, arthritis)

Suggestions for Use

See "Suggestions for Use" for "Pain" on pp. 310–311

Suggested Alternative Diagnosis

Pain

NOC Suggested Outcomes

Comfort Level: Feelings of physical and psychologic ease

Pain Control Behavior: Personal actions to control pain

Pain: Disruptive Effects: Observed or reported disruptive effects of pain on emotions and behavior

Pain Level: Amount of reported or demonstrated pain

Goals/Evaluation Criteria

Examples Using NOC Language

- Demonstrates **Pain: Disruptive Effects**, as evidenced by the following indicators (specify 1–5: severe, substantial, moderate, slight, or none):

    Impaired role performance or interpersonal relationships

    Compromised work, life enjoyment, or sense of control

    Impaired concentration

    Disrupted sleep

    Lack of appetite or difficulty eating

- Demonstrates **Pain Level**, as evidenced by the following indicators (specify 1–5: severe, substantial, moderate, slight, or none):

    No oral or facial expressions of pain

    No protective body positions

    No restlessness or muscle tension

    No appetite loss

    Frequency of pain and length of pain episodes reported as moderate or slight

Other Examples

- Verbalizes knowledge of alternative measures for pain relief
- Patient's level of pain is maintained at _____ or less (on scale of 0–10)
- Reports physical and psychologic well-being
- Recognizes factors that increase pain and takes preventive measures
- Appropriately uses analgesic and nonanalgesic relief measures

NIC Priority Interventions

Analgesic Administration: Use of pharmacologic agents to reduce or eliminate pain

Pain Management: Alleviation of pain or a reduction in pain to a level of comfort that is acceptable to the patient

Patient-Controlled Analgesia (PCA) Assistance: Facilitation of patient control of analgesic administration and regulation

Nursing Activities

Also refer to "Nursing Activities" for "Pain" on pp. 313–314

Assessments

- Assess and document effects of long-term medication use
- *(NIC) Pain Management:*
  Monitor patient satisfaction with pain management at specified
  intervals
  Determine the impact of the pain experience on quality of life
  (eg, sleep, appetite, activity, cognition, mood, relationships,
  performance of job, and role responsibilities)

Patient/Family Teaching

- Convey to patient that total pain relief may not be achievable

Collaborative Activities

- Initiate a multidisciplinary patient care planning conference
- *(NIC) Pain Management:*
  Consider referrals for patient, family, and significant others to
  support groups and other resources, as appropriate

Other

- Offer patient pain-relief measures to supplement pain medica-
  tion (eg, biofeedback, relaxation techniques, back rub)
- Assist patient in identifying reasonable and acceptable level of
  pain
- *(NIC) Pain Management:*
  Promote adequate rest/sleep to facilitate pain relief
  Medicate before an activity to increase participation but evalu-
  ate the hazard of sedation

Parent/Child Attachment, Risk for Altered (3.2.1.1.2.1) (1994)

Definition: Disruption of the interactive process between par-
ent/significant other and infant that fosters the development of
a protective and nurturing reciprocal relationship

Risk Factors

Anxiety associated with the parent role
Ill infant/child who is unable to effectively initiate parental contact
due to altered behavioral organization

Inability of parents to meet the child's personal needs
Lack of privacy
Physical barriers
Premature infant
Separation
Substance abuse

Suggestions for Use

Use this diagnosis when parent(s) are at risk for attachment problems. If actual signs of delayed attachment are observed, use *Risk for altered parenting related to Altered parent/infant/child attachment.*

Suggested Alternative Diagnoses

Parenting, altered
Parenting, risk for altered

NOC Suggested Outcomes

Child Development: 2, 4, 6, and 12 Months and 2, 3, 4, and 5 years: Milestones of physical, cognitive, and psychosocial progression by 2, 4, 6, and 12 months; and 2, 3, 4, and 5 years of age. [**NOTE:** NOC has separate outcomes and indicators for each age.]

Parent-Infant Attachment: Behaviors that demonstrate an enduring affectionate bond between a parent and infant

Parenting: Provision of an environment that promotes optimum growth and development of dependent children

Goals/Evaluation Criteria

Examples Using NOC Language

- Demonstrate **Parent-Infant Attachment**, as evidenced by the following indicators (specify 1–5: never, rarely, sometimes, often, or consistently demonstrated):

    Parent will:

    Practice healthy behaviors during pregnancy
    Assign specific attributes to fetus
    Prepare for infant prior to birth
    Hold, touch, stroke, pat, kiss, and smile at infant
    Talk to infant
    Use en face position and eye contact
    Play with infant

    Respond to infant cues

    Console/soothe infant

    Keep infant dry, clean, and warm

  Infant will do the following:

    Look at parent(s)

    Respond to parent(s)' cues

- Demonstrate **Parenting**, as evidenced by the following indicators (specify 1–5: not, slightly, moderately, substantially, or totally adequate):

    Stimulate child's cognitive and social development

    Facilitate the child's emotional and spiritual growth

    Demonstrate a loving relationship with child

    Verbalize positive attributes of child

NIC Priority Interventions

Attachment Promotion: Facilitation of the development of the parent-infant relationship

Environmental Management: Attachment Process: Manipulation of the patient's surroundings to facilitate the development of the parent-infant relationship

Parent Education: Childbearing Family: Preparing another to perform the role of parent

Teaching: Infant Care: Instruction on nurturing and physical care needed during the first year of life

Nursing Activities

Assessments

- Assess parent's learning needs
- Identify parent's readiness to learn about infant care
- Assess parent's ability to recognize infant's physiologic needs (eg, hunger cues)
- *(NIC) Attachment Promotion:*

    Ascertain before birth whether parent(s) has names picked out for both sexes

    Discuss parent's reaction to pregnancy

Patient/Family Teaching

- Teach/demonstrate care of newborn (eg, feeding, bathing)
- Teach parent(s) about child development
- Assist parents in interpreting infant/child's cues and changing needs (eg, nonverbal cues, crying, and vocalizations)

- Teach quieting techniques and support parent's ability to relieve child's distress
- *(NIC) Attachment Promotion:*
  Inform parent(s) of care being given to newborn
  Explain equipment used to monitor infant in nursery
  Demonstrate ways to touch infant confined to Isolette
  Share information gained from initial physical assessment of newborn with parent(s)
  Discuss infant behavioral characteristics with parent(s)

Other

Prenatal Period

- *(NIC) Attachment Promotion:*
  Provide parent(s) the opportunity to hear fetal heart tones as soon as possible
  Provide parent(s) the opportunity to see the ultrasound image of the fetus
  Encourage parent(s) to attend prenatal and/or parenting classes

Intrapartum Period

- *(NIC) Attachment Promotion:*
  Encourage father/significant other to participate in labor and delivery
  Place infant on mother's body immediately after birth
  Provide opportunity for parent(s) to see, hold, and examine newborn immediately after birth
  Provide family privacy during initial interaction with newborn
- *(NIC) Environmental Management: Attachment Process:*
  Limit number of people in delivery room
  Provide comfortable chair for father/significant other
  Maintain low level of stimuli in patient and family environment

Neonatal Period

- *(NIC) Attachment Promotion:*
  Assist parent(s) to participate in infant care
  Reinforce caregiver role behaviors
  Reinforce normal aspects of infant with defect
  Encourage parent(s) to bring personal items, such as toy or picture, to be put in Isolette or at bedside of infant
  Inform parent(s) of care being given to infant in another hospital
  Discuss infant behavioral characteristics with parent(s)
  Point out infant cues that show responsiveness to parent(s)

Keep infant with parent(s) after birth, when possible

Encourage parents to massage infant

Encourage parent(s) to touch and speak to newborn

- *(NIC) Environmental Management: Attachment Process:*

  Permit father/significant other to sleep in room with mother

  Reduce interruptions by hospital personnel

Parental Role Conflict
(3.2.3.1) (1988)

Definition: The state in which a parent experiences role confusion and conflict in response to crisis

Defining Characteristics

Subjective

Expressed concern about perceived loss of control over decisions relating to child

Expressed concern/feelings of inadequacy to provide for child's physical/emotional needs during hospitalization or in the home

Expressed concerns about changes in parental role, family functioning, family communication, family health

Verbalizes or demonstrates feelings of guilt, anger, fear, anxiety, and/or frustrations about effect of child's illness on family process

Objective

Demonstrated disruption in caretaking routines

Reluctance to participate in usual caretaking activities, even with encouragement and support

Related Factors

Change in marital status [eg, career, roles]

Financial crisis

Home care of a child with special needs [eg, apnea monitoring, postural drainage, hyperalimentation]

Interruptions in family life due to home care regimen [eg, treatments, caregivers, lack of respite]

Intimidation with invasive or restrictive modality [eg, isolation, intubation]

Specialized care centers, policies

Separation from child due to chronic illness

Suggestions for Use

Use this label when a situation causes unsatisfactory role performance by previously effective parents

Suggested Alternative Diagnoses

Caregiver role strain (actual/risk for)
Coping: family, ineffective, compromised
Family processes, altered
Parenting, altered
Parenting, risk for altered

NOC Suggested Outcomes

Caregiver Adaptation to Patient Institutionalization: Family caregiver adaptation of role when the care recipient is transferred outside the home

Caregiver Home Care Readiness: Preparedness to assume responsibility for the health care of a family member or significant other in the home

Coping: Actions to manage stressors that tax an individual's resources

Parenting: Provision of an environment that promotes optimum growth and development of dependent children

Psychosocial Adjustment: Life Change: Psychosocial adaptation of an individual to a life change

Role Performance: Congruence of an individual's role behavior with role expectations

Goals/Evaluation Criteria

Examples Using NOC Language

- *Parental role conflict* will be resolved or alleviated, as evidenced by satisfactory Caregiver Adaptation to Patient Institutionalization, Caregiver Home Care Readiness, Coping, Parenting, Psychosocial Adjustment: Life Change, and Role Performance.
- **Coping** will be demonstated, as evidenced by the following indicators (specify 1–5: never, rarely, sometimes, often, or consistently demonstrated):

     Uses available social supports
     Uses effective coping strategies
     Seeks professional help, as appropriate
     Seeks information concerning illness and treatment

- **Parenting will be demonstrated,** as evidenced by the following indicators (specify 1–5: not, slightly, moderately, substantially, or totally adequate):

  Provides for the child's physical needs

  Provides for the child's special needs

  Stimulates cognitive and social development

  Stimulates emotional and spiritual growth

  Demonstrates a loving relationship with child

- **Role Performance will be demonstrated**, as evidenced by the following indicators (specify 1–5: not, slightly, moderately, substantially, or totally adequate): performance of family and work role behaviors

Other Examples

The parent/caregiver will:

- Demonstrate ability to modify parenting role in response to crisis
- Express a sense of adequacy in providing for child's needs
- Be available to support child and give consent for treatments
- Develop trust in health care providers
- Express willingness to assume caregiving role
- Demonstrate knowledge of the child's illness, treatment regimen, and emergency care

NIC Priority Interventions

Crisis Intervention: Use of short-term counseling to help the patient cope with a crisis and resume a state of functioning comparable to or better than the precrisis state

Family Process Maintenance: Minimization of family process disruption effects

Role Enhancement: Assisting a patient, significant other, and/or family to improve relationships by clarifying and supplementing specific role behaviors

Nursing Activities

Assessment

- Ask parents to describe how they want to be involved in the care of their hospitalized child
- *(NIC) Family Process Maintenance:*

  Determine typical family processes

  Identify effects of role changes on family processes

Patient/Family Teaching

- Teach new role behaviors created by the crisis situation
- Explain rationale for treatments and encourage questions to minimize misunderstandings and maximize participation
- *(NIC) Family Process Maintenance:* Teach family time management/organization skills when performing patient home care, as needed

Collaborative Activities

- *(NIC) Family Process Maintenance:* Assist family members to use existing support mechanisms

Other

- Confront parents with their ineffective parenting behaviors (during this crisis) and discuss alternatives
- Help parents to identify personal strengths and coping skills that may be useful in resolving the crisis
- Discuss with parent(s) a strategy for meeting personal/family's current needs
- Give positive reinforcement for constructive parental actions
- *(NIC) Family Process Maintenance:*

  Keep opportunities for visiting flexible to meet needs of family members and patient

  Provide mechanisms for family members staying at health care agency to communicate with other family members (eg, telephones, tape recordings, open visiting, photographs, and videotapes)

  Assist family members to facilitate home visits by patient, when appropriate

Parenting, Altered
(3.2.1.1.1) (1978, 1998)

Definition: Inability of the primary caretaker to create, maintain, or regain an environment that promotes the optimum growth and development of the child

Defining Characteristic

Infant or Child

Objective

Behavioral disorders

Failure to thrive

Frequent accidents

Frequent illness

Incidence of physical and psychologic trauma or abuse

Lack of attachment

Lack of separation anxiety

Poor academic performance

Poor cognitive development

Poor social competence

Runaway

Parental

Subjective

Negative statements about child

Statements of inability to meet child's needs

Verbalization of role inadequacy frustration

Verbalization that cannot control child

Objective

Abandonment

Child abuse

Child neglect

High punitiveness

Inadequate child health maintenance

Inappropriate child-care arrangements

Inappropriate visual, tactile, and auditory stimulation

Inconsistent behavior management

Inconsistent care

Inflexibility to meet needs of child, situation

Insecure or lack of attachment to infant

Little cuddling

Maternal-child interaction deficit

Poor or inappropriate caretaking skills [eg, involving toilet training, sleep/rest, feeding, discipline]

Poor parent-child interaction

Rejection or hostility to child

Unsafe home environment

Other Defining Characteristics (non-NANDA)

Child care from multiple caretakers without consideration of infant's/child's needs

Compulsive seeking of role approval from others

Growth and development lag

Noncompliance with child's health appointments

Related Factors

Infant or Child

Altered perceptual abilities

Attention-deficit hyperactivity disorder

Difficult temperament

Handicapping condition or developmental delay

Illness

Lack of goodness of fit (ie, temperament) with parental expectations

Multiple births

Not gender desired

Premature birth

Prolonged separation from parent

Separation from parent at birth

Unplanned or unwanted child

Knowledge

Inability to recognize and act on infant cues

Lack of cognitive readiness for parenthood

Lack of knowledge about child development

Lack of knowledge about child health maintenance

Lack of knowledge about parenting skills

Limited cognitive functioning

Low educational level or attainment

Poor communication skills

Preference for physical punishment

Unrealistic expectation for self, infant, partner

Physiologic

Physical illness

Psychologic

Depression

Difficult labor and/or delivery

Disability

High number or closely spaced pregnancies

History of mental illness

History of substance abuse or dependencies

Lack of, or late, prenatal care

Multiple births

Separation from infant/child

Sleep deprivation or disruption

Young age, especially adolescent

Social

Change in family unit

Father of child not involved

Financial difficulties

History of being abused

History of being abusive

Inability to put child's needs before own

Inadequate child-care arrangements

Lack of access to resources

Lack of family cohesiveness

Lack of resources

Lack of social support networks

Lack of transportation

Lack of value of parenthood

Lack of, or poor, parental role model

Legal difficulties

Low self-esteem

Low socioeconomic class

Maladaptive coping strategies

Marital conflict, declining satisfaction

Poor home environments

Poor problem-solving skills

Poverty

Presence of stress (eg, financial, legal, recent crisis, cultural, move)

Relocations

Role strain or overload

Single parents

Social isolation

Unemployment or job problems

Unplanned or unwanted pregnancy

Suggestions for Use

Adjustment to parenting in general is a normal maturational process that elicits nursing behaviors of prevention of potential problems and health promotion" (NANDA 1999, p. 55). This label represents a less healthy level of functioning than *Parental role conflict,* in which a parent or parents have been functioning satisfactorily but face situational challenges (eg, divorce, illness) that create role conflict and confusion. Unresolved *Parental role conflict* may progress to *Altered parenting.*

Suggested Alternative Diagnoses

Caregiver role strain (actual/risk for)
Coping: family, ineffective, disabling
Development, risk for altered
Growth, risk for altered
Family processes, altered
Parental role conflict
Parenting, risk for altered
Role performance, altered

NOC Suggested Outcomes

Child Development (2, 4, 6, and 12 months; 2, 3, 4, and 5 years; 6–11 years, and 12–17 years): Milestones of physical, cognitive, and psychosocial progression by _____ age. [**NOTE:** NOC has separate outcomes and indicators for each age.]

Parent-Infant Attachment: Behaviors that demonstrate an enduring affectionate bond between a parent and infant

Parenting: Provision of an environment that promotes optimum growth

Parenting: Social Safety: Parental actions to avoid social relationships that might cause harm or injury

Role Performance: Congruence of an individual's role behavior with role expectations

Safety Behavior: Home Physical Environment: Individual or caregiver actions to minimize environmental factors that might cause physical harm or injury in the home

Social Support: Perceived availability and actual provision of reliable assistance from other persons

Goals/Evaluation Criteria

Also see "Goals/Evaluation Criteria" for "Altered Growth and Development," pp. 186–187, and "Risk for Altered Parenting," on page 334

Examples Using NOC Language

• Demonstrates **Parent-Infant Attachment**, as evidenced by the following indicators (specify 1–5: never, rarely, sometimes, often, or consistently demonstrated):

> Verbalize positive feelings toward infant
> Touch, stroke, pat, kiss, and smile at infant
> Visit nursery
> Talk to infant
> Use en face position and eye contact

- Demonstrates **Parenting**, as evidenced by the following indicators (specify 1–5: not, slightly, moderately, substantially, or totally adequate):

    Provides for the child's physical needs

    Stimulates cognitive and social development

    Stimulates emotional and spiritual growth

    Demonstrates a loving relationship with child

    Provides regular preventative and episodic health care

- Demonstrates **Role Performance**, as evidenced by the following indicators (specify 1–5: not, slightly, moderately, substantially, or totally adequate):

    Performance of family role behaviors

    Reported comfort with role expectation

- Demonstrates **Safety Behavior: Home Physical Environment**, as evidenced by the following indicators (specify 1–5: not, slightly, moderately, substantially, or totally adequate):

    Smoke detector maintenance

    Disposal of unused medicines

    Storage of firearms to prevent accidents

    Storage of hazardous materials to prevent injury

    Provision of a safe play area

    Use of electrical outlet covers

Other Examples

The parent(s) will:

- Demonstrate constructive discipline
- Identify effective ways to express anger/frustration that are not harmful to child
- Actively participate in counseling and/or parenting classes
- Identify/use community resources that assist with home care
- Identify people who can provide information and emotional support when needed
- Indicate willingness to ask others for help

    The child will:

- Achieve physical, cognitive, and psychosocial milestones at expected times. (Refer to appropriate age group for specific developmental norms.)

NIC Priority Interventions

Abuse Protection: Child: Identification of high-risk, dependent child relationships and actions to prevent possible or further infliction of physical, sexual, or emotional harm or neglect of basic necessities of life

Attachment Promotion: Facilitation of the development of the parent-infant relationship

Developmental Enhancement: Facilitating or teaching parents/caregivers to facilitate the optimal gross-motor, fine-motor, language, cognitive, social, and emotional growth of preschool and school-aged children

Family Integrity Promotion: Promotion of family cohesion and unity

Nursing Activities

Refer to "Nursing Activities" for "Parenting, Risk for Altered," pp. 335–337

Collaborative Activities

- Offer to make initial telephone call to appropriate community resources
- *(NIC) Abuse Protection: Child:*

    Refer families to human services and counseling professionals, as needed

    Provide parents with community resource information that includes addresses and phone numbers of agencies that provide respite care, emergency child care, housing assistance, substance abuse treatment, sliding-fee counseling services, food pantries, clothing distribution centers, health care, human services, hot lines, and domestic abuse shelters

    Report suspected abuse or neglect to proper authorities

    Refer parents to Parents Anonymous for group support, as appropriate

Other

- Encourage expression of feelings (eg, guilt, anger, ambivalence) regarding parenting role
- Help parent identify deficits/alterations in parenting skills
- Provide frequent opportunities for parent/child interaction
- Role model parenting skills
- Help identify realistic expectations of parenting role
- Acknowledge and reinforce parenting strengths and skills
- *(NIC) Family Integrity Promotion:*

    Establish trusting relationship with family members

    Assist family with conflict resolution

    Assist family to resolve feelings of guilt

    Facilitate a tone of togetherness within/among the family

    Facilitate open communications among family members

During Pregnancy

- *(NIC) Attachment Promotion:*

  Discuss parent's reaction to pregnancy

  Provide parent(s) the opportunity to hear fetal heart tones as soon as possible

  Discuss parent's reaction to hearing fetal heart tones, viewing ultrasound image, etc.

  Assist father/significant other during participation in labor and delivery

At Delivery

- *(NIC) Attachment Promotion:*

  Place infant on mother's body immediately after birth

  Provide father opportunity to hold newborn in delivery area

  Provide pain relief for mother

  Provide family privacy during initial interaction with newborn

  Encourage parents to touch and speak to newborn

Parenting, Risk for Altered
(3.2.1.1.2) (1978, 1998)

Definition: Risk for inability of the primary caretaker to create, maintain, or regain an environment that promotes the optimum growth and development of the child

Risk Factors

Infant or Child

Altered perceptual abilities

Attention-deficit hyperactivity disorder

Difficult temperament

Handicapping condition or developmental delay

Illness

Lack of goodness of fit (ie, temperament) with parental expectations

Multiple births

Not gender desired

Premature birth

Prolonged separation from parent

Separation from parent at birth

Unplanned or unwanted child

Knowledge

Inability to recognize and act on infant cues
Lack of cognitive readiness for parenthood
Lack of knowledge about child development
Lack of knowledge about child health maintenance
Lack of knowledge about parenting skills
Low cognitive functioning
Low educational level or attainment
Poor communication skills
Preference for physical punishment
Unrealistic expectations of child

Physiologic

Physical illness

Psychologic

Depression
Difficult labor and/or delivery
Disability
High number or closely spaced children
History of mental illness
History of substance abuse or dependence
Lack of, or late, prenatal care
Multiple births
Separation from infant/child
Sleep deprivation or disruption
Young ages, especially adolescent

Social

Change in family unit
Father of child not involved
Financial difficulties
History of being abused
History of being abusive
Inability to put child's needs before own
Inadequate child-care arrangements
Lack of access to resources
Lack of family cohesiveness
Lack of or poor parental role model
Lack of resources
Lack of social support network
Lack of transportation
Lack of value of parenthood
Legal difficulties

Low self-esteem
Low socioeconomic class
Maladaptive coping strategies
Marital conflict, declining satisfaction
Poor home environment
Poor problem-solving skills
Poverty
Relocation
Role strain/overload
Single parent
Social isolation
Stress
Unemployment or job problems
Unplanned or unwanted pregnancy

Suggestions for Use

NANDA states that, in general, adjustment to parenting is a normal maturational process that calls for nursing interventions to prevent potential problems and promote health.

Suggested Alternative Diagnoses

Caregiver role strain, risk for
Coping: family, ineffective, compromised
Coping: family, potential for growth
Family processes, altered
Parent/infant/child attachment, risk for altered
Parental role conflict
Role performance, altered

NOC Suggested Outcomes

Abuse Recovery: Emotional: Healing of psychologic injuries due to abuse

Caregiver Stressors: The extent of biopsychosocial pressure on a family care provider caring for a family member or significant other over an extended period of time

Coping: Actions to manage stressors that tax an individual's resources

Parent-Infant Attachment: Behaviors that demonstrate an enduring affectionate bond between a parent and infant

Parenting: Provision of an environment that promotes optimum growth and development of dependent children

Risk Control: Unintended Pregnancy: Actions to reduce the possibility of unintended pregnancy

Goals/Evaluation Criteria

Also see "Goals/Evaluation Criteria" for "Parenting, Altered," pp. 328–329

Examples Using NOC Language

- Demonstrates **Coping**, as evidenced by the following indicators (specify 1–5: never, rarely, sometimes, often, or consistently demonstrated):
  Employs behaviors to reduce stress
  Identifies and uses multiple, effective coping strategies
- Demonstrates **Parenting**, as evidenced by the following indicators (specify 1–5: not, slightly, moderately, substantially, or totally adequate):
  Uses appropriate discipline
  Has realistic expectations of parental role
  Verbalizes positive attributes of child
- Demonstrates **Parent-Infant Attachment** (during pregnancy), as evidenced by the following indicators (specify 1–5: never, rarely, sometimes, often, or consistently demonstrated):
  Practice healthy behaviors
  Assign specific attributes to fetus
  Prepare for infant prior to birth

Other Examples

Parent(s) will:
- Identify own risk factors that may lead to ineffective parenting
- Identify high-risk situations that may lead to ineffective parenting
- Recognize and compensate for physical, cognitive, and/or psychologic limitations for caregiving
- Demonstrate recovery from past emotional abuses (eg, verbalize confidence and self-esteem)
- Seek help for emotional problems/neuroses
- Verbalize a sense of control over own behaviors and life situation
- Report having positive interpersonal relationships

NIC Priority Interventions

Abuse Protection, Child: Identification of high-risk, dependent child relationships and actions to prevent possible or further infliction of physical, sexual, or emotional harm or neglect of basic necessities of life

Attachment Promotion: Facilitation of the development of the parent-infant relationship

Developmental Enhancement: Facilitating or teaching parents/caregivers to facilitate the optimal gross-motor, fine-motor, language, cognitive, social, and emotional growth of preschool and school-age children

Family Integrity Promotion: Promotion of family cohesion and unity

Normalization Promotion: Assisting parents and other family members of children with chronic illnesses or disabilities in providing normal life experiences for their children and families

Nursing Activities

Assessment

- Determine whether parents have unrealistic expectations for child's behavior or negative attributions for their child's behavior
- *(NIC) Abuse Protection: Child:*

    Identify parents who have had another child removed from the home or have placed previous children with relatives for extended periods

    Identify parents who have a history of substance abuse, depression, or major psychiatric illness

    Identify parents who have a history of domestic violence or a mother who has a history of numerous "accidental" injuries

    Identify crisis situations that may trigger abuse (eg, poverty, unemployment, divorce, homelessness, and domestic violence)

    Identify infants/children with high-care needs (eg, prematurity, low birth weight, colic, feeding intolerances, major health problems in the first year of life, developmental disabilities, hyperactivity, and attention-deficit disorders)

- *(NIC) Attachment Promotion:*

    Ascertain before birth whether parent(s) has names picked out for both sexes

    Monitor new parents' reactions to their infant, observing for feelings of disgust, fear, or disappointment in gender

    Determine parent's knowledge of infant/child basic care needs and provide appropriate child-care information, as indicated

- *(NIC) Family Integrity Promotion:*

    Determine typical family relationships

    Monitor current family relationships

- *(NIC) Normalization Promotion:*
  [For a child with a chronic illness] determine the following:
  Accessibility of activity and child's ability to participate in activity
  Need for respite care for parents or other care providers

Patient/Parent Teaching

- *(NIC) Abuse Protection:*
  Determine parent's knowledge of infant/child basic care needs
    and provide appropriate child-care information, as indicated
  Instruct parents on problem-solving, decision-making, and
    childrearing and parenting skills or refer parents to programs
    where these skills can be learned
  Provide parents with information on how to cope with protracted
    infant crying, emphasizing that they should not shake the baby
  Provide the parents with noncorporal punishment methods for
    disciplining children
- *(NIC) Attachment Promotion:*
  Demonstrate ways to touch infant confined to Isolette
  Discuss infant behavioral characteristics with parent(s)
  Instruct parent(s) on signs of overstimulation
- *(NIC) Developmental Enhancement:* Teach caregivers about nor-
  mal developmental milestones and associated behaviors

Collaborative Activities

- Refer to community support/educational programs to assist with
  development of parenting skills and provide anticipatory guidance
- *(NIC) Abuse Protection: Child:*
  Refer at-risk pregnant women and parents of newborns to nurse
    home visitation services
  Provide at-risk families with a public health nurse referral to
    ensure that the home environment is monitored, that siblings
    are assessed, and that families receive continued assistance
- *(NIC) Attachment Promotion:* Encourage parent(s) to attend pre-
  natal classes
- *(NIC) Family Integrity Promotion:* Refer for family therapy, as
  indicated

Other

- *(NIC) Attachment Promotion:*
  Encourage father/significant other to participate in labor and
    delivery
  Provide opportunity for parent(s) to see, hold, and examine
    newborn immediately after birth

Share information gained from initial physical assessment of newborn with parent(s)

Provide family privacy during initial interaction with newborn

Reinforce attachment behaviors (eg, eye contact)

Acknowledge and reinforce parenting strengths and skills

[For newborns who are premature or ill], explain equipment used to monitor infant in nursery, encourage parent(s) to visit infant in the nursery, place pictures of family in Isolette so infant can "see" the family, take picture of infant to leave with mother before transporting infant to another hospital, and reinforce normal aspects of infant with defect

- *(NIC) Family Integrity Promotion:*

  Be a listener for the family members

  Facilitate a tone of togetherness within/among the family

  Facilitate open communications among family members

- *(NIC) Normalization Promotion* [for ill child]:

  Encourage parents to have same parenting expectations and techniques for affected child as with other children in family, as appropriate

  Assist family in making changes in home environment that decrease reminders of child's special needs

Perioperative Positioning Injury, Risk for
(6.1.1.1.2) (1994)

Definition: A state in which the client is at risk for injury as a result of the environmental conditions found in the perioperative setting

Risk Factors

[Advanced age]

Disorientation

Edema

Emaciation

Immobilization, muscle weakness

Obesity

Sensory/perceptual disturbances due to anesthesia

Suggestions for Use

This diagnosis is a specific variation of *Risk for injury*. All patients have at least some risk for *Perioperative positioning injury* (PPI). For those with no preexisting risk factors, no etiology is needed because the perioperative positioning itself is the etiology. When there are preexisting risk factors (eg, edema, advanced age, diabetes, arthritis, vascular disease), include them as the etiology (eg, *Risk for Perioperative positioning injury related to generalized edema*). A long surgical procedure also increases the risk for PPI.

Actual PPI may be the etiology of other nursing diagnoses (eg, *Impaired skin integrity*).

Suggested Alternative Diagnoses

Peripheral neurovascular dysfunction, risk for
Skin integrity, risk for impaired
Trauma, risk for

NOC Suggested Outcomes

Body Positioning: Self-Initiated: Ability to change own body positions

Circulation Status: Extent to which blood flows unobstructed, unidirectionally, and at an appropriate pressure through large vessels of the systemic and pulmonary circuits

Cognitive Ability: Ability to execute complex mental processes

Cognitive Orientation: Ability to identify person, place, and time

Muscle Function: Adequacy of muscle contraction needed for movement

Tissue Perfusion: Peripheral: Extent to which blood flows through the small vessels of the extremities and maintains tissue function

Goals/Evaluation Criteria

Examples Using NOC Language

- Demonstrates **Body Positioning: Self-Initiated** (specify 1–5: dependent, does not participate; requires assistive person and device; requires assistive person; independent with assistive device; or completely independent)
- Demonstrates **Cognitive Ability** (specify 1–5: extremely, substantially, moderately, mildly, or not compromised)
- Demonstrates **Cognitive Orientation** (specify 1–5: never, rarely, sometimes, often, or consistently demonstrated)
- Demonstrates **Tissue Perfusion: Peripheral** (specify 1–5: extremely, substantially, moderately, mildly, or not compromised)
- Demonstrates **Circulation Status**, as evidenced by the following indicators (specify 1–5: extremely, substantially, moderately, mildly, or not compromised):

Peripheral tissue perfusion
Peripheral pulses strong and symmetric
Systolic and diastolic blood pressure in expected range

Other Examples

Patient will have:

- No skin, tissue, or neuromuscular injury as a result of perioperative positioning
- Brisk capillary refill
- Normal peripheral sensation
- Normal skin color and temperature
- Unimpaired muscle function
- No peripheral edema
- No localized extremity pain

NIC Priority Interventions

Positioning: Intraoperative: Moving the patient or body part to promote surgical exposure while reducing the risk of discomfort and complications

Skin Surveillance: Collection and analysis of patient data to maintain skin and mucous membrane integrity

Nursing Activities

Assessments

- Determine preexisting factors (eg, poor nutrition, diseases) that create risk for PPI
- *(NIC) Positioning: Intraoperative:*
  Determine patient's range of motion and stability of joints
  Check peripheral circulation and neurologic status
  Monitor patient's position intraoperatively
- *(NIC) Skin Surveillance (postoperative period)*
  Observe extremities for color, warmth, swelling, pulses, texture, edema, and ulcerations
  Monitor skin for areas of redness and breakdown
  Monitor skin color and temperature

Patient/Family Teaching

- *(NIC) Skin Surveillance:* Instruct family member/caregiver about signs of skin breakdown, as appropriate.

Collaborative Activities

- *(NIC) Positioning: Intraoperative:* Communicate to postanesthesia nurses any preexisting risk factors and/or any symptoms observed during the intraoperative period

Other

- Lift patient when positioning; do not slide or pull patient
- Always reposition patient slowly and gently
- Ensure that surgical team members do not lean on the patient
- *(NIC) Positioning: Intraoperative:*
  Use assistive devices [eg, leg restraint strap] for immobilization
  Use an adequate number of personnel to transfer patient
  Support the head and neck during transfer
  Protect IV lines, catheters, and breathing circuits
  Maintain patient's proper body alignment. [Refer to agency procedures or a surgical textbook for details of supine, prone, lateral, and lithotomy positions.]
  Elevate extremities, as appropriate
  Apply padding [eg, to bony prominences] to avoid pressure to superficial nerves
  Apply safety strap and arm restraint, as needed
  Protect the eyes, as appropriate

Peripheral Neurovascular Dysfunction, Risk for (6.1.1.1.1) (1992)

Definition: A state in which an individual is at risk of experiencing a disruption in circulation, sensation, or motion of an extremity

Risk Factors

Burns
Fractures
Immobilization
Mechanical compression (eg, tourniquet, cast, brace, dressing, or restraint)
Orthopedic surgery
Trauma
Vascular obstruction

Suggestions for Use

Use this label for situations nurses can prevent by reducing or eliminating causative factors (eg, *Risk for peripheral neurovascular dysfunction related to compression from restraints*). For situations requiring medical treatment (eg, thrombophlebitis), use a collaborative problem such as Potential Complication of thrombophlebitis in left leg: Peripheral neurovascular dysfunction.

Suggested Alternative Diagnosis

Perioperative positioning injury, risk for

NOC Suggested Outcomes

Circulation Status: Extent to which blood flows unobstructed, unidirectionally, and at an appropriate pressure through large vessels of the systemic and pulmonary circuits

Neurological Status: Extent to which the peripheral and central nervous systems receive, process, and respond to internal and external stimuli

Neurological Status: Cranial Sensory/Motor Function: Extent to which cranial nerves convey sensory and motor information

Neurological Status: Spinal Sensory/Motor Function: Extent to which spinal nerves convey sensory and motor information

Tissue Perfusion: Peripheral: Extent to which blood flows through the small vessels of the extremities and maintains tissue function

Goals/Evaluation Criteria

Examples Using NOC Language

- Demonstrates **Circulation Status**, as evidenced by the following indicators (specify 1–5: extremely, substantially, moderately, mildly, or not compromised):
    Peripheral tissue perfusion not compromised
    Peripheral pulses strong and symmetric
    Peripheral edema not present
- Demonstrates **Neurological Status**, as evidenced by the following indicators (specify 1–5: extremely, substantially, moderately, mildly, or not compromised):
    Neurological status: consciousness, central motor control, autonomic, and cranial and spinal sensory/motor function
- Demonstrates **Tissue Perfusion: Peripheral**, as evidenced by the following indicators (specify 1–5: extremely, substantially, moderately, mildly, or not compromised):
    Brisk capillary refill
    Intact muscle function
    Intact skin
    Warm extremity temperature
    Lack of localized extremity pain

Other Examples

Patient will:

- Recognize signs and symptoms of peripheral neurovascular dysfunction
- Remain free of injury from compression devices or restraints
- Demonstrate optimal healing and adaptation to cast, traction, or dressing
- Have good muscle tone and strong movement of extremities

NIC Priority Interventions

Circulatory Care: Promotion of arterial and venous circulation

Exercise Therapy: Joint Mobility: Use of active or passive body movement to maintain or restore joint flexibility

Peripheral Sensation Management: Prevention or minimization of injury or discomfort in the patient with altered sensation

Nursing Activities

Assessments

- Perform neurovascular assessments every hour for the first 24 hours following casting, injury, traction, or restraints. Then, if stable, perform the following activities q4 hours:

    Assess for and report increasing and progressive pain that is present on passive movement and not relieved by narcotics, which may be first sign of compartmental syndrome

    Assess motor function, movement, and strength of the involved peripheral nerve

- *(NIC) Circulatory Care:* Perform a comprehensive appraisal of peripheral circulation (eg, check peripheral pulses, edema, capillary refill, color, and temperature of extremity)

- *(NIC) Peripheral Sensation Management:*

    Monitor for paresthesia: numbness, tingling, hyperesthesia, and hypoesthesia

    Monitor sharp/dull and/or hot/cold discrimination

    Monitor fit of bracing devices, prosthesis, shoes, and clothing

    Check shoes, pockets, and clothing for wrinkles or foreign objects

    Monitor for thrombophlebitis and deep vein thrombosis

Patient/Family Teaching

- Teach patient/family routine cast care and measures to prevent complications
- Teach patient/family signs and symptoms of peripheral nerve injury and importance of immediate medical attention

- Teach patient/family to perform passive, assisted, or active range-of-motion exercises
- *(NIC) Circulatory Care:*
  Instruct the patient on proper foot care
  Instruct the patient on the importance of prevention of venous stasis (eg, not crossing legs, elevating feet without bending knees, and exercise)
- *(NIC) Peripheral Sensation Management:*
  Instruct patient to use timed intervals, rather than presence of discomfort, as a signal to alter position
  Instruct patient or family to use thermometer to test water temperature

Collaborative Activities

- Collaborate with physical therapist in developing and executing an exercise program

Other

- Avoid tight dressings and appliances to prevent ischemia
- Institute immediate treatment if compartmental syndrome is suspected: keep involved extremity at heart level; notify physician; and anticipate removal of anterior cast, occlusive bandages, and surgical intervention
- Recognize that restlessness, fussiness, and crying may be nonverbal cues of physical distress in infants, children, or adults with impaired verbal communication
- Assure that patient's clothing is not restrictive
- Perform passive or assisted range-of-motion exercises
- *(NIC) Circulatory Care:*
  Elevate affected limb 20 degrees or greater above the level of the heart to improve venous return, as appropriate
  Lower extremity to improve arterial circulation, as appropriate
  Maintain adequate hydration to prevent increased blood viscosity.
  Restrict smoking
  Change the patient's position at least every 2 hours, as appropriate
- *(NIC) Peripheral Sensation Management:*
  Avoid or carefully monitor use of heat or cold, such as heating pads, hot-water bottles, and ice packs
  Encourage patient to use the unaffected body part to identify location and texture of objects

Place cradle over affected body parts to keep bed clothes off affected areas

Encourage patient to wear well-fitting, low-heeled, soft shoes

Personal Identity Disturbance
(7.1.3) (1978)

Definition: Inability to distinguish between self and nonself

Defining Characteristics

To be developed by NANDA

Objective (non-NANDA)

Change in social involvement

Extension of body boundary to incorporate environmental objects

Grandiose behavior

Related Factors

To be developed by NANDA

non-NANDA

Chronic illness

Chronic pain

Congenital defects

Psychologic impairment (specify)

Situational crisis (specify)

Suggestions for Use

None

Suggested Alternative Diagnoses

Confusion, acute

Confusion, chronic

Self-esteem disturbance

Thought processes, altered

NOC Suggested Outcomes

Identity: Ability to distinguish between self and nonself and to characterize one's essence

Goals/Evaluation Criteria

Examples Using NOC Language

• Demonstrates **Identity**, as evidenced by the following indicators (specify 1–5: never, rarely, sometimes, often, or consistently demonstrated):

> Verbalizes clear sense of personal identity
> Verbalizes affirmations of personal identity
> Exhibits congruent verbal and nonverbal behavior about self
> Differentiates self from environment
> Differentiates self from other human beings
> Establishes personal boundaries

Other Examples

Patient will:

- Express willingness to use suggested resources upon discharge
- Identify personal strengths
- Maintain close personal relationships

NIC Priority Interventions

Decision-Making Support: Providing information and support for a patient who is making a decision regarding health care

Self-Esteem Enhancement: Assisting a patient to increase his/her personal judgment of self-worth

Nursing Activities

Also refer to "Nursing Activities" for "Self-Esteem, Chronic low," on pp. 397–398, and "Self-Esteem, Situational Low," on p. 400

Assessments

- Assess need for assistance from Social Services Department for planning care with patient/family
- *(NIC) Self-Esteem Enhancement:*
  Monitor patient's statements of self-worth
  Determine patient's confidence in own judgment
  Monitor frequency of self-negating verbalizations

Patient/Family Teaching

- *(NIC) Decision-Making Support:* Provide information requested by patient
- *(NIC) Self-Esteem Enhancement:* Instruct parents on the importance of their interest and support in their children's development of a positive self-concept

Collaborative Activities

- Offer to make initial phone call to appropriate community resources for patient/family
- Request psychiatric consultation

- *(NIC) Decision-Making Support:*
  Refer to support groups, as appropriate
  Refer to legal aid, as appropriate

Other

- Encourage patient to verbalize concerns about close personal relationships
- Encourage patient to verbalize consequences of physical and emotional changes that have influenced self-concept
- Encourage patient/family to air feelings and to grieve
- Provide care in a nonjudgmental manner, maintaining the patient's privacy and dignity
- *(NIC) Decision-Making Support:*
  Establish communication with patient early in admission
  Facilitate collaborative decision making
  Serve as a liaison between patient and family
- *(NIC) Self-Esteem Enhancement:*
  Encourage patient to identify strengths
  Provide experiences that increase patient's autonomy, as appropriate
  Refrain from negatively criticizing
  Convey confidence in patient's ability to handle situation
  Encourage the patient to evaluate own behavior

Poisoning, Risk for
(1.6.1.2) (1980)

Definition: Accentuated risk of accidental exposure to or ingestion of drugs or dangerous products in doses sufficient to cause poisoning

Risk Factors

Internal (Individual)

Cognitive or emotional difficulties
Insufficient finances
Lack of proper precautions
Lack of safety or drug education
Reduced vision
Verbalization of occupational setting without adequate safeguards

External (Environmental)

Availability of illicit drugs potentially contaminated by poisonous additives

Chemical contamination of food and water

Dangerous products placed or stored within the reach of children or confused persons

Flaking, peeling paint or plaster in presence of young children

Large supplies of drugs in house

Medicines stored in unlocked cabinets accessible to children or confused persons

Paint, lacquer, and so on in poorly ventilated areas or without effective protection

Presence of atmospheric pollutants

Presence of poisonous vegetation

Unprotected contact with heavy metals or chemicals

Suggestions for Use

Use the most specific label for which defining characteristics are present (ie, if required risk factors are present, use *Risk for poisoning* instead of *Risk for injury*)

Suggested Alternative Diagnoses

Home maintenance management, impaired

Injury, risk for

Parenting, altered

Violence: self-directed, risk for

NOC Suggested Outcomes

Knowledge Medication: Extent of understanding conveyed about the safe use of medication

Risk Control: Actions to eliminate or reduce actual, personal, and modifiable health threats

Risk Control: Drug Use: Actions to eliminate or reduce drug use that poses a threat to health

Risk Detection: Actions taken to identify personal health threats.

Goals/Evaluation Criteria

Examples Using NOC Language

- Demonstrates **Risk Control**, as evidenced by the following indicators (specify 1–5: never, rarely, sometimes, often, or consistently demonstrated):

    Monitors personal behavior risk factors

    Monitors environmental risk factors

    Follows selected risk-control strategies

Other Examples

Patient will:

- Develop strategies to prevent poisoning
- Demonstrate understanding of safe use of medication, as indicated by description of proper methods of administration, dosage, storage, and disposal
- Seek information about potential risks

NIC Priority Interventions

Environmental Management, Safety: Monitoring and manipulation of the physical environment to promote safety

Surveillance, Safety: Purposeful and ongoing collection and analysis of information about the patient and the environment for use in promoting and maintaining patient safety

Nursing Activities

Assessments

- *(NIC) Environmental Management: Safety:* Monitor the environment for changes in safety status
- *(NIC) Surveillance: Safety:*

  Monitor patient for alterations in physical or cognitive function that might lead to unsafe behavior

  Identify the safety needs of patient based on level of physical and cognitive function and past history of behavior

Patient/Family Teaching

- Provide educational materials related to safety strategies and countermeasures for poisons
- *(NIC) Environmental Management: Safety:*

  Educate high-risk individuals and groups about environmental hazards (eg, lead and radon)

  Provide patient with emergency phone numbers (eg, police, local health department, and poison control center)

Collaborative Activities

- Refer to community classes (eg, cardiopulmonary resuscitation [CPR], first aid)
- *(NIC) Environmental Management: Safety:* Collaborate with other agencies to improve environmental safety (eg, health department, police, and Environmental Protection Agency [EPA]

Other

- *(NIC) Environmental Management: Safety:*

  Modify the environment to minimize hazards and risk

  Use protective devices (eg, restraints, side rails, locked doors, fences, and gates) to physically limit mobility or access to harmful situations

  (NIC) Surveillance: Safety: Provide appropriate level of supervision/surveillance to monitor patient and to allow for therapeutic actions, as needed

Post-Trauma Syndrome
(9.2.3) (1986, 1998)

Definition: A sustained maladaptive response to a traumatic, overwhelming event

Defining Characteristics

Subjective

Anger and/or rage

Fear

Flashbacks

Guilt

Headaches

Intrusive thoughts

Numbing

Palpitations

Shame

Objective

Aggression

Alienation

Altered mood states

Anxiety

Avoidance

Compulsive behavior

Denial

Depression

Detachment

Difficulty concentrating

Enuresis (in children)

Exaggerated startle response

Gastric irritability
Grief
Hopelessness
Horror
Hypervigilant
Intrusive dreams
Irritability
Neurosensory irritability
Nightmares
Panic attacks
Psychogenic amnesia
Repression
Substance abuse

Related Factors

Being held prisoner of war or criminal victimization (torture)
Epidemics
Events outside the range of usual human experience
Industrial and motor vehicle accidents
Military combat
Natural disasters and/or man-made disasters
Physical and psychosocial abuse
Rape
Serious accidents
Serious threat or injury to self or loved ones
Sudden destruction of one's home or community
Tragic occurrence involving multiple deaths
Wars
Witnessing mutilation, violent death, or other horrors

Suggestions for Use

(1) If the related factor is rape, use one of the *Rape-trauma syndrome* diagnoses. (2) Because this is a syndrome diagnosis, the diagnostic statement does not need related factors and the second part of the statement (etiology) is omitted. (3) Other nursing diagnoses (eg, *Risk for suicide*) may be needed in addition to *Rape-trauma syndrome* in order to focus nursing interventions more specifically.

Suggested Alternative Diagnoses

Coping: family, ineffective, compromised/disabling
Coping: individual, ineffective

Rape-trauma syndrome: compound reaction
Rape-trauma syndrome: silent reaction
Self-mutilation, risk for
Violence: self directed, risk for

NOC Suggested Outcomes

Abuse Cessation: Evidence that the victim is no longer abused

Abuse Protection: Protection of self or dependent others from abuse

Abuse Recovery: Emotional: Healing of psychologic injuries due to abuse

Abuse Recovery: Sexual: Healing following sexual abuse or exploitation

Coping: Actions to manage stressors that tax an individual's resources

Impulse Control: Ability to self-restrain compulsive or impulsive behaviors

Self-Mutilation Restraint: Ability to refrain from intentional self-inflicted injury (nonlethal)

Goals/Evaluation Criteria

Examples Using NOC Language

- Demonstrates **Abuse Recovery: Sexual**, as evidenced by the following indicators (specify 1–5: none, limited, moderate, substantial, or extensive):

    Details of abuse
    Feelings about the abuse
    Appropriate and inappropriate guilt
    Accurate information about sexual functioning
    Confidence with sexual orientation
    Right to have been protected from abuse
    Hope

- Demonstrates **Abuse Recovery: Emotional**, as evidenced by the following indicators (specify 1–5: none, limited, moderate, substantial, or extensive):

    Demonstrates appropriate affect for situation
    Does not attempt suicide
    Reports feeling less depressed
    Is able to control impulses
    Reports satisfaction with social interactions

Other Examples

Patient will:
- Acknowledge value of counseling
- Identify feelings and situations that lead to impulsive actions
- Control destructive/harmful impulses without supervision
- Seek helps when unable to control impulses
- Report relief from physical symptoms (eg, headache, gastrointestinal upset)

NIC Priority Interventions

Counseling: Use of an interactive helping process focusing on the needs, problems, or feelings of the patient and significant others to enhance or support coping, problem-solving, and interpersonal relationships

Support System Enhancement: Facilitation of support to patient by family, friends, and community

Nursing Activities

Also refer to "Nursing Activities" for "Post-Trauma Syndrome, Risk for," p. 354

Collaborative Activities

- Follow hospital/agency policy regarding legal responsibility for reporting to authorities

Other

- Enhance patient's feeling of safety in the following ways:
  Monitor/hold phone calls at patient's request
  Monitor/limit visitation
  Consider private versus semiprivate assignment and choice of roommate
  Institute precautions to prevent physical harm to the patient or others
- *(NIC) Counseling:*
  Establish a therapeutic relationship based on trust and respect
  Demonstrate empathy, warmth, and genuineness
  Use techniques of reflection and clarification to facilitate expression of concerns
  Encourage expression of feelings in a nondestructive manner
  Reveal selected aspects of one's own experiences or personality to foster genuineness and trust, as appropriate
  Discourage decision making when the patient is under severe stress

Post-Trauma Syndrome, Risk for
(9.2.4) (1998)

Definition: A risk for sustained maladaptive response to a traumatic or overwhelming event

Risk Factors

Diminished ego strength
Displacement from home
Duration of the event
Exaggerated sense of responsibility
Inadequate social support
Nonsupportive environment
Occupation (eg, police, fire, rescue, corrections, emergency room staff, mental health)
Perception of event
Survivor's role in the event

Suggestions for Use

(1) As a rule, syndrome diagnoses are one-part diagnostic statements, omitting the related factors. However, because this is a "risk for" (potential) diagnosis, it is helpful to write a two-part statement with the related factors as the etiology (eg, *Risk for post-trauma syndrome related to inadequate social support to aid in coping with aftermath of surviving a fire in which friends died*). (2) If defining characteristics are present for any of the suggested alternative diagnoses, the nurse will need to decide whether it is more useful to write an actual diagnosis (eg, *Social isolation related to unacceptable social values*) or to use the alternative diagnosis as an etiology (eg, *Risk for post-trauma syndrome related to Social isolation*).

Suggested Alternative Diagnoses

Coping: community, ineffective
Coping: family, ineffective, compromised/disabling
Coping: individual, ineffective
Family processes, altered
Personal identity disturbance
Self-esteem disturbance
Social isolation
Spiritual distress

NOC Suggested Outcomes

To be developed

Goals/Evaluation Criteria

- Risk factors will be identified and controlled/eliminated so that *Post-trauma syndrome* does not occur.
  Patient will:
- Display adequate ego strength
- Have adequate social support
- Demonstrate appropriate affect for the situation
- Demonstrate adequate social interaction
- Identify and use effective coping strategies

NIC Priority Interventions

To be developed

Nursing Activities

Assessments

- Assess psychologic response to the trauma
- Assess adequacy and availability of support system and community resources
- Assess family situation

Patient/Family Teaching

- Explain to significant others how they can provide support

Collaborative Activities

- Provide information/referral on community resources (eg, rape counselors, clergy, crisis centers, support groups, mental health professionals, Social Services, Victims' Assistance, Survivors of Trauma)

Other

- Provide opportunity for social supports and problem solving (eg, participation in social and community activities)
- Encourage patient to verbalize account of the event
- Support the patient needing an invasive medical procedure, which may precipitate flashbacks:
  Explain necessity of procedure
  Premedicate if needed to minimize distress/discomfort
  Stay with patient during procedure
  Encourage patient to discuss feelings after procedure

Powerlessness
(7.3.2) (1982)

Definition: Perception that one's own action will not significantly affect an outcome; a perceived lack of control over a current situation or immediate happening

Defining Characteristics

Severe

Subjective
Verbal expressions of having no control or influence over situation, self-care, or outcome

Objective
Apathy
Depression over physical deterioration that occurs despite patient compliance with regimens

Moderate

Subjective
Anger
Expressions of dissatisfaction and frustration over inability to perform previous tasks and/or activities
Expression of doubt regarding role performance
Fear of alienation from caregivers
Guilt
Reluctance to express true feelings

Objective
Dependence on others that may result in irritability, resentment, anger, and guilt
No defense of self-care practices when challenged
No monitoring of progress
Inability to seek information regarding care
Nonparticipation in care or decision making when opportunities are provided
Passivity
Resentment

Low

Subjective
Expressions of uncertainty about fluctuating energy levels

Objective
Passivity

Related Factors

Health care environment
Illness-related regimen [eg, long-term, difficult, complex]
Interpersonal interaction
Lifestyle of helplessness
Chronic or terminal illness (non-NANDA)
Complications threatening pregnancy (non-NANDA)

Suggestions for Use

Differentiate between *Powerlessness* and *Hopelessness. Hopelessness* implies that the person believes there *is* no solution to his/her problem (ie, "no way out"). In *Powerlessness,* patients may know of a solution to their problem but believe it is beyond their control to achieve the solution. If *Powerlessness* is prolonged, it can lead to *Hopelessness*. Nurses should be careful to diagnose *Powerlessness* from the *patient's* perspective and not assume the patient perceives the situation as they would. Cultural and individual differences exist in a person's need to feel in control of a situation (eg, to be told they have a fatal illness).

Suggested Alternative Diagnoses

Coping: individual, ineffective
Disuse syndrome, risk for
Grieving, dysfunctional
Hopelessness
Rape-trauma syndrome: silent reaction
Self-esteem, chronic low
Spiritual distress

NOC Suggested Outcomes

Health Beliefs: Personal convictions that influence health behaviors
Health Beliefs: Perceived Ability to Perform: Personal conviction that one can carry out a given health behavior
Health Beliefs: Perceived Control: Personal conviction that one can influence an outcome
Health Beliefs: Perceived Resources: Personal conviction that one has adequate means to carry out a health behavior
Participation: Health Care Decisions: Personal involvement in selecting and evaluating health care options

Goals/Evaluation Criteria

Examples Using NOC Language

- Demonstrates Health Beliefs: Perceived Ability to Perform, Perceived Control, and Perceived Resources (specify 1–5: very weak, weak, moderate, strong, or very strong)
- Demonstrates **Participation: Health Care Decisions**, as evidenced by the following indicators (specify 1–5: never, rarely, sometimes, often, or consistently demonstrated):

  Identifies health outcome priorities

  Uses problem-solving techniques to achieve desired outcomes

  Negotiates for care preferences

Other Examples

Patient will:

- Verbalize any feelings of powerlessness
- Identify actions that are within his/her control
- Relate absence of barriers to action
- Verbalize ability to perform necessary actions
- Report adequate support from significant others, friends, and neighbors
- Report sufficient time, personal finances, and health insurance
- Report availability of equipment, supplies, services, and transportation

NIC Priority Interventions

Self-Esteem Enhancement: Assisting a patient to increase his/her personal judgment of self-worth

Self-Responsibility Facilitation: Encouraging a patient to assume more responsibility for own behavior

Nursing Activities

Assessments

- *(NIC) Self-Esteem Enhancement:*

  Determine patient's locus of control

  Determine patient's confidence in own judgment

  Monitor levels of self-esteem over time, as appropriate
- *(NIC) Self-Responsibility Facilitation:*

  Monitor level of responsibility that patient assumes

  Determine whether patient has adequate knowledge about health care condition

Collaborative Activities

- Initiate a multidisciplinary patient care conference to discuss and develop patient care routine

Other

- Help patient to identify factors that may contribute to powerlessness
- Discuss with patient realistic options in care, providing explanations for these options
- Involve patient in decision making about care routine
- Explain to patient the rationale for any change in the plan of care
- *(NIC) Self-Esteem Enhancement:*
  Explore previous achievements of success
  Reinforce the personal strengths that the patient identifies
  Convey confidence in patient's ability to handle situation
- *(NIC) Self-Responsibility Facilitation:*
  Encourage verbalizations of feelings, perceptions, and fears about assuming responsibility
  Encourage independence but assist patient when unable to perform

Protection, Altered
(1.6.2) (1990)

Definition: The state in which an individual experiences a decrease in the ability to guard self from internal or external threat such as illness or injury

Defining Characteristics

Subjective
Chilling
Dyspnea
Fatigue
Itching

Objective
Altered clotting
Anorexia
Cough
Deficient immunity
Disorientation
Immobility

Impaired healing
Insomnia
Maladaptive stress response
Neurosensory alteration
Perspiring
Pressure ulcers
Restlessness
Weakness

Related Factors

Abnormal blood profiles (eg, leukopenia, thrombocytopenia, ane-
    mia, coagulation)
Alcohol abuse
Diseases (eg, cancer, immune disorders)
Drug therapies (eg, antineoplastic, corticosteroid, immune, anti-
    coagulant, thrombolytic)
Extremes of age
Inadequate nutrition
Treatments (eg, surgery, radiation)
Abuse (non-NANDA)

Suggestions for Use

(1) When possible, use a more specific label such as *Risk for infection, Impaired skin integrity, Impaired tissue integrity, Altered oral
mucous membrane,* or *Fatigue.* (2) *Altered protection* should not be
used as a "catchall" diagnosis for patients who are immunosup-
pressed or who have abnormal clotting factors. (3) Although NOC
suggests Abuse Protection as an outcome, this author does not recommend using *Altered protection* to describe child or spousal abuse
situations. Instead, consider *Altered parenting, Ineffective family coping, Risk for violence,* or similar diagnoses. Likewise, although Intrapartum Fetal Monitoring is a NIC priority intervention, the author
does not recommend routine use of *Altered protection* during labor.

Suggested Alternative Diagnoses

Coping: family, ineffective, disabling
Infection, risk for
Injury, risk for
Parenting, altered
Perioperative positioning injury, risk for
Peripheral neurovascular dysfunction, risk for
Skin integrity, risk for impaired

NOC Suggested Outcomes

Abuse Protection: Protection of self or dependent others from abuse

Immune Status: Adequacy of natural and acquired appropriately targeted resistance to internal and external antigens

Goals/Evaluation Criteria

Examples Using NOC Language

- Demonstrates **Abuse Protection** (specify 1–5: not, slightly, moderately, substantially, or totally adequate)
- Demonstrates **Immune Status**. as evidenced by the following indicators (specify 1–5: extremely, substantially, moderately, mildly, or not compromised):

  Recurrent infections not present

  Chronic fatigue not present

  Immunizations current

  Antibody titers within normal limits (WNL)

  Differential white blood cell (WBC) values WNL

  T4-cell, T8-cell, and complement levels WNL

Other Examples

Patient will:

- Demonstrate behaviors that decrease risk of injury, infection, or bleeding
- Report early signs and symptoms of injury, infection, or bleeding
- Be free of signs and symptoms of injury, infection, or bleeding
- Verbalize a plan to provide safety for self and children (eg, obtaining a restraining order)

NIC Priority Interventions

Electronic Fetal Monitoring: Intrapartum: Electronic evaluation of fetal heart rate response to uterine contractions during intrapartal care

Environmental Management, Violence Prevention: Monitoring and manipulation of the physical environment to decrease the potential for violent behavior directed toward self, others, or environment

Infection Control: Minimizing the acquisition and transmission of infectious agents

Infection Protection: Prevention and early detection of infection in a patient at risk

Postanesthesia Care: Monitoring and management of the patient who has recently undergone general or regional anesthesia

Surgical Precautions: Minimizing the potential for iatrogenic injury to the patient related to a surgical procedure

Surveillance, Safety: Purposeful and ongoing collection and analysis of information about the patient and the environment for use in promoting and maintaining patient safety

Nursing Activities

Prevention of Infection

See "Nursing Activities" for "Risk for Infection," pp. 242–243

Prevention of Injury

See "Nursing Activities" for "Risk for Injury," pp. 247–248

Assessments

- *(NIC) Environmental Management, Violence Prevention:*

  Monitor the safety of items being brought to the environment by visitors

  Remove potential weapons from environment (eg, sharps and ropelike objects)

  Assign single room to patient with potential for violence toward others

  Lock utility and storage rooms

Prevention of Bleeding

Assessments

- Evaluate extent of patient's bleeding risk.

Patient/Family Teaching

- Advise patient to wear medical identification bracelet and to alert dentist or physician
- Instruct patient to avoid trauma (eg, from contact sports, sharp objects, stiff toothbrush)
- Teach patient signs and symptoms of bleeding and when to report it
- Teach patient first aid for bleeding

Intraoperative and Postoperative Periods

Also refer to "Nursing Activities" for "Perioperative Positioning Injury, Risk for," pp. 339–340

Assessments

- *(NIC) Postanesthesia Care:*

  Monitor oxygenation

  Ventilate, as appropriate

Monitor and record vital signs q15 minutes or more often, as appropriate

Monitor urinary output

Monitor level of consciousness

- Check surgical site, as appropriate.
- *(NIC) Surgical Precautions:*

Ensure documentation and communication of any allergies

Inspect the patient's skin at the site of grounding pad

Collaborative Activities

- *(NIC) Postanesthesia Care:*

Administer IV medication to control shivering, per agency protocol

Administer narcotic antagonists, as appropriate, per agency protocol

Other

- *(NIC) Postanesthesia Care:*

Restrain patient, as appropriate

Provide warm blankets, as appropriate

- *(NIC) Surgical Precautions:*

Verify the correct functioning of equipment

Count sponges, sharps, and instruments before, during, and after surgery, per agency policy

Inspect the patient's skin for injury after use of electrosurgery

Intrapartum

Assessments

- *(NIC) Electronic Fetal Monitoring: Intrapartum:*

Verify maternal and fetal heart rates before initiation of electronic fetal monitoring

Palpate [abdomen] to determine contraction intensity with tocotransducer use

Use intermittent or telemetry fetal monitoring, if available, to facilitate maternal ambulation and comfort

Apply internal fetal electrode after rupture of membranes when necessary for evaluation of short-term variability

Apply internal uterine pressure catheter after rupture of membranes when necessary for obtaining pressure data for uterine contractions and resting tone

Patient/Family Teaching

- *(NIC) Electronic Fetal Monitoring:*
  Instruct woman and support person(s) about the reason for electronic monitoring, as well as information to be obtained
  Discuss appearance of rhythm strip with mother and support person

Collaborative Activities

- *(NIC) Electronic Fetal Monitoring:* Keep physician informed of pertinent changes in the fetal heart rate, interventions for non-reassuring patterns, subsequent fetal response, labor progress, and maternal response to labor

Other

- *(NIC) Electronic Fetal Monitoring:*
  Adjust monitors to achieve and maintain clarity of the tracing
  Interpret strip when at least a 10-minute tracing has been obtained of the fetal heart and uterine activity signals
  Remove electronic monitors, as needed for ambulation, after verifying that the tracing is normal (ie, reassuring)
  Calibrate equipment, as appropriate, for internal monitoring with a spiral electrode and/or intrauterine pressure catheter

Restoration and Growth

Patient/Family Teaching

- Provide information on community resources/support groups

Collaborative Activities

- Consult dietitian for suggestions to improve nutrition
- Confer with social services to identify appropriate referral for counseling

Other

- Explore with patient ways to enhance sleep/rest
- Assist patient in achieving optimum sleep, rest, nutrition, activity, and stress management
- Discuss relaxation techniques with patient/family
- Assist patient/family in identifying and planning an appropriate exercise program

Rape-Trauma Syndrome
(9.2.3.1) (1980, 1998)

Definition: Sustained maladaptive response to a forced, violent sexual penetration against the victim's will and consent*

Defining Characteristics

Subjective
Anger
Confusion
Embarrassment
Guilt
Humiliation
Powerlessness
Self-blame
Shame

Objective
Aggression
Agitation
Anxiety
Change in relationships
Denial
Dependence
Depression
Disorganization
Dissociative disorders
Fear
Helplessness
Hyperalertness
Inability to make decisions
Loss of self-esteem
Mood swings
Muscle tension and/or spasms
Nightmares and sleep disturbances
Paranoia
Phobias
Physical trauma (eg, bruising, tissue irritation)
Revenge
Sexual dysfunction
Shock
Substance abuse
Suicide attempts
Vulnerability

Related Factors

Rape [patient's biopsychosocial response to event]

*This syndrome includes the following three subcomponents: Rape-Trauma, Compound Reaction, and Silent Reaction. In this text, each appears as a separate diagnosis.

Suggestions for Use

Use this diagnosis only if the specific diagnoses of *Rape-trauma syndrome: compound reaction and silent reaction* do not apply. This diagnosis does not need an etiology; the etiology, rape, is implied in the label itself.

Suggested Alternative Diagnoses

Rape-trauma syndrome: compound reaction
Rape-trauma syndrome: silent reaction

NOC Suggested Outcomes

Abuse Cessation: Evidence that the victim is no longer abused

Abuse Protection: Protection of self or dependent others from abuse

Abuse Recovery: Emotional: Healing of psychological injuries due to abuse

Abuse Recovery: Sexual: Healing following sexual abuse or exploitation

Coping: Actions to manage stressors that tax an individual's resources

Impulse Control: Ability to self-restrain compulsive or impulsive behaviors

Self-Mutilation Restraint: Ability to refrain from intentional self-inflicted injury (nonlethal)

Goals/Evaluation Criteria

Examples Using NOC Language

- Demonstrates **Abuse Recovery: Sexual**, as evidenced by the following indicators (specify 1–5: none, limited, moderate, substantial, or extensive):
    Verbalization of details of abuse
    Verbalization of feelings about the abuse
    Verbalization of appropriate and inappropriate guilt
    Verbalization of accurate information about sexual functioning
    Expressions of right to have been protected from abuse
    Expressions of hope
    Expressions of confidence with sexual orientation
    Freedom from sleep disturbances
    Evidence of appropriate same-sex and opposite-sex relationships
- Demonstrates **Coping**, as evidenced by the following indicators

(specify 1–5: never, rarely, sometimes, often, or consistently demonstrated):

Identifies and uses effective coping strategies

Uses available social support

Reports decrease in physical symptoms of stress

Reports decrease in negative feelings

Expresses feelings of empowerment

Other Examples

Patient will:
- Report cessation of sexual abuse
- Engage in positive interpersonal relationships
- Resolve feelings of depression
- Have appropriate affect for situation
- Obtain treatment for, and resolve, emotional problems and behaviors resulting from the trauma
- Be able to control negative/destructive impulses

NIC Priority Interventions

Crisis Intervention: Use of short-term counseling to help the patient cope with a crisis and resume a state of functioning comparable to or better than the precrisis state

Rape-Trauma Treatment: Provision of emotional and physical support immediately following an alleged rape

Nursing Activities

Assessments
- *(NIC) Crisis Intervention:* Determine whether patient presents safety risk to self or others
- *(NIC) Rape-Trauma Treatment:*

   Document whether patient has showered, douched, or bathed since incident

   Document mental state, physical state (clothing, dirt, and debris), history of incident, evidence of violence, and prior gynecologic history

   Determine presence of cuts, bruises, bleeding, lacerations, or other signs of physical injury

Patient/Family Teaching
- Support and educate significant others; discuss therapeutic response to victim and changes in victim's behaviors that can be anticipated

- *(NIC) Rape-Trauma Treatment:*
  Inform patient of HIV testing, as appropriate
  Give clear, written instructions about medication use, crisis support services, and legal support
  Explain legal proceedings available to patient

Collaborative Activities

- *(NIC) Rape-Trauma Treatment:*
  Refer patient to rape advocacy program
  Offer medication to prevent pregnancy, as appropriate
  Offer prophylactic antibiotic medication against venereal disease

Other

- Approach patient in a nonjudgmental and supportive manner
- Allow adequate time for patient to respond to even simple questions
- Counsel immediate family, spouse, or partner to maintain close relationship with victim, with attention to dispelling feelings of blame (eg, self or projected)
- Encourage patient/family to verbalize feelings
- *(NIC) Rape-Trauma Treatment:*
  Provide support person to stay with patient
  Use the term "alleged rape" in documentation
  Implement rape protocol (eg, label and save soiled clothing, vaginal secretions, and vaginal hair combings)
  Implement crisis intervention counseling

Rape-Trauma Syndrome: Compound Reaction (9.2.3.1.1) (1980)

Definition: Forced, violent sexual penetration against the victim's will and consent. The trauma syndrome that develops from this attack or attempted attack includes an acute phase of disorganization of the victim's lifestyle and a long-term process of reorganization of lifestyle

Defining Characteristics

Subjective

Emotional reaction (eg, anger, embarrassment, fear of physical violence and death, humiliation, revenge, self-blame in acute phase)

Objective

Change in lifestyle (eg, changes in residence, dealing with repetitive nightmares and phobias, seeking family support, seeking social network support in long-term phase)

Multiple physical symptoms (eg, gastrointestinal irritability, genitourinary discomfort, muscle tension, sleep pattern disturbance in acute phase)

Reactivated symptoms of such previous conditions (eg, physical illness, psychiatric illness in acute phase)

Reliance on alcohol and/or drugs in acute phase

Other Possible Defining Characteristics (non-NANDA)

Body image disturbance

Initiating period of celibacy

Physical trauma (eg, general soreness, bruises, lesions, trauma to mouth and rectum)

Promiscuity

Sexual fears

Suicidal/homicidal behavior

Related Factors

To be developed

Patient's biopsychosocial response to rape (non-NANDA)

Suggestions for Use

When appropriate, use this label instead of the more general diagnosis of *Rape-trauma syndrome*. This diagnosis does not need an etiology because the etiology (ie, rape) is implied by the label itself.

Suggested Alternative Diagnoses

Rape-trauma syndrome

Rape-trauma syndrome: silent reaction

NOC Suggested Outcomes

See "NOC Suggested Outcomes" for "Rape-Trauma Syndrome," p. 365

Goals/Evaluation Criteria

Examples Using NOC Language

See "Goals/Evaluation Criteria" for Rape-Trauma Syndrome," pp. 365–366

Other Examples

NOTE: In addition to the general goals for "Rape-Trauma Syndrome" on pp. 365–366, specific goals for this diagnosis depend on the extent to which the patient's previous psychiatric and/or medical conditions are reactivated and what those conditions are. It is not possible to address here all possibilities that might occur. Some examples are that the patient will:

- Be kept safe during reactivation of psychiatric and/or medical conditions
- Actively participate in rape counseling
- Not use alcohol/drugs as a coping mechanism
- Identify the existence of a relationship between his/her own psychiatric and/or medical conditions and the rape episode
- Return to previous level of biopsychosocial functioning

NIC Priority Interventions

Counseling: Use of an interactive helping process focusing on the needs, problems, or feelings of the patient and significant others to enhance or support coping, problem-solving, and interpersonal relationships

Rape-Trauma Treatment: Provision of emotional and physical support immediately following an alleged rape

Nursing Activities

NOTE: Refer to "Nursing Activities" for "Rape-Trauma Syndrome," pp. 366–367. In addition, the following apply:

Assessments

- Assess and document patient's orientation to person, place, time, and situation
- Perform physical assessment based on patient's complaints to determine presenting medical conditions
- Perform psychosocial assessment that focuses on rape
- *(NIC) Counseling:* Determine how family behavior affects patient

Patient/Family Teaching

- Educate significant others regarding psychiatric and/or medical conditions that reoccur. Discuss therapeutic response to victim and changed behaviors.

Collaborative Activities

- Refer patient/family for medical or psychiatric treatment, as needed

Other

- Establish a plan of care to stabilize medical/psychologic condition to proceed with rape-trauma counseling
- Provide necessary safety precautions indicated by suicide risk assessment
- Support significant others
- *(NIC) Counseling:*
  Establish a therapeutic relationship based on trust and respect
  Provide privacy and ensure confidentiality
  Discourage decision making when the patient is under severe stress

Rape-Trauma Syndrome: Silent Reaction (9.2.3.1.2) (1980)

Definition: Forced, violent sexual penetration against the victim's will and consent. The trauma syndrome that develops from this attack or attempted attack includes an acute phase of disorganization of the victim's lifestyle and a long-term process of reorganization of lifestyle.

Defining Characteristics

Subjective

Increase in nightmares

Increased anxiety during assessment interview (ie, blocking of associations, long periods of silence, minor stuttering, physical distress)

No verbalization of the occurrence of rape

Objective

Abrupt changes in relationships with men

Pronounced changes in sexual behavior

Sudden onset of phobic reactions

Other Possible Defining Characteristics (non-NANDA)

Avoidance of close relationships

Irritability toward gender of perpetrator

Persistently low self-confidence and self-esteem

Suspiciousness

Related Factors

To be developed

Suggestions for Use

If defining characteristics are present, use this label instead of the more general diagnosis of *Rape-trauma syndrome.* An etiology is not necessary for this diagnosis because the etiology (ie, rape) is implied in the label itself.

Suggested Alternative Diagnoses

Rape-trauma syndrome
Rape-trauma syndrome: compound reaction

NOC Suggested Outcomes

See "NOC Suggested Outcomes" for "Rape-Trauma Syndrome," p. 365

Goals/Evaluation Criteria

Examples Using NOC Language

See "Goals/Evaluation Criteria" for "Rape-Trauma Syndrome," pp. 365–366

Other Examples

NOTE: In addition to the general goals for "Rape-Trauma Syndrome" on pp. 365–366, specific goals for this diagnosis depend on the extent to which the patient's previous psychiatric and/or medical conditions are reactivated and what those conditions are. It is not possible to address here all possibilities that might occur. Some examples are that the patient will:

• Acknowledge the rape/attempted rape
• Verbalize details of the rape/attempted rape as a means of catharsis
• Verbalize feelings associated with rape/attempted rape
• Describe a plan that includes safety measures to reduce future risk
• Experience a decrease in stress response symptoms (eg, nightmares)
• Return to previous level of biopsychosocial functioning. Specify level

NIC Priority Interventions

Counseling: Use of an interactive helping process focusing on the needs, problems, or feelings of the patient and significant others to enhance or support coping, problem-solving, and interpersonal relationships

Rape-Trauma Treatment: Provision of emotional and physical support immediately following an alleged rape

Nursing Interventions

Also refer to "Nursing Activities" for "Rape-Trauma Syndrome," pp. 366–367, and for Rape-Trauma Syndrome: Compound Reaction, pp. 369–370

Other

- Confirm with patient that a traumatic event recently occurred and specifically identify it as "rape"
- Encourage patient to express thoughts, feelings, and behaviors
- Establish therapeutic relationship that will allow exploration of silent reaction
- Assist patient/family to establish support network
- *(NIC) Counseling:* Verbalize the discrepancy between the patient's feelings and behaviors

Relocation Stress Syndrome
(6.7) (1992)

Definition: Physiological and/or psychosocial disturbances as a result of transfer from one environment to another

Defining Characteristics

Subjective

Anxiety

Apprehension

Increased confusion [elderly population]

Loneliness

Increased verbalization of needs

Unfavorable comparison of post- to pretransfer staff

Verbalization of being concerned/upset about transfer

Verbalization of unwillingness to relocate

Objective

Change in environment/location

Depression

Change in eating habits

Dependency

Gastrointestinal disturbances

Insecurity

Lack of trust

Restlessness

Sad affect

Sleep disturbance

Vigilance

Weight change

Withdrawal

Related Factors

Decreased physical health status

Feeling of powerlessness

History and types of previous transfers

Impaired psychosocial health status

Lack of adequate support system

Little or no preparation for the impending move

Losses involved with decision to move

Moderate to high degree of environmental change

Past, concurrent, and recent losses

Suggestions for Use

Because this is a syndrome diagnosis, no etiology is needed in the diagnostic statement. A syndrome nursing diagnosis represents a group of other nursing diagnoses that are present together. If only one or two of the defining characteristics are present (eg, anxiety, loneliness), write separate nursing diagnoses for those responses (eg, *Anxiety*) instead of using *Relocation stress syndrome*.

Suggested Alternative Diagnoses

Anxiety

Confusion, acute

Grieving, dysfunctional

Hopelessness

Loneliness, risk for

Powerlessness

Sleep pattern disturbance
Sorrow, chronic
Spiritual distress

NOC Suggested Outcomes

Child Adaptation to Hospitalization: Child's adaptive response to hospitalization

Coping: Actions to manage stressors that tax an individual's resources

Psychosocial Adjustment: Life Change: Psychosocial adaptation of an individual to a life change

Quality of Life: An individual's expressed satisfaction with current life circumstances

Goals/Evaluation Criteria

Examples Using NOC Language

- Demonstrates **Coping**, as evidenced by the following indicators (specify 1–5: never, rarely, sometimes, often, or consistently demonstrated):

    Verbalizes acceptance of situation

    Reports decrease in negative feelings

    Reports decrease in physical symptoms of stress

    Modifies lifestyle, as needed

Other Examples

Patient will:
- Demonstrate ability to adjust to new environment
- Verbalize satisfaction with new living arrangements
- Express optimism
- Express satisfaction with life achievements
- Participate in diversions (eg, hobbies)
Child will:
- Adapt to hospitalization (eg, will not demonstrate agitation, regressive behaviors, anxiety, fear, or anger)
- Respond to play therapy and comfort measures
- Show resolution of separation anxiety

NIC Priority Interventions

Coping Enhancement: Assisting a patient to adapt to perceived stressors, changes, or threats which interfere with meeting life demands and roles

Discharge Planning: Preparation for moving a patient from one level of care to another within or outside the current health care agency

Hope Instillation: Facilitation of the development of a positive outlook in a given situation

Self-Responsibility Facilitation: Encouraging a patient to assume more responsibility for own behavior

Nursing Activities

Assessments

- Assess patient's orientation, mood (eg, depressed, angry, anxious), and physiologic status on admission and q _____.
- Identify patient's previous schedules and routines
- Assess readiness for discharge
- *(NIC) Coping Enhancement:* Appraise patient's needs/desires for social support
- *(NIC) Self-Responsibility Facilitation:* Monitor level of responsibility that patient assumes

Collaborative Activities

- Maintain consistency in caregivers and care routines as much as possible. Consider a case manager.
- Utilize other resources to assist in transition to new environment
- Coordinate referrals among health care providers and agencies to effect a smooth transfer/relocation

Other

- Orient patient to new environment as often as needed
- Establish new environment as close to previous environment as possible to maintain consistency in placement of personal belongings, furniture, pictures, and so on
- To ease the transfer, encourage family to stay with patient, bring familiar objects from home, and provide familiar socialization
- Avoid unplanned or abrupt transfers; also avoid transfers at night or at change of shift
- *(NIC) Coping Enhancement:*
  Assist the patient in developing an objective appraisal of the event
  Use a calm, reassuring approach
  Seek to understand the patient's perspective of a stressful situation
  Discourage decision making when the patient is under severe stress

Foster constructive outlets for anger and hostility

Arrange situations that encourage patient's autonomy

Introduce patient to persons (or groups) who have successfully undergone the same experience

Encourage verbalization of feelings, perceptions, and fears [about the relocation]

- *(NIC) Hope Instillation:*

Inform the patient about whether the current situation is a temporary state

Facilitate the patient's/family's reliving and savoring past achievements and experiences

Create an environment that facilitates patient practicing religion

Involve the patient actively in own care

- *(NIC) Self-Responsibility Facilitation:*

Encourage patient to take as much responsibility for own self-care as possible

Facilitate family support for new level of responsibility sought or attained by patient

Role Performance, Altered
(3.2.1) (1978, 1998)

Definition: The patterns of behavior and self-expression do not match the environmental context, norms, and expectations

Defining Characteristics

Subjective

Altered role perceptions

Anxiety or depression

Inadequate confidence

Inadequate motivation

Powerlessness

Role ambivalence, conflict, confusion, denial, dissatisfaction, overload, or strain

Uncertainty

Objective

Discrimination

Domestic violence

Harassment

Inadequate adaptation to change or transition

Inadequate external support for role enactment

Inadequate knowledge

Inadequate opportunities for role enactment

Inadequate role competency and skills

Inappropriate developmental expectations

Related Factors

Knowledge

Developmental transitions

Education attainment level

Inadequate role preparation (eg, role transition, skill, rehearsal, validation)

Lack of knowledge about role

Lack of knowledge about role skills

Lack of opportunity for role rehearsal

Lack of or inadequate role model

Role transition

Unrealistic role expectations

Physiologic

Body image alteration

Cognitive deficits

Depression

Fatigue

Health alterations (eg, physical health, body image, self-esteem, mental health, psychosocial health, cognition, learning style, neurologic health)

Inadequate/inappropriate linkage with health care system

Low self-esteem

Mental illness

Pain

Physical illness

Substance abuse

Social

Domestic violence

Family conflict

Inadequate or inappropriate linkage with health care system

Inadequate role socialization (eg, role model, expectations, responsibilities)

Inadequate support system

Job schedule demands

Lack of resources

Lack of rewards

Low socioeconomic status

Poverty

Stress and conflict

Young age, developmental level

Suggestions for Use

When applicable, use more specific labels such as *Parental role conflict, Sexual dysfunction, and Altered family processes*. Some degree of role conflict and disruption is present for everyone. If the patient is having difficulty with role performance, consider using *Altered role performance* as the etiology of another diagnosis that describes the impact on functioning (eg, *Impaired home maintenance management related to Altered role performance*).

"There is a typology of roles [that applies to this diagnosis]: sociopersonal (eg, friendship, family, marital, parenting, community), home management, intimacy (eg, sexuality, relationship building), leisure/exercise/recreation, self-management, socialization (eg, developmental transitions), community contributor, and religious)." (NANDA, 1999, pp. 52–53).

Suggested Alternative Diagnoses

Caregiver role strain, actual/risk for

Family processes, altered

Home maintenance management, impaired

Parental role conflict

Self-esteem, situational low

NOC Suggested Outcomes

Caregiver Lifestyle Disruption: Disturbances in the lifestyle of a family member due to caregiving

Psychosocial Adjustment: Life Change: Psychosocial adaptation of an individual to a life change

Role Performance: Congruence of an individual's role behavior with role expectations

Goals/Evaluation Criteria

Examples Using NOC Language

• Demonstrates **Role Performance**, as evidenced by the following indicators (specify 1–5: not, slightly, moderately, substantially, or totally adequate):

   Ability to meet role expectations

   Knowledge of role transition periods

Performance of family, community, work, intimate, and friendship role behaviors

Reported strategies for role change(s)

Other Examples

Patient will:

- Acknowledge impact of situation on existing personal relation-
ships, lifestyle, and role performance
- Describe actual change in function
- Express willingness to use resources upon discharge
- Verbalize feelings of productivity and usefulness
- Demonstrate ability to manage finances

NIC Priority Interventions

Role Enhancement: Assisting a patient, significant other, and/or
family to improve relationships by clarifying and supplementing
specific role behaviors

Nursing Activities

Assessments

- Assess need for assistance from Social Services Department for
planning care with patient/family

Patient/Family Teaching

- *(NIC) Role Enhancement:* Teach new behaviors needed by
patient/parent to fulfill a role

Other

- Assist patient in identifying personal strengths
- Actively listen to patient/family and acknowledge reality of con-
cerns
- Encourage patient/family to air feelings and to grieve
- *(NIC) Role Enhancement:*

Assist patient to identify various roles in life

Assist patient to identify usual role in family

Assist patient to identify role insufficiency

Assist adult children to accept elderly parent's dependency and
the role changes involved, as appropriate

Facilitate discussion of how siblings' roles will change with newborn's arrival, as appropriate

Facilitate discussion of role adaptations related to children leaving home (ie, empty-nest syndrome), as appropriate

Self-Care Deficit—Discussion

Self-care deficit describes a state in which a person experiences impaired ability to perform self-care activities such as bathing, dressing, eating, and toileting. If the person is unable to perform any self-care, the situation is described as *Total self-care deficit.* However, the diagnoses are classified into more specific problems, each with its own defining characteristics; these problems can exist alone or in various combinations, such as *Feeding self-care deficit* and *Feeding and bathing/hygiene self-care deficit.*

Self-care deficits are often caused by *Activity intolerance, Impaired physical mobility, Pain, Anxiety,* or perceptual or cognitive impairment (eg, *Feeding self-care deficit +2 related to disorientation*). As an etiology, *Self-care deficit* can cause depression, *Fear* of becoming dependent, and *Powerlessness* (eg, *Fear of becoming totally dependent related to total self-care deficit +2 secondary to residual weakness from CVA*).

Self-care deficit should be used to label only those conditions in which the focus is to support or improve the patient's self-care abilities. Outcome and evaluation criteria for these labels must reflect improved functioning. Therefore, if the diagnosis is used for states not amenable to treatment, there is no hope of achieving the stated outcomes. The focus of nursing interventions in this case is twofold: (1) to increase the patient's ability to perform self-care and (2) to help patients with limitations and perform care the patient cannot do.

Self-Care Deficit: Bathing/Hygiene (Specify Level) (6.5.2) (1980, 1998)

Definition: Impaired ability to perform or complete bathing/hygiene activities for oneself

Defining Characteristics

Objective

Inability to [perform the following tasks]:

Dry body

Get bath supplies

Get in and out of bathroom

Obtain or get to water source

Regulate temperature or flow of bathwater

Wash body or body parts

Related Factors

Decreased or lack of motivation

Environmental barriers

Inability to perceive body part or spatial relationship

Neuromuscular impairment

Pain

Perceptual or cognitive impairment

Severe anxiety

Weakness and tiredness

Other Related Factors (non-NANDA)

Decreased strength and endurance

Depression

Developmental disability

Intolerance to activity

Medically imposed restrictions

Musculoskeletal impairment

Psychologic impairment (specify)

Suggestions for Use

See "Self-Care Deficits—Discussion" on p. 380

In order to promote efforts to restore functioning, the patient's functional level must be classified. NANDA uses the following scale.

0 = Completely independent
1 = Requires use of equipment or device
2 = Requires help from another person for assistance, supervision, or teaching
3 = Requires help from another person and equipment or device
4 = Dependent, does not participate in activity

The following definitions and descriptors may be helpful in determining which number to assign to a patient's functional level:

Table 5

	Totally Dependent (+4)	**Moderately Dependent (+3)**	**Semi-dependent (+2)**
Bathing	Patient needs complete bath; cannot assist at all.	Nurse supplies all equipment; positions patient; washes back, legs, perineum, and all other parts, as needed. Patient can assist.	Nurse provides all equipment; positions patient in bed/bathroom. Patient completes bath, except for back and feet.
Oral Hygiene	Nurse completes entire procedure.	Nurse prepares brush, rinses, mouth, positions patient.	Nurse provides equipment; patient does task.

Suggested Alternative Diagnoses

Activity intolerance
Physical mobility, impaired
Sensory/perceptual alterations
Thought processes, altered
Total self-care deficit

NOC Suggested Outcomes

Self-Care: Activities of Daily Living (ADLs): Ability to perform the most basic physical tasks and personal care activities
Self-Care: Bathing: Ability to cleanse own body
Self-Care: Hygiene: Ability to maintain own hygiene

Goals/Evaluation Criteria

Examples Using NOC Language

- Demonstrates **Self-Care: Activities of Daily Living (ADLs)**, as evidenced by the following indicators (specify 1–5: dependent (does not participate), requires assistive person and device, requires assistive person, independent with assistive device, or is completely independent):

    Bathing

    Hygiene

Other Examples

Patient will:

- Accept assistance or total care by caregiver, if needed
- Verbalize satisfactory body cleanliness and oral hygiene
- Maintain mobility needed to get to bathroom and get bath supplies
- Be able to turn on and regulate water temperature and flow
- Wash and dry body
- Perform mouth care
- Apply deodorant

NIC Priority Interventions

Bathing: Cleaning of the body for the purposes of relaxation, cleanliness, and healing

Self-Care Assistance, Bathing/Hygiene: Assisting patient to perform personal hygiene

Nursing Activities

Assessments

- Assess ability to use assistive devices
- Assess oral mucous membranes and body cleanliness daily
- Assess skin condition during bath
- Monitor for changes in functional abilities
- *(NIC) Self-Care Assistance: Bathing/Hygiene:* Monitor cleaning of nails, according to patient's self-care ability

Patient/Family Teaching

- Instruct patient/family in alternative methods for bathing and oral hygiene

Collaborative Activities

- Offer pain medications prior to bathing
- Refer patient and family to social services for home care

- Use occupational and physical therapy as resources in planning patient care activities

Other

- Encourage independence in bathing and oral hygiene, assisting patient only as necessary
- Encourage patient to set own pace during self-care
- Include family in provision of care
- *(NIC) Self-Care Assistance: Bathing/Hygiene:*
  Provide assistance until patient is fully able to assume self-care
  Place towels, soap, deodorant, shaving equipment, and other needed accessories at bedside/bathroom
  Wash hair, as needed and desired
  Shave patient, as indicated
  Offer hand washing after toileting and before meals

Self-Care Deficit: Dressing/Grooming (Specify Level) (6.5.3) (1980, 1998)

Definition: An impaired ability to perform or complete dressing and grooming activities for oneself

Defining Characteristics

Objective

Impaired ability to:
  Fasten clothing
  Obtain or replace articles of clothing
  Put on or take off necessary items of clothing

Inability to:
  Choose clothing
  Maintain appearance at a satisfactory level
  Pick up clothing
  Put on clothing on lower body
  Put on clothing on upper body
  Put on shoes
  Put on socks
  Remove clothes
  Use assistive devices
  Use zippers

Related Factors

Decreased or lack of motivation

Discomfort

Environmental barriers

Musculoskeletal impairment

Neuromuscular impairment

Perceptual or cognitive impairment

Severe anxiety

Weakness or tiredness

Other Related Factors (non-NANDA)

Depression

Developmental disability

Intolerance to activity

Psychologic impairment (specify)

Suggestions for Use

See "Self-Care Deficits—Discussion" on p. 380. NANDA uses the following scale to classify patient's functional level:

0	=	Completely independent
1	=	Requires use of equipment or device
2	=	Requires help from another person for assistance, supervision, or teaching
3	=	Requires help from another person and equipment or device
4	=	Dependent; does not participate in activity

The following definitions and descriptors may be helpful in determining which number to assign to a patient's functional level:

Table 6

	Totally Dependent (+4)	**Moderately Dependent (+3)**	**Semi-dependent (+2)**
Dressing/ Grooming	Patient needs to be dressed and cannot assist the nurse; nurse combs patient's hair.	Nurse combs patient's hair, assists with dressing, buttons and zips clothing, ties shoes.	Nurse gathers items for patient; may button, zip or tie clothing. Patient dresses self.

Suggested Alternative Diagnoses

Activity intolerance
Fatigue
Physical mobility, impaired
Sensory/perceptual alterations
Thought processes, altered
Total self-care deficit

NOC Suggested Outcomes

Self-Care: Activities of Daily Living (ADLs): Ability to perform the most basic physical tasks and personal care activities
Self-Care: Dressing: Ability to dress self
Self-Care: Grooming: Ability to maintain kempt appearance
Self-Care: Hygiene: Ability to maintain own hygiene

Goals/Evaluation Criteria

Examples Using NOC Language

- Demonstrates **Self-Care: Activities of Daily Living (ADLs)**, as evidenced by the following indicators (specify 1–5: dependent (does not participate), requires assistive person and device, requires assistive person, independent with assistive device, or completely independent):
  Dressing
  Grooming

Other Examples

  Patient will:
- Accept care by caregiver
- Express satisfaction with dressing and hair grooming
- Dress and comb hair independently
- Use adaptive devices to facilitate dressing
- Choose clothes and obtain them from closet or drawers
- Zip and button clothing
- Be neatly dressed
- Be able to remove clothing, socks, and shoes
- Have clean, neat hair
- Apply makeup

NIC Priority Interventions

Dressing: Choosing, putting on, and removing clothes for a person who cannot do this for self

Hair Care: Promotion of neat, clean, attractive hair
Self-Care Assistance: Dressing/Grooming: Assisting patient with
 clothes and makeup

Nursing Activities

Assessments

- Assess ability to use assistive devices
- Monitor energy level and activity tolerance
- Monitor for improved or deteriorating ability to dress and per-
 form hair care
- Monitor for sensory, cognitive, or physical deficits that may
 make dressing difficult for the patient

Patient/Family Teaching

- Demonstrate use of assistive devices and adaptive activities
- Instruct patient in alternative methods for dressing and hair
 care. Specify methods.

Collaborative Activities

- Offer pain medications prior to dressing and grooming
- Refer patient and family to social services for obtaining home
 health aide, as needed
- Use occupational and physical therapy as resource in planning
 patient care activities
- *(NIC) Self-Care Assistance: Dressing/Grooming:* Facilitate assistance of a barber or beautician, as necessary

Other

- Encourage independence in dressing/grooming, assisting
 patient only as necessary
- Accommodate cognitive deficits in the following ways:
  Use nonverbal cues (eg, give patient one article of clothing at
   a time, in the order needed)
  Speak slowly and keep directions simple
- Use Velcro fasteners and closures when possible
- Create opportunities for small successes. Specify
- Encourage patient to set own pace during dressing/grooming
- Help patient choose clothing that is loose fitting and easy to put on
- Provide for safety by keeping environment uncluttered and well-
 lighted
- *(NIC) Self-Care Assistance: Dressing/Grooming:*
  Provide patient's clothes in accessible area (eg, at bedside) [and
   in the order they will be needed for dressing]

Facilitate patient's combing hair, as appropriate

Maintain privacy while the patient is dressing

Help with laces, buttons, and zippers, as needed

Use extension equipment [eg, long-handled shoehorn, button-hook, zipper pull] for pulling on clothing, if appropriate

Reinforce efforts to dress self

Self-Care Deficit: Feeding (Specify Level) (6.5.1) (1980, 1998)

Definition: An impaired ability to perform or complete feeding activities

Defining Characteristics

Objective

Inability to:

Bring food from a receptacle to the mouth

Chew food

Complete a meal

Get food onto utensil

Handle utensils

Ingest food in a socially acceptable manner

Ingest food safely

Ingest sufficient food

Manipulate food in mouth

Open containers

Pick up cup or glass

Prepare food for ingestion

Swallow food

Use assistive device

Related Factors

Decreased or lack of motivation

Discomfort

Environmental barriers

Musculoskeletal impairment

Neuromuscular impairment

Pain

Perceptual or cognitive impairment

Severe anxiety
Weakness or tiredness

Other Related Factors (non-NANDA)
Depression
Developmental disability
Intolerance to activity
Psychologic impairment

Suggestions for Use

Feeding self-care deficit may be the etiology (ie, related factor) for *Altered nutrition: less than body requirements*. Also see "Self-Care Deficits—Discussion" on p. 380. NANDA uses the following scale to classify patient's functional level:

0 = Completely independent
1 = Requires use of equipment or device
2 = Requires help from another person for assistance, supervision, or teaching
3 = Requires help from another person and equipment or device
4 = Dependent, does not participate in activity

The following definitions and descriptors may be helpful in determining which number to assign to a patient's functional level:

Table 7

	Totally Dependent (+4)	**Moderately Dependent (+3)**	**Semi-dependent (+2)**
Feeding	Patient needs to be fed totally.	Nurse cuts food, opens containers, positions patient, monitors and encourages eating	Nurse positions patient, gathers supplies, monitors eating.

Suggested Alternative Diagnoses

Activity intolerance
Physical mobility, impaired
Sensory/perceptual alterations
Thought processes, altered
Total self-care deficit

NOC Suggested Outcomes

Self-Care: Activities of Daily Living (ADLs): Ability to perform the most basic physical tasks and personal care activities

Self-Care: Eating: Ability to prepare and ingest food

Goals/Evaluation Criteria

Examples Using NOC Language

- Demonstrates **Self-Care: Activities of Daily Living (ADLs)**, as evidenced by the following indicator (specify 1–5: dependent (does not participate), requires assistive person and device, requires assistive person, independent with assistive device, or completely independent):

  Feeding

Other Examples

Patient will:

- Accept feeding by caregiver
- Be able to feed self independently (or specify level)
- Express satisfaction with eating and with ability to feed self
- Demonstrate adequate intake of food and fluids
- Use adaptive devices to eat
- Open containers and prepare food

NIC Priority Interventions

Feeding: Providing nutritional intake for patient who is unable to feed self

Self-Care Assistance: Feeding: Assisting a person to eat

Nursing Activities

Assessments

- Assess ability to use assistive devices
- Assess energy level and activity tolerance
- Assess for improved or deteriorating ability to feed self
- Assess for sensory, cognitive, or physical deficits that may make self-feeding difficult
- Assess ability to chew and swallow
- Assess intake for nutritional adequacy

Patient/Family Teaching

- Demonstrate use of assistive devices and adaptive activities
- Instruct patient in alternative methods for eating/drinking. Specify method and teaching plan.

Collaborative Activities

- Refer patient and family to social services for obtaining home health aide
- Use occupational and physical therapy as resources in planning patient care activities
- *(NIC) Self-Care Assistance: Feeding:* Provide for adequate pain relief before meals, as appropriate

Other

- Accommodate cognitive deficits in the following ways:
    Avoid using sharp eating utensils (eg, steak knives)
    Check for food in cheeks
    Have meals in quiet environment to limit distraction from task
    Keep verbal communication short and simple
- Serve one food at a time in small amounts
- Acknowledge and reinforce patient's accomplishments
- Encourage independence in eating and drinking, assisting patient only as necessary
- Encourage patient to wear dentures and eyeglasses
- Provide for privacy while eating if patient is embarrassed
- When feeding, allow patient to determine order of foods
- Sit down while feeding; do not hurry
- Serve finger foods (eg, fruit, bread) to promote independence
- Include parents/family in feeding/meals
- *(NIC) Self-Care Assistance: Feeding:*
    Create a pleasant environment during mealtime (eg, put bedpans, urinals, and suctioning equipment out of sight)
    Provide for oral hygiene before meals
    Fix food on tray, as necessary, such as cutting meat or peeling an egg
    Avoid placing food on a person's blind side
    Provide a drinking straw, as needed or desired
    Provide adaptive devices to facilitate patient's feeding self (eg, long handles, handle with large circumference, or small strap on utensils), as needed
    Provide frequent cuing and close supervision, as appropriate

Self-Care Deficit: Toileting (Specify Level) (6.5.4) (1980, 1998)

Definition: An impaired ability to perform or complete own toileting activities

Defining Characteristics

Objective
Unable to get to toilet or commode
Unable to sit on or rise from toilet or commode
Inability to manipulate clothing
Unable to carry out proper toilet hygiene
Unable to flush toilet or commode

Related Factors

Decreased or lack of motivation
Environmental barriers
Impaired mobility status
Impaired transfer ability
Musculoskeletal impairment
Neuromuscular impairment
Pain
Perceptual or cognitive impairment
Severe anxiety
Weakness or tiredness

Other Possible Defining Characteristics (non-NANDA)
Depression
Developmental disability
Intolerance to activity
Medically imposed restrictions
Psychologic impairment (specify)

Suggestions for Use

Self-care deficit: toileting may be an etiology (ie, related factor) for *Impaired skin integrity* and/or *Social isolation*. Also see "Self-Care Deficits—Discussion" on p. 380. NANDA uses the following scale to classify functional levels:

 0 = Completely independent
 1 = Requires use of equipment or device
 2 = Requires help from another person for assistance, supervision, or teaching

3 = Requires help from another person and equipment or device

4 = Dependent, does not participate in activity

The following definitions and descriptors may be helpful in determining which number to assign to a patient's functional level:

Table 8

	Totally Dependent (+4)	**Moderately Dependent (+3)**	**Semi-dependent (+2)**
Toileting	Patient is incontinent; nurse places patient on bedpan or commode.	Nurse provides bedpan, positions patient on or off bedpan, places patient on commode.	Patient can walk to bathroom/commode with assistance; nurse helps with clothing.

Suggested Alternative Diagnoses

Activity intolerance

Fatigue

Incontinence, bowel

Incontinence, urinary (functional, stress, total, urge)

Incontinence: urinary, urge, risk for

Physical mobility, impaired

Sensory/perceptual alterations

Thought processes, altered

Total self-care deficit

Transfer ability, impaired

NOC Suggested Outcomes

Self-Care: Activities of Daily Living (ADLs): Ability to perform the most basic physical and personal care activities

Self-Care: Toileting: Ability to toilet self

Goals/Evaluation Criteria

Examples Using NOC Language

• Demonstrates **Self-Care: Activities of Daily Living (ADLs)**, as evidenced by the following indicators (specify 1–5: dependent (does not participate), requires assistive person and device, requires assistive person, independent with assistive device, or completely independent):

Toileting

Other Examples

Patient will:

- Accept help from caregiver
- Recognize/acknowledge need for help with toileting
- Recognize and respond to urge to urinate and/or defecate
- Be able to get to and from toilet
- Wipe self after toileting

NIC Priority Interventions

Environmental Management: Manipulation of the patient's surroundings for therapeutic benefit

Self-Care Assistance: Toileting: Assisting another with elimination

Nursing Activities

Also see "Nursing Activities" for "Bowel Incontinence" on pp. 210–212 and for Urinary Incontinence: Functional, Reflex, Stress, Total, and Urge" on pp. 213–224.

Assessments

- Assess ability to ambulate independently and safely
- Assess ability to use assistive devices (eg, walkers, canes)
- Monitor energy level and activity tolerance
- Assess for improved or deteriorating ability to toilet self
- Assess for sensory, cognitive, or physical deficits that may limit self-toileting

Patient/Family Teaching

- Instruct patient and family in transfer and ambulation techniques
- Demonstrate use of assistive equipment and adaptive activities
- *(NIC) Self-Care Assistance: Toileting:* Instruct patient/appropriate others in toileting routine
- *(NIC) Environmental Management:* Provide family/significant other with information about making home environment safe for patient

Collaborative Activities

- Offer pain medications prior to toileting
- Refer patient and family to social services for obtaining home health aide
- Use occupational and physical therapy as resources in planning patient care activities and obtaining necessary equipment

Other

- Specify functional level and assist with toileting or provide basic care, as needed
- Accommodate cognitive deficits (eg, keep verbal instructions short and simple)
- Allow sufficient time for toileting to avoid fatigue and frustration
- Avoid use of indwelling catheters and condom catheters if possible
- Encourage patient to wear clothes that are easy to manage; assist with clothing, as needed
- Keep bedpan or urinal within patient's reach
- *(NIC) Self-Care Assistance: Toileting:*
  Assist patient to toilet/commode/bedpan/fracture pan/urinal [specify] at specified intervals
  Facilitate toilet hygiene after completion of elimination
  Flush toilet; cleanse elimination utensil
  Replace patient's clothing after elimination
  Provide privacy during elimination
- *(NIC) Environmental Management:*
  Remove environmental hazards (eg, loose rugs and small, movable furniture)
  Provide room deodorizers, as needed
  Provide immediate and continuous means to summon nurse and let the patient and family know they will be answered immediately

Self-Esteem, Chronic Low
(7.1.2.1) (1988, 1996)

Definition: Long-standing, negative self-evaluation/feelings about self or self-capabilities

Defining Characteristics

Subjective

Evaluates self as unable to deal with events (long-standing or chronic)

Expressions of shame/guilt (long-standing or chronic)

Rationalizes away/rejects positive feedback and exaggerates negative feedback about self (long-standing or chronic)

Self-negating verbalization (long-standing or chronic)

Objective

Dependent on others' opinions

Excessively seeks reassurance

Frequent lack of success in work or other life events

Hesitant to try new things/situations (long-standing or chronic)

Indecisive

Lack of eye contact

Nonassertive/passive

Overly conforming

Other Possible Defining Characteristics (non-NANDA)

Projection of blame/responsibility for problems

Self-destructive behaviors (eg, alcohol, drug abuse)

Self-neglect

Related Factors

To be developed

Related Factors (non-NANDA)

Chronic illness

Congenital anomaly

Psychologic impairment (specify)

Repeated unmet expectations

Suggestions for Use

Chronic low self-esteem is different from *Situational low self-esteem* in that the symptoms are long-standing and seem to result from frequent, actual or perceived lack of success in work or role performance. Initially, if the nurse does not have enough clinical data to validate one of the self-esteem diagnoses, the more general non-NANDA diagnosis of *Self-concept disturbance* can be used (Carpenito 1997b).

Suggested Alternative Diagnoses

Hopelessness

Individual coping, ineffective

Powerlessness

Self-concept disturbance (non-NANDA)

Self-esteem, situational low

Self-esteem disturbance

NOC Suggested Outcomes

Self-Esteem: Personal judgment of self-worth

Goals/Evaluation Criteria
Examples Using NOC Language
- Demonstrates **Self-Esteem**, as evidenced by the following indicators (specify 1–5: never, rarely, sometimes, often, or consistently demonstrated):
    Verbalization of self-acceptance
    Maintenance of erect posture
    Maintenance of eye contact
    Maintenance of grooming/hygiene
    Acceptance of compliments from others
    Description of success in work, school, and/or social groups

Other Examples
  Patient will:
- Acknowledge personal strengths
- Express a willingness to seek counseling
- Participate in making decisions regarding plan of care
- Practice behaviors that generate self-confidence

NIC Priority Interventions
Self-Esteem Enhancement: Assisting a patient to increase his/her personal judgment of self-worth

Nursing Activities
Assessments
- *(NIC) Self-Esteem Enhancement:*
    Monitor patient's statements of self-worth
    Determine patient's confidence in own judgment
    Monitor frequency of self-negating verbalizations

Patient/Family Teaching
- Provide information about the value of counseling and available community resources
- Teach positive behavioral skills through role play, role modeling, discussion, and so on
- *(NIC) Self-Esteem Enhancement:*
    Instruct parents on the importance of their interest and support in their children's development of a positive self-concept

Collaborative Activities
- Seek assistance from hospital resources (eg, social workers, psychiatric clinical specialist, pastoral care services), as needed

Other

- Set limits about negative verbalization (eg, regarding frequency, content, audience)
- *(NIC) Self-Esteem Enhancement:*
  Reinforce the personal strengths that patient identifies
  Assist patient to identify positive responses from others
  Refrain from teasing
  Assist in setting realistic goals to achieve higher self-esteem
  Assist patient to reexamine negative perceptions of self
  Assist the patient to identify the impact of peer group on feelings of self-worth
  Explore previous achievements of success
  Reward or praise patient's progress toward reaching goals
  Facilitate an environment and activities that will increase self-esteem

Self-Esteem, Situational Low
(7.1.2.2) (1988, 1996)

Definition: Negative self-evaluation/feelings about self that develop in response to a loss or change in an individual who previously had a positive self-evaluation

Defining Characteristics

Subjective
Expressions of shame/guilt
Self-negating verbalizations
Verbalization of negative feelings about self (eg, helplessness, uselessness)

Objective
Episodic occurrence of negative self-appraisal in response to life events in a person with a previous positive self-evaluation
Evaluates self as unable to handle situations/events
Difficulty in making decisions

Related Factors

To be developed

Related Factors (non-NANDA)
Situational crisis (specify)

Suggestions for Use

Situational low self-esteem can be differentiated from *Chronic low self-esteem* in that the symptoms are episodic. Symptoms occur in a person with previously good self-esteem and are in response to some actual or perceived event or situation. Goals and nursing activities, therefore, may focus on problem solving the situation in addition to building the patient's self-esteem.

Suggested Alternative Diagnoses

Adjustment, impaired
Body image disturbance
Individual coping, ineffective
Personal identity disturbance
Individual coping, ineffective
Self-esteem, chronic low
Self-esteem disturbance

NOC Suggested Outcomes

Decision Making: Ability to choose between two or more alternatives
Self-Esteem: Personal judgment of self-worth

Goals/Evaluation Criteria

Examples Using NOC Language

- Demonstrates **Self-Esteem**, as evidenced by the following indicators (specify 1–5: never, rarely, sometimes, often, or consistently demonstrated):
    Verbalization of self-acceptance
    Open communication
    Fulfillment of personally significant roles
    Acceptance of compliments from others
    Willingness to confront others
    Description of success in work, school, and social groups
- Demonstrates **Decision/Making**, as evidenced by the following indicators (specify 1–5: never, rarely, sometimes, often, or consistently demonstrated):
    Identifies alternatives and potential consequences of each
    Identifies resources necessary to support each alternative
    Weighs and chooses among alternatives

Other Examples

Patient will:
- Acknowledge personal strengths

- Practice behaviors that generate self-confidence
- Verbalize episodic change/loss

NIC Priority Interventions

Self-Esteem Enhancement: Assisting a patient to increase his/her personal judgment of self-worth

Nursing Activities

Also refer to "Nursing Activities" for "Self-Esteem, Chronic Low" on pp. 397–398

Patient/Family Teaching

- Teach positive behavioral skills through role play, role modeling, discussion, and so on

Collaborative Activities

- Refer to appropriate community resources
- Seek assistance from hospital resources (social worker, clinical nurse specialist, pastoral care services), as needed

Other

- Explore recent changes with patient that may have influenced low self-esteem
- *(NIC) Self-Esteem Enhancement:*
  Convey confidence in patient's ability to handle situation
  Encourage increased responsibility for self, as appropriate
  Explore reasons for self-criticism or guilt
  Encourage patient to accept new challenges

Self-Esteem Disturbance
(7.1.2) (1978, 1988, 1996)

Definition: Negative self-evaluation/feelings about self or self-capabilities, which may be directly or indirectly expressed

Defining Characteristics

Subjective
Expressions of shame/guilt
Self-negating verbalizations
Objective
Denial of problems obvious to others

Rationalizes away/rejects positive feedback and exaggerates negative feedback about self

Evaluates self as unable to deal with events

Grandiosity

Hesitant to try new things/situations

Hypersensitivity to slight or criticism

Projection of blame/responsibility for problems

Rationalization of personal failures

Other Possible Defining Characteristics (non-NANDA)

Difficulty in making decisions

Lack of eye contact

Lack of follow-through

Nonparticipation in therapy

Verbalization of negative feelings about self

Related Factors

To be developed

Related Factors (Non-NANDA)

Assumption of new role

Chronic illness

Chronic pain

Congenital anomalies

Psychologic impairment (specify)

Situational crisis (specify)

Unmet expectations for child

Unmet expectations for childbirth

Unmet expectations for pregnancy

Suggestions for Use

This label has some defining characteristics in common with *Body image disturbance*; however, the diagnoses can be differentiated by the presence, in *Body image disturbance*, of preoccupation with change in or loss of a body part or function. *Body image disturbance* is specific, but it may contribute to the broader, more pervasive *Self-esteem disturbance*. When you have adequate supporting clinical data, use more specific labels such as *Chronic Low or Situational low self-esteem* instead of *Self-esteem disturbance*.

Suggested Alternative Diagnoses

Body image disturbance

Hopelessness

Personal identity disturbance

Powerlessness
Self-esteem, chronic low
Self-esteem , situational low

NOC Suggested Outcomes

Child Development: 2, 3, 4, 5 Years; Middle Childhood (6–11 Years), and Adolescence (12–17 Years): Milestones of physical, cognitive, and psychosocial progression by (specify) years of age. [**NOTE:** NOC lists each age as a separate outcome.]

Self-Esteem: Personal judgment of self-worth

Goals/Evaluation Criteria

Examples Using NOC Language

Also see NOC "Goals/Evaluation Criteria" for "Self-Esteem, Chronic Low" on p. 397

- Demonstrates **Child Development: 2, 3, 4, 5 Years; Middle Childhood (6–11 Years), and Adolescence (12–17 Years).** [Refer to pediatrics text or NOC manual for age-specific indicators; an exhaustive list is beyond the scope of this text.] Examples of indicators (specify 1–5: extreme, substantial, moderate, mild, or no delay from expected range):

    2 years—Indicates wants verbally; interacts with adults in simple games

    3 years—Gives own first name; plays interactive games with peers

    4 years—Gives first and last name; describes a recent experience

    5 years—Follows rules of interactive games with peers

Other Examples

Patient will:
- Acknowledge impact of situation on existing personal relationships, lifestyle, and role performance
- Express willingness to use resources upon discharge
- Identify personal strengths
- Maintain close personal relationships

NIC Priority Interventions

Self-Esteem Enhancement: Assisting a patient to increase his/her personal judgment of self-worth

Nursing Activities

Refer to "Nursing Activities" for "Self-Esteem, Chronic Low" on pp. 397–398 and for "Self-Esteem, Situational Low" on p. 400

Self-Mutilation, Risk for
(9.2.2.1) (1992)

Definition: A state in which an individual is at risk to perform an act upon the self to injure, not kill, which produces tissue damage and tension relief

Risk Factors
Command hallucinations
Emotionally disturbed and/or battered children
Feelings of depression, rejection, self-hatred, separation anxiety, guilt, and depersonalization
Fluctuating emotions
Inability to cope with increased psychologic/physiologic tension in a healthy manner
Mentally retarded and autistic children
Need for sensory stimuli
Parental emotional deprivation
Patients in psychotic state—frequently males in young adulthood
Patients with a history of self-injury
Patients with borderline personality disorder, especially females from 16 to 25 years of age
History of physical, emotional, or sexual abuse

Suggestions for Use
Risk for self-mutilation is a more specific diagnosis than *Risk for self-directed violence*, although the two diagnoses have some of the same defining characteristics (ie, risk factors). *Risk for self-directed violence* includes actions such as drug and alcohol abuse and high-risk lifestyle (eg, driving fast), which are not included in *Risk for self-mutilation*.

Suggested Alternative Diagnoses
Self-directed violence, risk for
Suicide, risk for

NOC Suggested Outcomes
Aggression Control: Ability to restrain assaultive, combative, or destructive behavior toward others. [**AUTHOR'S NOTE:** This outcome refers to behavior toward others; however, the diagnosis of *Risk for self-mutilation* refers to acts that are harmful to

oneself. Therefore, I do not recommend Aggression Control as an outcome for self-mutilation.]

Impulse Control: Ability to self-restrain compulsive or impulsive behaviors

Risk Detection: Actions taken to identify personal health threats

Self-Mutilation Restraint: Ability to refrain from intentional self-inflicted injury (non-lethal)

Goals/Evaluation Criteria

Examples Using NOC Language

- Demonstrates **Self-Mutilation Restraint**, as evidenced by the following indicators (specify 1–5: never, rarely, sometimes, often, or consistently demonstrated):

    Seeks help when feeling urge to injure self

    Upholds contract to not harm self

    Refrains from gathering means for self-injury

    Maintains self-control without supervision

Other Examples

Patient will:

- Be free from self-injury
- Verbalize reduction or absence of command hallucinations and/or delusions
- Identify feelings that lead to impulsive actions
- Identify and avoid high-risk environments and situations

NIC Priority Interventions

Anger Control Assistance: Facilitation of the expression of anger in an adaptive nonviolent manner

Behavior Management: Self-Harm: Assisting the patient to decrease or eliminate self-mutilating or self-abusive behaviors

Environmental Management, Safety: Monitoring and manipulation of the physical environment to promote safety

Nursing Activities

For All Patients

Assessments

- Assess patient for history of self-injury behaviors, including methods used, known triggers, and so on
- *(NIC) Anger Control Assistance:* Monitor potential for inappropriate aggression and intervene before its expression

- *(NIC) Behavior Management: Self-Harm:* Determine the motive/reason for the behaviors

Patient/Family Teaching

- Provide support and education to family regarding patient status and methods of treatment
- *(NIC) Behavior Management: Self-Harm:* Instruct patient in coping strategies (eg, assertiveness training, impulse control training, and progressive muscle relaxation, as appropriate)

Other

- Provide patient safety, using least restrictive measures (eg, environmental manipulation, assign roommate, assign patient room close to nursing station, family/visitor restriction, patient within eyesight at all times, patient within arm's length, other interventions specific to patient)
- Accompany patient to activities outside of the unit, as needed
- *(NIC) Behavior Management: Self-Harm:*

  Develop appropriate behavioral expectations and consequences, given the patient's level of cognitive functioning and capacity for self-control

  Remove dangerous items from the patient's environment

  Use a calm, nonpunitive approach when dealing with self-harmful behaviors
- *(NIC) Anger Control Assistance:*

  Use external controls (eg, physical or manual restraint, time-outs) as needed to calm patient who is expressing anger in a maladaptive manner

  Identify consequences of inappropriate expression of anger

  Establish basic trust and rapport with patient

Psychotic Patients

Assessments

- Observe for behavioral changes from baseline assessment (eg, increased withdrawal, agitation)
- Assess patient for morbid preoccupation with suicide, self-mutilation, hopelessness, and worthlessness
- Assess patient with command hallucinations to determine content and source (eg, ask patient, "Whose voice is it? What is the voice telling you to do? Is the voice telling you to hurt yourself and how? Does the voice have control over you?")
- Monitor intensity of hallucinations/delusions and attempt reality testing q _____

- Assess patient for religious and/or persecutory delusions that may lead to self-injury
- Assess patient for somatic delusions that may lead to self-injury (eg, beliefs that part of body is diseased, rotten, or unnecessary)

Collaborative Activities

- Obtain physician order if intervention is a denial of rights
- *(NIC) Behavior Management: Self-Harm:* Administer medications, as appropriate, to decrease anxiety, stabilize mood, and decrease self-stimulation

Other

- If patient exhibits calmness abruptly following a period of agitation, provide increased safety measures to prevent self-injury
- Assist patient to differentiate internal stimuli from outside world
- Encourage patient to verbalize thoughts and impulses instead of storing up tension
- Search patient as needed for potentially harmful items
- Trim patient's fingernails/toenails to prevent scratching
- Encourage physical activity
- Contract with patient to not injure self
- If patient is unable to make contract or follow directions, stay with patient at all times until either patient reports a decrease in command hallucinations, delusions, or self-mutilation impulses, or until seclusion/restraint is used
- *(NIC) Behavior Management: Self-Harm:*
  Place patient in a more protective environment (eg, area restriction and seclusion) if self-harmful impulses/behaviors escalate
  Apply, as appropriate, mitts, splints, helmets, or restraints to limit mobility and ability to initiate self-harm
  Assist patient to identify trigger situations and feelings that prompt self-harmful behavior

Personality Disorder Patients

Assessments

- Assess patient's level of impulsivity and frustration tolerance

Patient/Family Teaching

- Teach patient alternative stress-tension-relieving measures (eg, relaxation techniques; physical exercise; journal writing; self-affirmations and distracting techniques such as music, television, and conversation)

- Provide family/significant other with guidelines explaining how self-harmful behavior can be managed outside the care environment
- *(NIC) Behavior Management: Self-Harm:* Provide illness teaching to patient/significant others if self-harmful behavior is illness-based (eg, borderline personality disorder or autism)

Collaborative Activities

- Consider antianxiety or neuroleptic medications according to physician order
- Provide consistent responses to patient by collaborating closely with other health care providers. Review treatment plan frequently to prevent staff splitting and conflict regarding treatment goals.

Other

- Encourage patient to seek out staff and peers instead of using alcohol or drugs
- Establish regular and frequent check-in times with assigned staff
- *(NIC) Behavior Management: Self-Harm:*
  Contract with patient, as appropriate, for "no self-harm"
  Provide predetermined consequences if patient is engaging in self-harmful behaviors

Retarded/Autistic Patients

Assessments

- Assess patient's response to environment to determine if there is a stressor that may lead to self-injury

Patient/Family Teaching

- *(NIC) Behavior Management: Self-Harm:* Provide illness teaching to patient/significant others if self-harmful behavior is illness-based (eg, borderline personality disorder or autism)

Other

- Alter environmental situations that may produce stress that provokes self-injury behaviors
- Remove reinforcement that may induce self-injury behavior (eg, comforting patient after headbanging, excusing patient from perceived unpleasant tasks
- Develop behavioral plan that will prevent or decrease incidence of self-injury
- Use protective devices to prevent self-injury (eg, mitts, helmet, jacket restraint, protective clothing)

Sensory/Perceptual Alterations (Specify: auditory, gustatory, kinesthetic, olfactory, tactile, visual) (7.2) (1978, 1980, 1998)

Definition: A state in which an individual experiences a change in the amount or patterning of incoming stimuli, accompanied by a diminished, exaggerated, distorted, or impaired response to such stimuli

Defining Characteristics

Subjective
Auditory distortions
Reported change in sensory acuity
Visual distortions

Objective
Altered communication patterns
Change in behavior pattern
Change in problem-solving abilities
Change in usual response to stimuli
Disoriented in time, in place, or with people
Hallucinations
Irritability
Measured change in sensory acuity
Poor concentration
Restlessness

Other Possible Defining Characteristics (non-NANDA)
Alteration in posture
Altered abstraction
Anxiety
Apathy
Change in muscular tension
Inappropriate responses
Indication of alteration in body image

Related Factors

Altered sensory perception
Altered sensory reception, transmission, and/or integration
Biochemical imbalance
Biochemical imbalances for sensory distortion (eg, illusions, hallucinations)

Electrolyte imbalance
Excessive environmental stimuli
Insufficient environmental stimuli
Psychological stress

Suggestions for Use

A diagnosis of *Sensory/perceptual alterations* represents a change from the individual's usual response to stimuli; the changes in response are not a result of mental or personality disorders. Use this label to describe patients whose perceptions have been influenced by physiologic factors such as pain, sleep deprivation, or immobility or by disease states such as cerebrovascular accident (CVA), brain trauma, and increased intracranial pressure.

Altered cognition and perception can be symptoms of both *Sensory/perceptual alterations* and *Altered thought processes*. When a person's ability to interpret stimuli is affected by physical or physiologic factors, use *Sensory/perceptual alterations*; when the ability to interpret stimuli is affected by mental disorders, use *Altered thought processes*. To further help differentiate between the two diagnoses, note that the following defining characteristics and related factors may be present in *Altered thought processes* but not in *Sensory/perceptual alterations*:

Obsessive thinking
Loss of memory
Impaired judgment

In addition, the following defining characteristics are present in *Sensory/perceptual alterations*, but not in *Altered thought processes*:

Visual and auditory distortions
Discoordinated motor activity
Changes in sensory acuity

Sensory/perceptual alterations may be more useful as the etiology of other problems, for example the following:

Risk for injury related to visual sensory/perceptual alterations
Self-care deficit related to visual sensory/perceptual alterations
Impaired communication related to auditory sensory/perceptual alterations
Risk for injury related to kinesthetic or tactile sensory/perceptual alterations
Altered nutrition related to olfactory or gustatory sensory/perceptual alterations

When *Sensory/perceptual alterations* exists as a result of immobility, consider using *Risk for disuse syndrome*.

Suggested Alternative Diagnoses

Confusion, acute/chronic
Disuse syndrome, risk for
Environmental interpretation syndrome, impaired
Peripheral neurovascular dysfunction, risk for
Thought processes, altered
Unilateral neglect

NOC Suggested Outcomes

Anxiety Control: Ability to eliminate or reduce feelings of apprehension and tension from an unidentifiable source

Body Image: Positive perception of own appearance and body functions

Cognitive Ability: Ability to execute complex mental processes

Cognitive Orientation: Ability to identify person, place, and time

Distorted Thought Control: Ability to self-restrict disruption in perception, thought processes, and thought content

Energy Conservation: Extent of active management of energy to initiate and sustain activity

Goals/Evaluation Criteria

Examples Using NOC Language

- Demonstrates **Anxiety Control**, as evidenced by the following indicators (specify 1–5: never, rarely, sometimes, often, or consistently demonstrated):

  Reports absence of physical and behavioral manifestations of anxiety

  Reports absence of sensory perceptual distortions

- Demonstrates **Body Image**, as evidenced by the following indicators (specify 1–5: never, rarely, sometimes, often, or consistently positive):

  Congruence between body reality, body ideal, and body presentation

- Demonstrates **Cognitive Ability**, as evidenced by the following indicators (specify 1–5: extremely, substantially, moderately, mildly, or not compromised):

  Attentiveness, concentration, and orientation

  Demonstrates immediate, recent, and remote memory

  Makes appropriate decisions

  Communicates clearly and appropriately for age and ability

- Demonstrates **Cognitive Orientation**, as evidenced by the following indicators (specify 1–5: never, rarely, sometimes, often, or consistently demonstrated): Identifies self, significant other, current place, and correct day, month, year, and season

Other Examples

Patient will:

- Interact appropriately with others and with the environment
- Exhibit logical organization of thoughts
- Correctly interpret ideas communicated by others
- Compensate for sensory deficits by maximizing the use of unimpaired senses

NOTE: Consider other outcomes specific to the particular deficit (ie, visual, auditory, kinesthetic, gustatory, tactile, olfactory)

NIC Priority Interventions

Auditory

Communication Enhancement, Hearing Deficit: Assistance in accepting and learning alternate methods for living with diminished hearing

Gustatory, Olfactory

Nutrition Management: Assisting with or providing a balanced dietary intake of foods and fluids

Kinesthetic

Body Mechanics Promotion: Facilitating the use of posture and movement in daily activities to prevent fatigue and musculoskeletal strain or injury

Olfactory

Nutrition Management: Assisting with or providing a balanced dietary intake of foods and fluids

Weight Management: Facilitating maintenance of optimal body weight and percent body fat

Tactile

Peripheral Sensation Management: Prevention or minimization of injury or discomfort in the patient with altered sensation

Surveillance, Safety: Purposeful and ongoing collection and analysis of information about the patient and the environment for use in promoting and maintaining patient safety

Visual

Communication Enhancement, Visual Deficit: Assistance in accepting and learning alternate methods for living with diminished vision

Environmental Management: Manipulation of the patient's surroundings for therapeutic benefit

Nursing Activities

Assessments

- Monitor and document changes in patient's neurologic status
- Monitor patient's level of consciousness
- Identify factors that contribute to sensory/perceptual alterations, such as sleep deprivation, chemical dependence, medications, treatments, electrolyte imbalance, and so on
- *(NIC) Peripheral Sensation Management:*
  Monitor sharp/dull and/or hot/cold discrimination
  Monitor for paresthesia: numbness, tingling, hyperesthesia, and hypoesthesia
- *(NIC) Surveillance: Safety:*
  Monitor patient for alterations in physical or cognitive function that might lead to unsafe behavior
  Monitor environment for potential safety hazards

Patient/Family Teaching

- *(NIC) Communication Enhancement: Hearing Deficit:* Teach patient that sounds will be experienced differently with the use of a hearing aid
- *(NIC) Peripheral Sensation Management:* Instruct patient or family to examine skin daily for alteration in skin integrity

Collaborative Activities

- Initiate occupational therapy referral, as appropriate

Other

- Ensure access to and use of sensory assistive devices, such as hearing aid and glasses
- Increase number of stimuli to achieve appropriate sensory input (eg, increase social interaction; schedule contacts; provide radio, television, clock with large numbers)
- Reduce number of stimuli to achieve appropriate sensory input (eg, dim lights, provide a private room, limit visitors, establish rest periods for patient)
- Orient to person, place, time, and situation with each interaction
- Reassure patient/family that sensory/perceptual deficit is temporary, whenever appropriate
- *(NIC) Communication Enhancement: Hearing Deficit:*
  Give one simple direction at a time
  Increase voice volume, as appropriate
  Obtain patient's attention through touch

Do not cover your mouth, smoke, talk with a full mouth, or chew
gum when speaking

Refrain from shouting at patient with communication disorders

- *(NIC) Communication Enhancement: Visual Deficit:*

Identify yourself when you enter the patient's space

Build on patient's remaining vision, as appropriate

Do not move items in patient's room without informing patient.

- *(NIC) Nutrition Management:*

Provide patient with high-protein, high-calorie, nutritious finger foods and drinks that can be readily consumed, as appropriate

Provide food selection

- *(NIC) Peripheral Sensation Management:*

Avoid or carefully monitor use of heat or cold, such as heating
pads, hot-water bottles, and ice packs

Instruct patient to visually monitor position of body parts, if
proprioception is impaired

Sexual Dysfunction
(3.2.1.2.1) (1980)

Definition: The state in which an individual experiences a change
in sexual function that is viewed as unsatisfying, unrewarding,
or inadequate

Defining Characteristics

Subjective

Alteration in achieving sexual satisfaction

Change of interest in self or others

Inability to achieve desired satisfaction

Seeking confirmation of desirability

Verbalization of problem

Objective

Actual or perceived limitations imposed by disease and/or therapy

Alterations in achieving perceived sex role

Alteration in relationship with significant other

Conflicts involving values

Other Possible Defining Characteristics (non-NANDA)

Alteration in orgasm/ejaculation

Change in sexual desire

Concern over adequacy in meeting sexual desire of partner
Impotence
Painful coitus
Phobic avoidance of sexual experience
Vaginal dryness

Related Factors

Altered body function or structure (eg, pregnancy, recent childbirth, drugs, surgery, anomalies, disease process, trauma, radiation)
Biopsychosocial alteration of sexuality
Ineffectual or absent role models
Lack of knowledge
Lack of privacy
Lack of significant other
Misinformation
Medical treatment
Physical abuse
Psychosocial abuse (eg, harmful relationships)
Values conflict
Vulnerability

Other Possible Related Factors (non-NANDA)
Body image disturbance
Disturbance in self-esteem
Hormonal changes
Impaired relationship
Pain
Sexual trauma/exploitation
Unrealistic expectations of self and partner

Suggestions for Use

If patient data does not fit the defining characteristics, consider the more general label *Altered sexuality patterns*. **NOTE:** *Sexual dysfunction* may be a symptom of other diagnoses, such as *Rape-trauma syndrome.*

Suggested Alternative Diagnoses

Body image disturbance
Rape-trauma syndrome: silent reaction
Self-esteem disturbance
Sexuality patterns, altered

NOC Suggested Outcomes

Abuse Recovery: Sexual: Healing following sexual abuse or exploitation

Child Development: Adolescence (12–17 Years): Milestones of physical, cognitive, and psychosocial progression between 12 and 17 years of age

Physical Aging Status: Physical changes that commonly occur with adult aging

Risk Control: Sexually Transmitted Diseases (STDs): Actions to eliminate or reduce behaviors associated with sexually transmitted disease

Goals/Evaluation Criteria

Examples Using NOC Language

- Demonstrates **Abuse Recovery: Sexual**, as evidenced by the following indicators (specify 1–5: none, limited, moderate, substantial, or extensive):

    Evidence of appropriate same-sex relationships

    Evidence of appropriate opposite-sex relationships

    Expressions of confidence with gender identity and sexual orientation

- Demonstrates **Child Development: Adolescence (12–17 Years)**, as evidenced by the following indicators (specify 1–5: extreme, substantial, moderate, mild, or no delay from expected range):

    Describes sexual development

    Expresses comfort with own sexual identity

    Maintains good peer relationships with same gender

    Maintains good peer relationships with opposite gender

    Demonstrates capacity for intimacy

    Practices responsible sexual behaviors

Other Examples

Patient/partner will:

- Demonstrate willingness to discuss changes in sexual function
- Request needed information about changes in sexual function
- Verbalize understanding of medically imposed restrictions
- Adapt modes of sexual expression to accommodate age- or illness-related physical changes
- Verbalize ways to avoid sexually transmitted diseases

NIC Priority Interventions

Sexual Counseling: Use of an interactive helping process focusing on the need to make adjustments in sexual practice or to enhance coping with a sexual event/disorder

Nursing Activities

Assessments

- Monitor for indicators of resolution of *Sexual dysfunction* (eg, capacity for intimacy)
- *(NIC) Sexual Counseling:*
  Preface questions about sexuality with a statement that tells the patient that many people experience sexual difficulties
  Determine amount of sexual guilt associated with the patient's perception of the illness

Patient/Family Teaching

- Provide information necessary to enhance sexual function (eg, anticipatory guidance, educational materials, stress-reduction exercises, sensation-enhancing exercises, prosthetics, implants, focused counseling)
- *(NIC) Sexual Counseling:*
  Discuss the effect of the illness/health situation/medication on sexuality, as appropriate [eg, medication side effects; normal aspects of aging; postsurgical adjustments, especially after surgery on sexual organs or ostomy; postmyocardial infarction]
  Discuss the necessary modifications in sexual activity, as appropriate
  Inform patient initially that sexuality is an important part of life and that illness, medications, and stress (or other problems/events the patient is experiencing) often alter sexual functioning
  Provide factual information about sexual myths and misinformation that patient may verbalize
  Instruct the patient only on techniques compatible with values/beliefs

Collaborative Activities

- Encourage continuation of counseling after discharge
- *(NIC) Sexual Counseling:*
  Provide referral/consultation with other members of the health care team, as appropriate
  Refer the patient to a sex therapist, as appropriate

Other

- Encourage verbalization of sexual concerns by utilizing caregivers who have an established rapport with patient and are comfortable discussing patient's sexual concerns. Specify caregiver.
- Allow time and privacy to address patient's sexual concerns
- Alert patient/partner to possibility of disinterest in, decreased capacity for, or discomfort during sexual activity
- *(NIC) Sexual Counseling:*

  Encourage patient to verbalize fears and to ask questions

  Help patient to express grief and anger about alterations in body functioning/appearance, as appropriate

  Include the spouse/sexual partner in the counseling as much as possible, as appropriate

  Introduce patient to positive role models who have successfully conquered a similar problem, as appropriate

  Provide reassurance and permission to experiment with alternative forms of sexual expression, as appropriate

Sexuality Patterns, Altered
(3.3) (1986)

Definition: The state in which an individual expresses concern regarding his/her sexuality

Defining Characteristics

Subjective

Reported difficulties, limitations, or changes in sexual behaviors or activities

Related Factors

Conflicts with sexual orientation or variant preferences

Fear of pregnancy or acquiring sexually transmitted disease

Impaired relationship with significant other

Ineffective or absent role models

Knowledge/skill deficit about alternative responses to health-related transitions, altered body function or structure, illness, or medical condition

Lack of privacy

Lack of significant other

Other Possible Related Factors (non-NANDA)
Body image disturbance
Disturbance in self-esteem
Illness or medical treatments

Suggestions for Use

When possible, use a more specific label, such as *Sexual dysfunction.*

Suggested Alternative Diagnoses

Body image disturbance
Rape-trauma syndrome: silent reaction
Self-esteem disturbance
Sexual dysfunction

NOC Suggested Outcomes

Abuse Recovery: Sexual: Healing following sexual abuse or exploitation

Body Image: Positive perception of own appearance and body function

Child Development: Middle Childhood (6–11 Years): Milestones of physical, cognitive, and psychosocial progression between 6 and 11 years of age

Child Development: Adolescence (12–17 Years): Milestones of physical, cognitive, and psychosocial progression between 12 and 17 years of age

Role Performance: Congruence of an individual's role behavior with role expectations

Self-Esteem: Personal judgment of self-worth

Goals/Evaluation Criteria

Examples Using NOC Language

- Demonstrates **Abuse Recovery: Sexual**: (See "Goals/Evaluation Criteria" for "Sexual Dysfunction," p. 415.)
- Demonstrates **Child Development: Adolescence (12–17 Years).** (Also see "Goals/Evaluation Criteria" for "Sexual Dysfunction," p. 415.)
- Demonstrates **Child Development: Middle Childhood (6–11 Years),** as evidenced by the following indicators (specify 1–5: extreme, substantial, moderate, mild, or no delay from expected range):

    Identifies with same-sex peer group
    Develops close friendships

Other Examples

Patient/partner will:

- Actively participate in counseling
- Request needed information about sexuality
- Acknowledge importance of discussing sexual issues with partner
- Discuss concerns about sexuality
- Express satisfaction with sexuality

NIC Priority Interventions

Sexual Counseling: Use of an interactive helping process focusing on the need to make adjustments in sexual practice or to enhance coping with a sexual event/disorder

Nursing Activities

Refer to "Nursing Activities" for "Sexual Dysfunction," pp. 416–417

Skin Integrity, Impaired [Specify]
(1.6.2.1.2.1) (1975, 1998)

Definition: A state in which an individual has altered epidermis and/or dermis

Defining Characteristics

Objective

Disruption of skin surface (epidermis)

Destruction of skin layers (dermis)

Invasion of body structures

Related Factors

External [Environmental]

Chemical substance

Humidity

Hyperthermia

Hypothermia

Mechanical factors (eg, shearing forces, pressure, restraint)

Medications

Physical immobilization

Radiation

Internal [Somatic]

Altered circulation

Alterations in turgor (changes in elasticity)
Altered fluid status
Altered metabolic state
Altered nutritional state (eg, obesity, emaciation)
Altered pigmentation
Altered sensation
Developmental factors
Extremes in age
Immunologic deficit
Skeletal prominence

Suggestions for Use

Impaired skin integrity is rather nonspecific. A disruption of the skin surface could be a surgical incision, abrasion, blisters, or decubitus ulcers. When this label is used, the type of disruption should be specified in the problem, not in the etiology. **NOTE:** In the following example, the dermal ulcer is a specific *type* of *Impaired skin integrity*, not a *cause* of *Impaired skin integrity*:

> **Correct**: *Impaired skin integrity: dermal ulcer related to complete immobility*

> **Incorrect**: *Impaired skin integrity related to dermal ulcer*

When an ulcer is deeper than the epidermis, use *Impaired tissue integrity* instead of *Impaired skin integrity*. Deeper ulcers may require a collaborative approach (ie, surgical treatment). Do not use *Impaired skin integrity* as a label for a surgical incision because there are no independent nursing actions to treat this type of "impairment" and the condition is usually self-limiting. The usual nursing care for a surgical incision is to prevent and detect infection; therefore, a diagnosis of *Risk for infection of surgical incision* or the collaborative problem Potential Complication of surgery: Incision infection might be used instead of *Impaired skin integrity*.

Suggested Alternative Diagnoses

Infection, risk for
Skin integrity, risk for impaired
Tissue integrity, impaired

NOC Suggested Outcomes

Tissue Integrity: Skin and Mucous Membranes: Structural intactness and normal physiologic function of skin and mucous membranes
Wound Healing: Primary Intention: The extent to which cells and tissues have regenerated following intentional closure

Wound Healing: Secondary Intention: The extent to which cells and tissues in an open wound have regenerated

Goals/Evaluation Criteria

Examples Using NOC Language

- Demonstrates **Tissue Integrity: Skin and Mucous Membranes,** as evidenced by the following indicators (specify 1–5: extremely, substantially, moderately, mildly, or not compromised):

   Tissue temperature, elasticity, hydration, pigmentation, and color in expected range

   Tissue lesion-free

   Skin intactness

- Demonstrates **Wound Healing: Primary Intention**, as evidenced by the following indicators (specify 1–5: none, slight, moderate, substantial, or complete):

   Skin approximation

   Resolution of drainage from wound and/or drain

   Resolution of surrounding skin erythema

   Resolution of wound odor

- Demonstrates **Wound Healing: Secondary Intention**, as evidenced by the following indicators (specify 1–5: none, slight, moderate, substantial, or complete):

   Purulent (or other) drainage and/or wound odor

   Blistered or macerated skin

   Necrosis, sloughing, tunneling, undermining, and/or sinus tract formation

   Skin and periwound erythema

   Wound size

Other Examples

- Patient/family demonstrate optimal skin/wound care routine

NIC Priority Interventions

Incision Site Care: Cleansing, monitoring, and promotion of healing in a wound that is closed with sutures, clips, or staples

Skin Surveillance: Collection and analysis of patient data to maintain skin and mucous membrane integrity

Wound Care: Prevention of wound complications and promotion of wound healing

Nursing Activities

Also see "Nursing Activities" for "Skin Integrity, Risk for Impaired" pp. 426–428

Assessments

- Assess functioning of equipment such as pressure-relieving devices, including static-air mattress, low-air loss therapy, air-fluidized therapy, and water bed
- *(NIC) Incision Site Care:* Inspect the incision site for redness, swelling, or signs of dehiscence or evisceration
- *(NIC) Wound Care:*
  Inspect the wound with each dressing change

NOTE: Characteristics of the wound should include the following:

- Location, dimensions and depth of wound
- Presence and character of exudate, including tenacity, color, and odor
- Presence or absence of granulation/epithelialization
- Presence or absence of necrotic tissue. Describe color, odor, amount.
- Presence or absence of symptoms of local wound infection (eg, pain on palpation, edema, pruritus, induration, warmth, foul odor, eschar, exudate)
- Presence or absence of undermining and/or sinus-tract formation]

Patient/Family Teaching

- Instruct in care of surgical incision, including signs and symptoms of infection, ways to keep incision dry during bath, and minimization of stress on the incision
- *(NIC) Skin Surveillance:* Instruct family member/caregiver about signs of skin breakdown, as appropriate
- *(NIC) Wound Care:* Teach patient or family member(s) wound care procedures

Collaborative Activities

- Consult dietitian for foods high in proteins, minerals, calories, and vitamins
- Consult physician regarding implementation of enteral feedings or parenteral nutrition to increase wound healing potential
- Refer to enterostomal therapy nurse for assistance with assessment, staging, treatment, and documentation of wound care/skin breakdown
- *(NIC) Wound Care:* Apply TENS (transcutaneous electrical nerve stimulation) unit for wound healing enhancement, as appropriate

Other

- Evaluate topical dressing/treatment measures, which may

include hydrocolloid dressings, hydrophilic dressings, absorbent dressings, and so forth
- Establish a wound/skin care routine, which may include the following:
    Frequently turn and reposition patient
    Keep surrounding tissue free from excess moisture and drainage
    Protect patient from fecal/urinary contamination
    Protect patient from other wound and drain-tube excretions into wound
- Clean and dress surgical incision site using the following principles of sterility or medical asepsis, as appropriate:
    Wear disposable gloves (sterile, if needed)
    Clean incision from "clean to dirty," using one swab for each wipe
    Clean around staples/sutures, using sterile cotton-tipped applicator
    Clean around drain last, moving from center outward in a circular motion
    Apply antiseptic ointment, as ordered
    Change dressing at appropriate intervals or leave open to air according to order
- *(NIC) Wound Care:*
    Remove adhesive tape and debris
    Clean with antibacterial soap, as appropriate
    Place affected area in a whirlpool bath, as appropriate
    Administer IV site, Hickman line, or central venous line site care, as appropriate
    Massage the area around the wound to stimulate circulation
    Administer skin ulcer care, as needed
    Position to avoid placing tension on the wound, as appropriate

Skin Integrity, Risk for Impaired
(1.6.2.1.2.2) (1975, 1998)

Definition: A state in which the individual's skin is at risk of being adversely altered. **NOTE:** Risk should be determined by the use of a risk assessment tool (eg, Braden Scale).

Risk Factors

External [Environmental]
Chemical substance
Excretions/secretions

Extremes of age
Humidity
Hyperthermia
Hypothermia
Mechanical factors (eg, shearing forces, pressure, restraint)
Medications
Moisture
Physical immobilization
Radiation

Internal [Somatic]
Alterations in nutritional state (eg, obesity, emaciation)
Alterations in skin turgor (ie, changes in elasticity)
Altered circulation
Altered metabolic state
Altered pigmentation
Altered sensation
Developmental factors
Immunologic [deficit]
Psychogenic
Skeletal prominence

Suggestions for Use

Use this diagnosis for patients who have no symptoms but who are at risk of developing disruption of skin surface or destruction of skin layers if preventive measures are not instituted. The presence of more than one risk factor increases the likelihood of skin damage. When *Risk for impaired skin integrity* occurs as a result of immobility and when other body systems are also at risk for impairment, consider using *Risk for disuse syndrome*.

Suggested Alternative Diagnosis

Disuse syndrome, risk for
Skin integrity, impaired

NOC Suggested Outcomes

Child Development: Adolescence (12–17 Years): Milestones of physical, cognitive, and psychosocial progression between 12 and 17 years of age

Immobility Consequences: Physiologic: Compromise in physiologic functioning due to impaired physical mobility

Nutritional Status: Extent to which nutrients are available to meet metabolic needs

Risk Control: Actions to eliminate or reduce actual, personal, and modifiable health threats

Self-Mutilation Restraint: Ability to refrain from intentional self-inflicted injury (nonlethal)

Tissue Perfusion: Peripheral: Extent to which blood flows through the small vessels of the extremities and maintains tissue function

Goals/Evaluation Criteria

Examples Using NOC Language

- Demonstrates **Immobility Consequences: Physiological**, as evidenced by the following indicators (specify 1–5: severe, substantial, moderate, slight, or none):

    Pressure sores

    Decreased nutrition status

- Demonstrates **Risk Control**, as evidenced by the following indicators (specify 1–5: never, rarely, sometimes, often, or consistently demonstrated):

    Monitors environmental and behavioral risk factors [that contribute to *Impaired skin integrity*]

    Follows selected risk-control strategies

    Recognizes changes in health status [that affect skin]

- Demonstrates **Self-Mutilation Restraint** (specify 1–5: never, rarely, sometimes, often, or consistently demonstrated).

- Demonstrates **Tissue Perfusion: Peripheral**, as evidenced by the following indicators (specify 1–5: extremely, substantially, moderately, mildly, or not compromised):

    Capillary refill brisk

    Distal and proximal pulses strong and symmetric

    Skin color and sensation level normal

    Extremity temperature warm

    Localized extremity pain not present

Other Examples

Patient/family will:

- Have intact skin
- Demonstrate effective skin care routine
- Ingest foods adequate to promote skin integrity

NIC Priority Interventions

Pressure Management: Minimizing pressure to body parts

Pressure Ulcer Prevention: Prevention of decubitus ulcers for a patient at high risk for developing them

Skin Surveillance: Collection and analysis of patient data to maintain skin and mucous membrane integrity

Nursing Activities
All Patients at Risk
Assessments

- On admission and whenever physical condition changes, assess for risk factors that may lead to skin breakdown (eg, bed/chair confinement, inability to move, loss of bowel/bladder control, poor nutrition, and lowered mental awareness)
- Identify sources of pressure and friction (eg, cast, bedding, clothing)
- *(NIC) Pressure Ulcer Prevention:*
  Use an established risk assessment tool to monitor patient's risk factors (eg, Braden scale)
  Inspect skin over bony prominences and other pressure points when repositioning or at least daily
- *(NIC) Skin Surveillance:*
  Monitor skin for the following:
  Rashes and abrasions
  Color and temperature
  Excessive dryness and moistness
  Areas of redness and breakdown

Collaborative Activities

- Refer to enterostomal therapy nurse for assistance with prevention, assessment, and treatment of skin breakdown/wounds

Other

- Use a pressure-reducing mattress (eg, polyurethane foam pad)
- Avoid massage over bony prominences
- *(NIC) Pressure Ulcer Prevention:*
  Apply elbow and heel protectors, as appropriate
  Keep bed linens clean, dry, and wrinkle-free

Patients with Mobility/Activity Deficit
Assessments

- Assess for extent of limitations in ability to transfer or move about in bed

Other

- Pad cast edges and traction connections

For chair-bound individuals:
- Consider postural alignment; distribution of weight, balance, and stability; and pressure relief when positioning individuals in chairs or wheelchairs
- Have patient shift weight q 15 minutes if able
- Use pressure-reducing devices for seating surfaces. *Do not use donut-type devices.*
  For bed-bound individuals:
- Avoid positioning directly on the trochanter
- Elevate the head of the bed as little and for as short a time as possible
- Use a pressure-reducing mattress/bed (eg, foam, air, egg-crate)
- Use proper positioning, transferring, and turning techniques
- Use lifting devices to move, rather than drag, individuals during transfers and position changes
- *(NIC) Pressure Ulcer Prevention:*
  Turn q 1 to 2 hours continuously, as appropriate
  Provide trapeze to assist patient in shifting weight frequently
  Position with pillows to elevate pressure points off the bed
  Apply elbow and heel protectors, as appropriate

Patients with Incontinence or Presence of Moisture

Assessments
- Assess need for indwelling or condom catheter
- Check for urinary or fecal incontinence q ____

Other
- Cleanse skin at time of soiling
- Individualize bathing schedule, avoid hot water, use mild cleansing agent
- Minimize skin exposure to moisture
- *(NIC) Pressure Ulcer Prevention:*
  Remove excessive moisture on the skin resulting from perspiration, wound drainage, and fecal or urinary incontinence
  Apply protective barriers, such as creams or moisture-absorbing pads, to remove excess moisture, as appropriate
  Apply transparent film occlusive dressing to areas at risk to protect skin from wetness
  Turn with care to prevent injury to fragile skin

Patients with Nutritional Deficit

Assessments
- Monitor nutritional status and food intake

Collaborative Activities

- Consult dietitian for foods high in protein, minerals, and vitamins
- Request physician order for serum albumin level, packed-cell volume, and transferrin levels

Other

- Compare actual weight to ideal body weight
- Investigate factors that compromise an apparently well-nourished individual's dietary intake (especially protein or calories) and offer support with eating
- *(NIC) Pressure Ulcer Prevention:* Ensure adequate nutrition, especially protein, vitamins B and C, iron, and calories, using supplements, as appropriate

Sleep Deprivation
(6.2.1.1) (1998)

Definition: Prolonged periods of time without sustained natural, periodic suspension of relative unconsciousness

Defining Characteristics

Subjective

Anxious

Daytime drowsiness

Hallucinations

Heightened sensitivity to pain

Malaise

Perceptual disorders (eg, disturbed body sensation, delusions, feeling afloat)

Objective

Acute confusion

Agitated or combative

Apathy

Decreased ability to function

Hand tremors

Listlessness

Inability to concentrate

Irritability

Lethargy

Mild, fleeting nystagmus

Restlessness
Slowed reaction
Tiredness
Transient paranoia

Related Factors

Aging-related sleep stage shifts
Dementia
Familial sleep paralysis
Idiopathic central nervous system hypersomnolence
Inadequate daytime activity
Narcolepsy
Nightmares
Nonsleep-inducing parenting practices
Periodic limb movement (eg, restless leg syndrome, nocturnal
   myoclonus)
Prolonged physical discomfort
Prolonged psychologic discomfort
Prolonged use of pharmacologic or dietary antisoporifics
Sleep apnea
Sleep terror
Sleepwalking
Sleep-related enuresis
Sleep-related painful erections
Sundowner's syndrome
Sustained circadian asynchrony
Sustained environmental stimulation
Sustained inadequate sleep hygiene
Sustained unfamiliar or uncomfortable sleep environment

Suggestions for Use

Because *Sleep deprivation* represents a lack of sleep that continues over long periods of time, the defining characteristics are
more varied and more severe than those for *Sleep pattern disturbance*, which is a short-term lack of sleep that might occur, for
example, during a brief hospitalization. Therefore, in addition to
measures to promote and restore sleep, nursing activities for *Sleep
deprivation* will focus on relieving symptoms, such as paranoia,
restlessness, and confusion. *Sleep deprivation* can be the etiology
of other nursing diagnoses, for example, *Anxiety, Acute confusion,
Altered thought processes, Impaired memory,* and *Sensory/percep-
tual alterations.*

Suggested Alternative Diagnoses

Activity intolerance

Confusion, acute

Fatigue

Sleep pattern disturbance

NOC Suggested Outcomes

This is a new diagnosis, so NOC has not yet published suggested outcomes. However, the following outcomes seem to be appropriate choices:

Rest: Extent and pattern of diminished activity for mental and physical rejuvenation

Sleep: Extent and pattern of sleep for mental and physical rejuvenation

Well-Being: An individual's expressed satisfaction with health status

Goals/Evaluation Criteria

Examples Using NOC Language

- Demonstrates **Sleep**, as evidenced by the following indicators (specify 1–5: extremely, substantially, moderately, mildly, or not compromised):

    Feelings of rejuvenation after sleep

    Sleep pattern, quality, and routine not compromised

    Hours of sleep not compromised

    Wakeful at appropriate times

Other Examples

The patient will:

- Report relief from symptoms of *Sleep deprivation* (eg, confusion, anxiety, daytime drowsiness, perceptual disorders, and tiredness)
- Identify and use measures that will increase rest/sleep
- Identify factors that contribute to *Sleep deprivation* (eg, pain, inadequate daytime activity)

NIC Priority Interventions

This is a new diagnosis, so priority interventions are not yet available from NIC. The following seems to be an appropriate intervention:

Sleep Enhancement: Facilitation of regular sleep/wake cycles

Nursing Activities

See "Nursing Activities" for "Sleep Pattern Disturbance," on pp. 435–436

Assessments

- Assess for symptoms of *Sleep deprivation*, such as *Acute confusion*, agitation, *Anxiety*, perceptual disorders, slowed reactions, and irritability

Patient Teaching

- Teach patient/family about factors that interfere with sleep (eg, stress, hectic lifestyle, shift work, room temperature too cold or too hot)

Collaborative Activities

- Confer with physician regarding need to revise medication regimen when it interferes with sleep
- Confer with physician regarding use of sleep medications that do not suppress REM sleep
- Make referrals as needed for treatment of severe symptoms of *Sleep deprivation* (eg, *Acute confusion*, agitation, or *Anxiety*)

Other

- Treat symptoms of *Sleep deprivation*, as needed (eg, *Anxiety*, restlessness, transient paranoia, inability to concentrate); these will vary with individual patients

Sleep Pattern Disturbance
(6.2.1) (1980, 1998)

Definition: Time-limited disruption of sleep (natural, periodic suspension of consciousness) amount and quality

Defining Characteristics

Subjective

Awakening earlier or later than desired

Dissatisfaction with sleep

Verbal complaints of difficulty in falling asleep

Verbal complaints of not feeling well-rested

Objective

Decreased ability to function

Decreased proportion of REM sleep (eg, REM rebound, hyperactivity, emotional lability, agitation and impulsivity, atypical polysomnographic features)

Decreased proportion of stages 3 and 4 sleep (eg, hyporesponsiveness, excess sleepiness, decreased motivation)

Early-morning insomnia

Increased proportion of stage 1 sleep

Less than age-normed total sleep time

Prolonged awakenings

Self-induced impairment of normal pattern

Sleep maintenance insomnia

Sleep onset greater than 30 minutes

Three or more nighttime awakenings

Other Possible Defining Characteristics (non-NANDA)

Dark circles under eyes

Decreased attention span

Flat affect

Frequent daytime napping

Frequent yawning

Interrupted sleep

Irritability

Lethargy

Listlessness

Mood alterations

Ptosis of eyelid

Restlessness

Slight hand tremor

Thick speech with mispronunciation and incorrect words

Related Factors

Psychologic

Aging-related sleep shifts

Anticipation

Anxiety

Biochemical agents

Body temperature

Boredom

Childhood onset

Circadian asynchrony

Daylight/darkness exposure

Daytime activity pattern

Delayed or advanced sleep phase syndrome

Depression

Dietary
Fatigue
Fear
Fear of insomnia
Frequent travel across time zones
Frequently changing sleep/wake schedule
Grief
Inadequate sleep hygiene
Loneliness
Loss of sleep partner, life change
Maladaptive conditioned wakefulness
Periodic gender-related hormonal shifts
Preoccupation with trying to sleep
Ruminative presleep thoughts
Separation from significant others
Shift work
Social schedule inconsistent with chronotype
Sustained use of antisleep agents
Temperament
Thinking about home

Environmental

Ambient temperature, humidity
Excessive stimulation
Lack of sleep privacy/control
Lighting
Medications [eg, depressants or stimulants]
Noise
Noxious odors
Nurse [who wakens patient] for therapeutics, monitoring, lab tests
Other-generated awakening
Physical restraint
Sleep partner
Unfamiliar sleep furnishings

Parental

Mother's emotional support
Mother's sleep/wake pattern
Parent-infant interaction

Physiologic

Fever
Gastroesophageal reflux
Nausea
Position

Shortness of breath
Stasis of secretions
Urinary urgency
Wet

Other Possible Related Factors (Non-NANDA)
Anxiety
Inactivity
Pain/discomfort
Unfamiliar surroundings

Suggestions for Use

Sleep pattern disturbance is used when disruption of sleep causes discomfort or interferes with the patient's desired lifestyle. *Sleep pattern disturbance* is a general diagnosis. The etiologic factors can sometimes make it specific enough to direct nursing intervention, as in *Sleep pattern disturbance related to frequent awakening of infant during the night.* When possible, the specific type of *Sleep pattern disturbance* should be identified (on the problem side of the diagnosis) in order to better direct nursing care. Following are examples of appropriate diagnoses:

*Sleep pattern disturbance (**early awakening**) related to depression*
*Sleep pattern disturbance (**delayed onset of sleep**) related to overstimulation prior to bedtime*

Suggested Alternative Diagnoses

Activity intolerance
Fatigue
Sleep deprivation

NOC Suggested Outcomes

Comfort Level: Feelings of physical and psychologic ease
Pain Level: Amount of reported or demonstrated pain
Psychosocial Adjustment: Life Change: Psychosocial adaptation of an individual to a life change
Quality of Life: An individual's expressed satisfaction with current life circumstances
Rest: Extent and pattern of diminished activity for mental and physical rejuvenation
Sleep: Extent and pattern of sleep for mental and physical rejuvenation
Well-Being: An individual's expressed satisfaction with health status

Goals/Evaluation Criteria

Examples Using NOC Language

- Patient demonstrates **Sleep**, as evidenced by the following indicators (specify 1–5: extremely, substantially, moderately, mildly, or not compromised):

    Hours of sleep not compromised

    Sleep pattern, quality, and routine not compromised

    Feelings of rejuvenation after sleep and/or rest

    Napping appropriate for age

    Wakeful at appropriate times

Other Examples

Patient will:

- Identify measures that will increase rest/sleep
- Demonstrate physical and psychologic well-being

NIC Priority Interventions

Sleep Enhancement: Facilitation of regular sleep/wake cycles

Nursing Activities

Assessments

- *(NIC) Sleep Enhancement:*

    Determine the effects of the patient's medications on sleep pattern

    Monitor patient's sleep pattern and note physical (eg, sleep apnea, obstructed airway, pain/discomfort, and urinary frequency) and/or psychologic (eg, fear or anxiety) circumstances that interrupt sleep

Patient/Family Teaching

- *(NIC) Sleep Enhancement:*

    Explain the importance of adequate sleep during pregnancy, illness, psychosocial stresses, etc.

    Instruct the patient and significant others about factors (eg, physiologic, psychologic, lifestyle, frequent work-shift changes, rapid time-zone changes, excessively long work hours, and other environmental factors) that contribute to sleep pattern disturbances

Collaborative Activities

- Confer with physician regarding need to revise medication regimen when it interferes with sleep pattern
- *(NIC) Sleep Enhancement:* Encourage use of sleep medications that do not contain REM-sleep suppressors

Other

- Avoid loud noises and use of overhead lights during nighttime sleep, providing a quiet, peaceful environment and minimizing interruptions
- Find a compatible roommate for the patient, if possible
- Help patient identify possible underlying causes of sleeplessness, such as fear, unresolved problems, and conflicts
- Reassure patient that irritability and mood alterations are common consequences of sleep deprivation
- *(NIC) Sleep Enhancement:*

    Facilitate maintenance of patient's usual bedtime routine, presleep cues/props, and familiar objects (eg, for children, a favorite blanket/toy, rocking, pacifier, or story; for adults, a book to read, etc.), as appropriate

    Instruct patient to avoid bedtime foods and beverages that interfere with sleep

    Assist patient to limit daytime sleep by providing activity that promotes wakefulness, as appropriate

    Initiate/implement comfort measures of massage, positioning, and affective touch

    Provide for naps during the day, if indicated, to meet sleep requirements

    Group care activities to minimize number of awakenings; allow for sleep cycles of at least 90 minutes

Social Interaction, Impaired
(3.1.1) (1986)

Definition: The state in which an individual participates in an insufficient or excessive quantity or ineffective quality of social exchange

Defining Characteristics

Subjective

Family report of change of style or pattern of interaction

Verbalized or observed discomfort in social situations

Verbalization or observed inability to receive or communicate a satisfying sense of belonging, caring, interest, or shared history

Objective

Dysfunctional interaction with peers, family, and/or others

Observed use of unsuccessful social interaction behaviors

Related Factors

Absence of available significant others/peers
Altered thought processes
Communication barriers
Environmental barriers
Knowledge/skill deficit about ways to enhance mutuality
Limited physical mobility
Self-concept disturbance
Sociocultural dissonance
Therapeutic isolation

Other Related Factors (non-NANDA)
Chemical dependence
Developmental disability
Psychologic impairment (specify)

Suggestions for Use

Differentiate between *Impaired social interaction* and *Social isolation*. A diagnosis of *Impaired social interaction* focuses more on the patient's social skills and abilities, whereas *Social isolation* focuses on the patient's feelings of aloneness and may not be a result of her/his ineffective social skills. Compare the defining characteristics and related factors in Table 9 in "Suggestions for Use" for "Social Isolation," p. 441.

Suggested Alternative Diagnoses

Communication, impaired verbal
Self-esteem disturbance
Social isolation
Thought processes, altered

NOC Suggested Outcomes

Child Development: 2, 4, 6, and 12 Months; 2, 3, 4, and 5 Years, Middle Childhood (6–11 Years), and Adolescence (12–17 Years): Milestones of physical, cognitive, and psychosocial progression by years of age. [NOC lists each age as a separate outcome.]

Play Participation: Use of activities as needed for enjoyment, entertainment, and development by children

Role Performance: Congruence of an individual's role behavior with role expectations

Social Interaction Skills: An individual's use of effective interaction behaviors

Social Involvement: Frequency of an individual's social interactions with persons, groups, or organizations

Goals/Evaluation Criteria

Examples Using NOC Language

- Demonstrates **Play Participation** (specify 1–5: not, slightly, moderately, substantially, or totally adequate)
- Demonstrates **Social Interaction Skills** (specify 1–5: none, limited, moderate, substantial, or extensive)
- Demonstrates **Child Development**, as evidenced by the following indicators (specify 1–5: extreme, substantial, moderate, mild, or no delay from expected range). [Refer to pediatrics text or NOC manual for age-specific indicators; an exhaustive list is beyond the scope of this text.]

    2 Months: Shows pleasure in interactions, especially with primary caregivers

    4 Months: Recognizes parents' voices and touch

    6 Months: Comforts self

    12 Months: Waves bye-bye

    2 Years: Interacts with adults in simple games

    3 Years: Plays interactive games with peers

    4 Years: Describes a recent experience

    5 Years: Follows rules of interactive games with peers

    6–11 Years: Plays in groups

    12–17 Years: Uses social interaction skills

- Demonstrates **Role Performance**, as evidenced by the following indicators (specify 1–5: not, slightly, moderately, substantially, or totally adequate): Performance of family, community, work, friendship, and intimate role behaviors
- Demonstrates **Social Involvement**, as evidenced by the following indicators (specify 1–5: none, limited, moderate, substantial, or extensive): Interaction with close friends, neighbors, family members, and members of work group(s)

Other Examples

Patient will:
- Acknowledge the effect of own behavior on social interactions
- Demonstrate behaviors that may increase/improve social interactions
- Acquire/improve social interaction skills (eg, disclosure, cooperation, sensitivity, assertiveness, genuineness, compromise)
- Express a desire for social contact with others
- Participate in and enjoy appropriate play

NIC Priority Interventions

Socialization Enhancement: Facilitation of another person's ability to interact with others

Nursing Activities

Assessments

- Assess established pattern of interaction between patient and others

Patient/Family Teaching

- Provide information on community resources that will assist the patient to continue with increasing social interaction after discharge

Collaborative Activities

- Confer with other disciplines and patient to establish, implement, and evaluate a plan to increase/improve the patient's interactions with others
- *(NIC) Socialization Enhancement:* Refer patient to transactional analysis group or program in which understanding of transactions can be increased, as appropriate

Other

- Assign scheduled interactions
- Identify specific behavior change
- Identify tasks that will increase or improve social interactions
- Involve supportive peers in giving feedback to patient on social interactions
- Mediate between patient and others when patient exhibits negative behavior
- *(NIC) Socialization Enhancement:*
  Encourage honesty in presenting oneself to others
  Encourage respect for the rights of others
  Encourage patience in developing new relationships
  Help patient increase awareness of strengths and limitations in communicating with others
  Use role playing to practice improved communication skills and techniques
  Request and expect verbal communication
  Give positive feedback when patient reaches out to others
  Facilitate patient input and planning of future activities

Social Isolation
(3.1.2) (1982)

Definition: Aloneness experienced by the individual and perceived as imposed by others and as a negative or threatened state

Defining Characteristics

Subjective
Expressed feelings of aloneness imposed by others
Experiences feelings of differences from others
Expressed feelings of rejection
Expresses values acceptable to the subculture but unacceptable to the dominant cultural group
Projects hostility in voice, behavior

Objective
Absence of supportive significant others (eg, family, friends, group)
Evidence of physical/mental handicap or altered state of wellness
Inability to meet expectations of others
Inadequate or absent significant purpose in life
Inappropriate or immature activities/interests for developmental stage
Insecurity in public
No eye contact
Preoccupation with own thoughts
Repetitive meaningless actions
Sad, dull affect
Seeks to be alone or exists in a subculture
Shows behavior unacceptable to dominant cultural group
Uncommunicative
Withdrawal

Related Factors

Alterations in physical appearance
Altered state of wellness
Factors contributing to the absence of satisfying personal relationships (eg, delay in accomplishing developmental tasks)
Immature interests
Inability to engage in satisfying personal relationships
Inadequate personal resources
Unaccepted social behavior or values

<u>Other Related Factors (non-NANDA)</u>
Chemical dependence
Psychologic impairment (specify)
Treatment-imposed isolation

Suggestions for Use

Differentiate between *Social isolation* and *Impaired social interaction.* A diagnosis of *Impaired social interaction* focuses more on the patient's social skills and abilities, whereas *Social isolation* focuses on the patient's feelings of aloneness and may not be a result of her/his ineffective social skills. Table 9 compares the defining characteristics and related factors of *Impaired social interaction* to *Social isolation.*

Table 9

	Impaired Social Interaction	**Social Isolation**
Shared Defining Characteristics	Verbalized or observed discomfort in social situations	Verbalized or observed discomfort in social situations
Differentiating Defining Characteristics	Ineffective social behaviors Feelings of rejection	Feelings of aloneness imposed by others
Related Factors	Lack of knowledge of social skills Communication barriers	Mental impairment Physical disabilities

Suggested Alternative Diagnoses

Communication, impaired verbal
Post-trauma syndrome
Relocation stress syndrome
Social interaction, impaired
Thought processes, altered

NOC Suggested Outcomes

Loneliness: The extent of emotional, social, or existential isolation response
Mood Equilibrium: Appropriate adjustment of prevailing emotional tone in response to circumstance

Play Participation: Use of activities as needed for enjoyment, entertainment, and development by children

Social Interaction Skills: An individual's use of effective interaction behaviors

Social Involvement: Frequency of an individual's social interactions with persons, groups, or organizations

Social Support: Perceived availability and actual provision of reliable assistance from other persons

Well-Being: An individual's expressed satisfaction with health status

Goals/Evaluation Criteria

Examples Using NOC Language

- Demonstrates **Social Involvement**, as evidenced by the following indicators (specify 1–5: none, limited, moderate, substantial, or extensive):

    Reports interaction with close friends, neighbors, family members, and/or work groups

    Reports participation as member of church, club, or volunteer group

    Participates in leisure activities

Other Examples

Patient will:

- Identify and accept personal characteristics and/or behaviors that contribute to social isolation
- Identify community resources that will assist in decreasing social isolation after discharge
- Verbalize fewer feelings/experiences of being excluded
- Begin to establish contact with others
- Develop a mutual relationship
- Exhibit affect appropriate to situation
- Develop social skills that decrease isolation (eg, cooperation, compromise, consideration, warmth, and engagement)
- Report increasing social support (eg, help from others in the form of emotional help, time, money, labor, or information)

NIC Priority Interventions

Socialization Enhancement: Facilitation of another person's ability to interact with others

Nursing Activities

Also see "Nursing Activities" for "Social Interaction, Impaired," p. 439

Other

- Assist patient to distinguish reality from perceptions
- Identify with patient those factors that may be contributing to feelings of social isolation
- Reduce stigma of isolation by respecting patient's dignity
- Reduce visitor anxiety by explaining reason for isolation precautions and/or equipment
- Reinforce efforts by patient, family, friends to establish interactions
- *(NIC) Socialization Enhancement:*
  Encourage relationships with persons who have common interests and goals
  Allow testing of interpersonal limits
  Give feedback about improvement in care of personal appearance or other activities
  Confront patient about impaired judgment, when appropriate
  Encourage patient to change environment, such as going outside for walks and movies

Sorrow, Chronic
(9.2.1.3) (1998)

Definition: A cyclical, recurring, and potentially progressive pattern of pervasive sadness that is experienced by a client (parent or caregiver, or individual with chronic illness or disability) in response to continual loss, throughout the trajectory of an illness or disability

Defining Characteristics

Subjective

Feelings that vary in intensity, are periodic, may progress and intensify over time, and may interfere with the client's ability to reach his/her highest level of personal and social well-being

Client expresses periodic, recurrent feelings of sadness

Client expresses one or more of the following feelings: anger, being misunderstood, confusion, depression, disappointment, emptiness, fear, frustration, guilt/self-blame, helplessness, hopelessness, loneliness, low self-esteem, recurring loss, overwhelmed

Related Factors

Death of a loved one

Person experiences chronic physical or mental illness or disability such as: mental retardation, multiple sclerosis, prematurity, spina bifida or other birth defects, chronic mental illness, infertility, cancer, Parkinson's disease

Person experiences one or more trigger events (eg, crises in management of the illness, crises related to developmental stages and missed opportunities or milestones that bring comparisons with developmental, social, or personal norms)

Unending caregiving as a constant reminder of loss

Suggestions for Use

Compared to normal grieving that occurs in response to loss, *Chronic sorrow* does not subside with time—in part, because the loss continues unabated (as it does in a chronic disability) and the condition remains as a constant reminder of loss. *Chronic sorrow* demonstrates coping that is more effective than that which occurs with *Dysfunctional grieving*.

Several of the defining characteristics of *Chronic sorrow* are, themselves, nursing diagnoses. When more than one of the following diagnoses are present, a diagnosis of *Chronic sorrow* may be more useful: *Fear, Hopelessness, Loneliness, Chronic low self-esteem* and *Powerlessness*.

Suggested Alternative Diagnoses

Death anxiety
Fear
Grieving, anticipatory
Grieving, dysfunctional
Hopelessness
Loneliness, risk for
Powerlessness
Self-esteem, chronic low
Spiritual distress

NOC Suggested Outcomes

To be developed

Goals/Evaluation Criteria

Patient will:
- Express feelings of guilt, anger, or sorrow
- Identify and use effective coping strategies
- Verbalize the impact of the loss(es)
- Seek information about illness and treatment

- Identify and use available social supports, including significant others
- Work toward acceptance of the loss(es)
- Draw upon spiritual beliefs for comfort

NIC Priority Interventions

To be developed

Nursing Activities

Refer to "Nursing Activities" for "Spiritual Distress" on pp. 448–449.

For patients for whom *Fear* is an etiology, refer to "Nursing Activities" for "Fear" on pp. 158–159.

For patients for whom *Chronic low self-esteem* is an etiology, refer to "Nursing Activities" for "Self-Esteem, Chronic Low" on pp. 397–398.

For patients for whom *Hopelessness* is an etiology, refer to "Nursing Activities" for "Hopelessness" on pp. 201–202.

For patients for whom *Powerlessness* is an etiology, refer to "Nursing Activities" for "Powerlessness" on pp. 357–358.

Assessments

- Assess and document the presence and source of patient's sorrow

Patient/Family Teaching

- Discuss characteristics of normal and abnormal grieving
- Provide patient/family with information about hospital and community resources, such as self-help groups

Collaborative Activities

- Initiate a patient care conference to review patient/family needs related to their stage of the grieving process and to establish a plan of care

Other

- Acknowledge patient's and family's grief reactions while continuing necessary care activities
- Discuss with patient/family the impact of the loss on the family and its functioning
- Establish a schedule for contact with patient
- Establish a trusting relationship with patient and family
- Provide a safe, secure, and private environment to facilitate patient/family grieving process

- Recognize and reinforce the strength of each family member.
- *(NIC) Grief Work Facilitation:*
  Assist the patient to identify the nature of the attachment to the lost object or person
  Include significant others in discussions and decisions, as appropriate
  Encourage patient to implement cultural, religious, and social customs associated with the loss
  Encourage expression of feelings about the loss
  Answer children's questions associated with the loss
  Encourage expression of feelings in ways comfortable to the child, such as writing, drawing, or playing
  Assist the child to clarify misconceptions

Spiritual Distress
(4.1.1) (1978)

Definition: Disruption in the life principle that pervades a person's entire being and that integrates and transcends one's biological and psychosocial nature

Defining Characteristics

Subjective
Description of nightmares/sleep disturbances
Expresses concern with meaning of life/death and/or belief system
Gallows humor
Questions meaning of suffering
Questions meaning of own existence
Questions moral/ethical implications of therapeutic regimen
Verbalizes concern about relationship with deity
Verbalizes inner conflict about beliefs

Objective
Alteration in behavior/mood evidenced by anger, crying, withdrawal, preoccupation, anxiety, hostility, apathy, etc.
Anger toward God
Displacement of anger toward religious representatives
Seeks spiritual assurance
Unable to participate in usual religious practices

Other Defining Characteristics (Non-NANDA)
Spiritual questioning (eg, "Why did this happen to me?")

Feelings of hopelessness/abandonment
Questioning of existence or fairness of deity
Refusal to accept visits from priest, minister, or rabbi

Related Factors

Challenge to belief and value system (eg, due to moral/ethical
    implications of therapy or intense suffering)
Separation from religious/cultural ties

Other Related Factors (Non-NANDA)
Discrepancy between spiritual beliefs and prescribed treatment

Suggestions for Use

(1) Spiritual well-being should be thought of in a broad sense and
not limited to religion. All people are religious in the sense that they
need something to give meaning to their lives. For some it is belief in
God in the traditional sense; for others, it is a feeling of harmony with
the universe; for still others, it may be family and children. When the
patient believes that life has no meaning or purpose, in whatever
sense, then *Spiritual distress* is present. (2) Some of the following
suggested alternative diagnoses may lead to *Spiritual distress*.

Suggested Alternative Diagnoses

Anxiety, death
Decisional conflict
Individual coping, ineffective
Sorrow, chronic
Spiritual distress, risk for

NOC Suggested Outcomes

Dignified Dying: Maintaining personal control and comfort with
    the approaching end of life
Hope: Presence of internal state of optimism that is personally sat-
    isfying and life-supporting
Spiritual Well-Being: Personal expressions of connectedness with
    self, others, higher power, all life, nature, and the universe that
    transcend and empower the self

Goals/Evaluation Criteria

Examples Using NOC Language

- Demonstrates **Hope**, as evidenced by the following indicators
    (specify 1–5: none, limited, moderate, substantial, or extensive):
    Expression of faith, meaning in life, and inner peace.

- Demonstrates **Spiritual Well-Being**, as evidenced by the following indicators (specify 1–5: extremely, substantially, moderately, mildly, or not compromised):

  Meaning and purpose in life

  Spiritual world view

  Serenity, love, and forgiveness

  Prayer, worship, and/or meditation

  Interaction with spiritual leaders

  Connectedness with inner self

  Connectedness with others to share thoughts, feelings, and beliefs

Other Examples

Patient will:
- Acknowledge that illness is a challenge to belief system
- Acknowledge that treatment conflicts with belief system
- Demonstrate coping techniques to deal with spiritual distress
- Express acceptance of limited religious/cultural ties
- Discuss spiritual practices and concerns

Dying patient will:
- Express acceptance/readiness for death
- Reconcile previous relationships
- Express affection toward significant others

NIC Priority Interventions

Spiritual Support: Assisting the patient to feel balance and connection with a greater power

Nursing Activities

Assessments

- For patients who indicate a religious affiliation, assess for direct indicators of patient's spiritual status by asking questions such as the following:

  Do you feel your faith is helpful to you? In what ways is it important to you right now?

  How can I help you carry out your faith? For example, would you like me to read your prayer book to you?

  Would you like a visit from your spiritual counselor or the hospital chaplain?

  Please tell me about any particular religious practices that are important to you.

- Make indirect assessments of the patient's spiritual status by doing the following:

Determine patient's concept of "God" by observing the books at the bedside or the programs he/she watches on television. Also note whether the patient's life seems to have meaning, value, and purpose.

Determine the patient's source of hope and strength. Is it God in the traditional sense, a family member, or an "inner source" of strength? Note who the patient talks about most. Or ask, "Who is important to you?"

Observe whether the patient seems to be praying when you enter the room, before meals, or during procedures

Look for items such as religious literature, rosaries, and religious get-well cards at the bedside

Listen for patient's thoughts about the relationship between spiritual beliefs and his/her state of health—particularly for statements such as, "Why did God let this happen to me" or "If I have faith, I will get well."

Collaborative Activities

- Communicate dietary needs (eg, kosher food, vegetarian diet, pork-free diet) to dietitian
- Request spiritual consultation to help patient/family determine posthospitalization needs and community resources for support
- *(NIC) Spiritual Support:* Refer to spiritual advisor of patient's choice

Other

- Explain limitations that hospitalization imposes on religious observances
- Make immediate changes necessary to accommodate patient's needs (eg, encourage patient's family or friends to bring special food)
- Provide privacy and time for patient to observe religious practices
- *(NIC) Spiritual Support:*

  Be open to patient's expressions of loneliness and powerlessness

  Use values clarification techniques to help patient clarify beliefs and values, as appropriate

  Express empathy with patient's feelings

  Listen carefully to patient's communication and develop a sense of timing for prayer or spiritual rituals

  Assure patient that nurse will be available to support patient in times of suffering

  Encourage chapel service attendance, if desired

  Provide desired spiritual articles, according to patient preference

Spiritual Distress, Risk for
(4.1.2) (1998)

Definition: At risk for an altered sense of harmonious connectedness with all of life and the universe in which dimensions that transcend and empower the self may be disrupted

Risk Factors

Blocks to self-love
Energy-consuming anxiety
Inability to forgive
Loss of loved one
Low self-esteem
Maturational losses
Mental illness

Natural disasters
Physical illness
Physical or psychologic stress
Poor relationships
Situational losses
Substance abuse

Suggestions for Use

See "Suggestions for Use" for "Spiritual Distress," p. 447

Suggested Alternative Diagnoses

Anxiety, death
Decisional conflict
Grieving, dysfunctional
Individual coping, ineffective
Sorrow, chronic
Spiritual distress

NOC Suggested Outcomes

Not yet developed; the following seems appropriate:
Spiritual Well-Being: Personal expressions of connectedness with self, others, higher power, all life, nature, and the universe that transcend and empower the self

Goals/Evaluation Criteria

See "Goals/Evaluation Criteria" for "Spiritual Distress" on pp. 447–448

NIC Priority Interventions

Not yet identified. The following is a possible choice:
Spiritual Support: Assisting the patient to feel balance and connection with a greater power

Nursing Activities

See "Nursing Activities" for "Spiritual Distress" pp. 448–449

Assessments

- Assess for situations that might lead to spiritual distress (eg, low self-esteem, anxiety, lack of supportive relationships)

Other

- Institute the following measures to promote self-esteem:
  Assist patient in identifying personal strengths
  Encourage patient to verbalize concerns about close relationships
  Encourage patient/family to air feelings and to grieve
  Provide care in a nonjudgmental manner, maintaining the patient's privacy and dignity
- *(NIC) Spiritual Support:*
  Use values clarification techniques to help patient clarify beliefs and values, as appropriate
  Listen carefully to patient's communication and develop a sense of timing for prayer or spiritual rituals

Spiritual Well-Being, Potential for Enhanced (4.2) (1994)

Definition: Spiritual well-being is the process of an individual's developing/unfolding of mystery through harmonious interconnectedness that springs from inner strengths

Defining Characteristics

Inner Strengths: A sense of awareness, self-consciousness, sacred source, unifying force, inner core, and transcendence

Unfolding Mystery: One's experience about life's purpose and meaning, mystery, uncertainty, and struggles

Harmonious Interconnectedness: Relatedness, connectedness, and harmony with self, others, higher power/God, and the environment

Suggestions for Use

Because this is a wellness diagnosis, an etiology (eg, related factors) is not needed. If situations exist that pose a risk to spiritual development, use *Risk for spiritual distress.*

Suggested Alternative Diagnosis

Spiritual distress, risk for

NOC Suggested Outcomes

Hope: Presence of internal state of optimism that is personally satisfying and life-supporting

Quality of Life: An individual's expressed satisfaction with current life circumstances

Spiritual Well-Being: Personal expressions of connectedness with self, others, higher power, all life, nature, and the universe that transcend and empower the self

Well-Being: An individual's expressed satisfaction with health status

Goals/Evaluation Criteria

Examples Using NOC Language

See "Examples Using NOC Language" for "Spiritual Distress," pp. 447–448

Other examples

Patient will:

- Continue and enhance spiritual growth
- Verbalize feelings of peace and harmony with the universe
- Verbalize satisfaction with sociocultural circumstances and interpersonal relationships
- Report satisfaction with self-concept and achievement of life goals
- Indicate happiness and satisfaction with spiritual life

NIC Priority Interventions

Spiritual Support: Assisting the patient to feel balance and connection with a greater power

Nursing Activities

Also see "Nursing Activities" for "Spiritual Distress," pp. 448–449

Collaborative Activities

- *(NIC) Spiritual Support:* Encourage chapel service attendance, if desired

Other

- *(NIC) Spiritual Support:*

  Be open to patient's feelings about illness and death

  Assist patient to properly express and relieve anger in appropriate ways

  Be available to listen to patient's feelings

  Facilitate patient's use of meditation, prayer, and other religious traditions and rituals

Spontaneous Ventilation, Inability to Sustain (1.5.1.3.1) (1992)

Definition: A state in which the response pattern of decreased energy reserves results in an individual's inability to maintain breathing adequate to support life

Defining Characteristics

Subjective

Dyspnea

Objective

Apprehension

Decreased cooperation

Decreased SaO_2

Decreased PO_2

Decreased tidal volume

Increased heart rate

Increased metabolic rate

Increased PCO_2

Increased restlessness

Increased use of accessory muscles

Related Factors

Metabolic factors [eg, alkalemia, hypokalemia, hypochloremia, hypophosphatemia, anemia]

Respiratory muscle fatigue

Suggestions for Use

Impaired gas exchange is one of the defining characteristics for this label. When blood gases are altered but the patient is able to breathe without mechanical assistance, a diagnosis of *Impaired gas exchange* should be made instead of *Inability to sustain spontaneous ventilation.*

The author does not recommend use of this label as a nursing diagnosis. When breathing is "inadequate to support life," an emergency exists; the interventions are physician-prescribed, including resuscitation and mechanical ventilation. The nurse is accountable for monitoring changes in the patient's condition and performing interventions according to agency protocols. Goals and interventions are included in this text only because NOC and NIC standardized language includes them.

Suggested Alternative Diagnoses

Airway clearance, ineffective
Breathing patterns, ineffective
Dysfunctional ventilatory weaning response (DVWR)
Gas exchange, impaired

NOC Suggested Outcomes

Endurance: Extent that energy enables a person's activity
Muscle Function: Adequacy of muscle contraction needed for movement
Neurologic Status: Central Motor Control: Extent to which skeletal muscle activity (ie, body movement) is coordinated by the central nervous system
Vital Signs Status: Temperature, pulse, respiration, and blood pressure within expected range for the individual

Goals/Evaluation Criteria

Examples Using NOC Language

• Demonstrates **Vital Signs Status**, as evidenced by the following indicators (specify 1–5: extreme, substantial, moderate, mild, or no deviation from expected range): temperature, pulse, respirations, and blood pressure

Other Examples

Patient will:
• Have adequate energy level and muscle function to sustain spontaneous breathing

- Receive adequate nutrition prior to, during, and following weaning process
- Have arterial blood gases/oxygen saturation within acceptable range
- Demonstrate neurologic status adequate to sustain spontaneous breathing

NIC Priority Interventions

Artificial Airway Management: Maintenance of endotracheal and tracheostomy tubes and preventing complications associated with their use

Mechanical Ventilation: Use of an artificial device to assist a patient to breathe

Respiratory Monitoring: Collection and analysis of patient data to ensure airway patency and adequate gas exchange

Resuscitation: Neonate: Administering emergency measures to support newborn adaptation to extrauterine life

Ventilation Assistance: Promotion of an optimal spontaneous breathing pattern that maximizes oxygen and carbon dioxide exchange in the lungs

Nursing Activities

Assessments

- For patients requiring artificial airway: Monitor tube placement, Check cuff inflation q4h and whenever it is deflated and reinflated
- *(NIC) Mechanical Ventilation:*
  Monitor for impending respiratory failure
  Monitor for decrease in exhale volume and increase in inspiratory pressure in patients receiving mechanical ventilation
  Monitor the effectiveness of mechanical ventilation on patient's physiologic and psychologic status
  Monitor for adverse effects of mechanical ventilation: infection, barotrauma, and reduced cardiac output
  Monitor effects of ventilator changes on oxygenation: ABG, SaO_2, SvO_2, end-tidal CO_2, Q_{sp}/Qt, and $A\text{-}aDO_2$ levels and patient's subjective response
  Monitor degree of shunt, vital capacity, V_d/V_T, MVV, inspiratory force, FEV_1 for, and readiness to wean from mechanical ventilation, based on agency protocol

- *(NIC) Respiratory Monitoring:*

  Note location of trachea

  Auscultate breath sounds, noting areas of decreased/absent ventilation and presence of adventitious sounds

  Determine the need for suctioning by auscultating for crackles and rhonchi over major airways

  Monitor for increased restlessness, anxiety, and air hunger

  Monitor for crepitus, as appropriate

Patient/Family Teaching

- Instruct patient/family about weaning process and goals, including the following:

  How patient may feel as process evolves

  Participation required by patient

  Reasons why weaning is necessary

- *(NIC) Mechanical Ventilation:* Instruct the patient and family about the rationale and expected sensations associated with use of mechanical ventilators

Collaborative Activities

- *(NIC) Mechanical Ventilation:*

  Consult with other health care personnel in selection of a ventilator mode

  Administer muscle-paralyzing agents, sedatives, and narcotic analgesics, as appropriate

Other

- Initiate calming techniques, as appropriate
- *(NIC) Mechanical Ventilation:*

  Initiate setup and application of the ventilator

  Ensure that ventilator alarms are on

  Provide patient with a means for communication (eg, paper and pencil or alphabet board)

  Perform suctioning, based on presence of adventitious sounds and/or increased ventilatory pressures

  Provide routine oral care

  For patients requiring an artificial airway:
- Provide artificial airway management according to agency procedures/protocols, which may include the following:

  Provide oral care at least q4hr

  Rotate endotracheal tube from side to side daily

  Tape endotracheal tube securely; change tapes/ties q24hr

Administer sedation, utilize mitts or wrist restraints, if necessary, to prevent unplanned extubation

Clean stoma and tracheal cannula q4hr (according to agency
protocol)

Suction oropharynx, as needed

NOTE: For in-depth information about artificial airway management, refer to med-surg text, nursing techniques/skills manual,
and/or agency protocols

For neonates requiring resuscitation:
- Refer to maternity or pediatric nursing texts for full details of
  resuscitation procedure
- Have resuscitation equipment available at birth
- Calmly explain procedures to parents to minimize anxiety
- Prepare for neonatal transfer or transport

For patients requiring ventilatory weaning:
- Refer to "Nursing Activities" for "Ventilatory Weaning Response,
  Dysfunctional (DVWR)," pp. 510–512

Suffocation, Risk for
(1.6.1.1) (1980)

Definition: Accentuated risk of accidental suffocation (ie, inadequate air available for inhalation)

Risk Factors
Internal (Individual)
Cognitive or emotional difficulties

Disease or injury process

Lack of safety education

Lack of safety precautions

Reduced motor abilities

Reduced olfactory sensation

External (Environmental)
Children left unattended in bathtubs or pools

Children playing with plastic bags or inserting small objects into
their mouths or noses

Discarded or unused refrigerators or freezers without removed
doors

Household gas leaks

Low-strung clothesline
Pacifier hung around infant's head
Person who eats large mouthfuls of food
Pillow placed in an infant's crib
Propped bottle placed in an infant's crib
Smoking in bed
Use of fuel-burning heaters not vented to outside
Vehicle warming in closed garage

Suggestions for Use

Use the most specific label that matches the patient's defining characteristics. This label is more specific than *Risk for injury* or *Risk for trauma*, for example.

Suggested Alternative Diagnoses

Injury, risk for
Trauma, risk for

NOC Suggested Outcomes

Knowledge: Personal Safety: Extent of understanding conveyed about preventing unintentional injuries
Risk Detection: Actions taken to identify personal health threats
Safety Behavior: Home Physical Environment: Individual or caregiver actions to minimize environmental factors that might cause physical harm or injury in the home
Substance Addiction Consequences: Compromise in health status and social functioning due to substance addiction

Goals/Evaluation Criteria

Examples Using NOC Language

- Demonstrates **Safety Behavior: Home Physical Environment**, as evidenced by the following indicators (specify 1–5: not, slightly, moderately, substantially, or totally adequate):

    Safe disposal of hazardous materials
    Removal of unused refrigerator and freezer doors
    Provision of age-appropriate toys

Other Examples

Patient will:
- Identify appropriate safety factors that protect individual/child from suffocation
- Recognize signs of substance abuse/addiction
- Verbalize knowledge of emergency procedures

NIC Priority Interventions

Airway Management: Facilitation of patency of air passages

Environmental Management, Safety: Monitoring and manipulation of the physical environment to promote safety

Respiratory Monitoring: Collection and analysis of patient data to ensure airway patency and adequate gas exchange

Nursing Activities

Assessments

- *(NIC) Environmental Management: Safety:* Identify safety hazards in the environment (ie, physical, biologic, and chemical)
- *(NIC) Respiratory Monitoring:*
  Monitor rate, rhythm, depth, and effort of respirations
  Monitor for hoarseness and voice changes every hour in patients with facial burns
  Institute resuscitation efforts, as needed

Patient/Family Teaching

- Provide educational materials related to strategies and countermeasures for preventing suffocation and to emergency measures for dealing with it
- Provide information on environmental hazards and characteristics (eg, stairs, windows, cupboard locks, swimming pools, streets, gates)
- *(NIC) Environmental Management: Safety:* Provide patient with emergency phone numbers (eg, health department, environmental services, EPA [Environmental Protection Agency], and police)

Collaborative Activities

- Refer patient to educational classes in the community (CPR [cardiopulmonary resuscitation], first aid, swimming classes)
- *(NIC) Environmental Management: Safety:* Notify agencies authorized to protect the environment (eg, health department, environmental services, EPA, and police)

Other

- *(NIC): Airway Management:* Position the patient to maximize ventilation potential
- *(NIC) Environmental Management: Safety:* Modify the environment to minimize hazards and risks

Surgical Recovery, Delayed
(6.4.2.1) (1998)

Definition: An extension of the number of postoperative days required for individuals to initiate and perform on their own behalf activities that maintain life, health, and well-being

Defining Characteristics

Difficulty in moving about

Evidence of interrupted healing of surgical area (eg, red, indurated, draining, immobile)

Fatigue

Loss of appetite with or without nausea

Perception more time is needed to recover

Postpones resumption of work/employment activities

Report of pain/discomfort

Requires help to complete self-care

Related Factors

To be developed

Suggestions for Use

The defining characteristics for this diagnosis represent several other nursing diagnoses: *Impaired skin integrity, Risk for altered nutrition, Nausea, Impaired mobility, Self-care deficit, Fatigue,* and *Pain.* If only one or two of the defining characteristics are present, use those individual diagnoses. If several are present, *Delayed surgical recovery* may be used. Note, however, that this label is not yet fully developed.

Suggested Alternative Diagnoses

Activity intolerance

Fatigue

Impaired mobility

Impaired skin integrity

Pain

Risk for altered nutrition: less than body requirements

Self-care deficit

NOC Suggested Outcomes

To be developed

Goals/Evaluation Criteria

The patient will:

- Recognize and cope effectively with surgery-related anxiety
- Regain presurgery energy level, as evidenced by rested appearance, ability to concentrate, and statements that exhaustion is not present
- Regain presurgery mobility
- Demonstrate healing of surgical incision: edges approximated and no drainage, redness, or induration
- Experience timely resolution of pain, progressing to oral analgesics by (<u>date</u>) and requiring no pain medications by (<u>date</u>)
- Meet all discharge criteria by the date of "expected stay" for his/her particular surgery

NIC Priority Interventions

NIC has not yet published priority interventions for this nursing diagnosis. However, the following might be appropriate.

Bowel Management: Establishment and maintenance of a regular pattern of bowel elimination

Energy Management: Regulating energy use to treat or prevent fatigue and optimize function

Nutritional Management: Assisting with or providing a balanced dietary intake of foods and fluids

Pain Management: Alleviation of pain or a reduction in pain to a level of comfort that is acceptable to the patient

Self-Care Assistance: Assisting another to perform activities of daily living

Surveillance: Purposeful and ongoing acquisition, interpretation, and synthesis of patient data for clinical decision making

Urinary Elimination Management: Maintenance of an optimum urinary elimination pattern

Wound Care: Prevention of wound complications and promotion of wound healing

Nursing Activities

NOTE[1]: The following nursing activities are general because the nursing diagnosis is nonspecific. It does not specify any particular type of surgery, and it includes several different nursing diagnoses (see the preceding "Suggestions for Use").

NOTE[2]: For more specific nursing activities, refer to "Nursing Activities" for the nursing diagnoses *Activity intolerance, Fatigue,*

Nausea, Impaired mobility, Impaired skin integrity, Pain, Risk for altered nutrition: less than body requirements, and *Self-care deficit.*

Assessments

- Monitor nature and location of pain
- Assess patient's self-care abilities (eg, consider mobility, sedation, and level of consciousness)
- *(NIC) Surveillance:*

  Select appropriate patient indices for ongoing monitoring, based on patient's condition

  Establish the frequency of data collection and interpretation, as indicated by status of the patient

  Monitor neurologic status

  Monitor vital signs, as appropriate

  Monitor for signs and symptoms of fluid and electrolyte imbalance

  Monitor tissue perfusion, as appropriate

  Monitor for infection, as appropriate

  Monitor nutritional status, as appropriate

  Monitor gastrointestinal function, as appropriate

  Monitor elimination patterns, as appropriate

  Monitor for bleeding tendencies in high-risk patient

  Note type and amount of drainage from tubes and orifices and notify the physician of significant changes
- *(NIC) Bowel Management:*

  Monitor bowel sounds

  Note date of last bowel movement
- *(NIC) Energy Management:*

  Determine causes of fatigue (eg, treatments, pain, and medications)

  Monitor patient for evidence of excess physical and emotional fatigue

  Monitor cardiorespiratory response to activity (eg, tachycardia, other dysrhythmias, dyspnea, diaphoresis, pallor, hemodynamic pressures, and respiratory rate)

  Monitor/record patient's sleep pattern and number of sleep hours
- *(NIC) Nutrition Management:* Ascertain patient's food preferences
- *(NIC) Wound Care:* Inspect the wound with each dressing change

Patient Teaching

- *(NIC) Energy Management:* Teach patient and significant other techniques of self-care that will minimize oxygen consumption (eg, self-monitoring and pacing techniques for performance of activities of daily living)

Collaborative Activities

- *(NIC) Bowel Management:* Report diminished bowel sounds
- *(NIC) Nutrition Management:* Determine—in collaboration with dietitian, as appropriate—number of calories and type of nutrients needed to meet nutrition requirements
- *(NIC) Surveillance:*

  Analyze physician orders in conjunction with patient status to ensure safety of the patient

  Obtain consultation from the appropriate health care worker to initiate new treatment or change existing treatments

Other

- Ensure that the patient receives appropriate analgesic care
- Consider cultural influences on pain response
- Reduce or eliminate factors that precipitate or increase the pain experience (eg, fear, fatigue, monotony, and lack of knowledge)
- Provide assistance until patient is fully able to assume self-care
- Encourage independence but intervene when patient is unable to perform activities
- Compare current status with previous status to detect improvements and deterioration in patient's condition
- *(NIC) Energy Management:*

  Determine what and how much activity is required to build endurance

  Use passive and/or active range-of-motion exercises to relieve muscle tension

  Avoid care activities during scheduled rest periods

  Institute appropriate treatment, using standing protocols
- *(NIC) Wound Care:*

  Provide incision site care, as needed

  Administer IV site care, as appropriate

  Maintain patency of any drainage tubes

  Bandage appropriately

  Position to avoid placing tension on the wound, as appropriate

Swallowing, Impaired
(6.5.1.1) (1986, 1998)

Definition: Abnormal functioning of the swallowing mechanism associated with deficits in oral, pharyngeal, or esophageal structure or function

Defining Characteristics

Pharyngeal Phase Impairment

Abnormality in pharyngeal phase by swallow study
Altered head positions
Choking, coughing, or gagging
Delayed swallow
Food refusal
Gurgly voice quality
Inadequate laryngeal elevation
Multiple swallows
Nasal reflux
Recurrent pulmonary infections
Unexplained fevers

Esophageal Phase Impairment

Abnormality in esophageal phase by swallow study
Acidic-smelling breath
Bruxism
Complaints of "something stuck"
Food refusal or volume limiting
Heartburn or epigastric pain
Hematemesis
Hyperextension of head, arching during or after meals
Nighttime coughing or awakening
Observed evidence of difficulty in swallowing (eg, stasis of food in oral cavity, coughing/choking)
Odynophagia
Regurgitation of gastric contents or wet burps
Repetitive swallowing or ruminating
Unexplained irritability surrounding mealtime
Vomiting
Vomitus on pillow

Oral Phase Impairment

Abnormality in oral phase of swallow study
Coughing, choking, gagging before a swallow

Food falls from mouth
Food pushed out of mouth
Inability to clear oral cavity
Incomplete lip closure
Lack of chewing
Lack of tongue action to form bolus
Long meals with little consumption
Nasal reflux
Piecemeal deglutition
Pooling in lateral sulci
Premature entry of bolus
Sialorrhea or drooling
Slow bolus formation
Weak suck, resulting in inefficient nippling

Related Factors

Achalasia
Acquired anatomic defects
Behavioral feeding problems
Cerebral palsy
Conditions with significant hypotonia
Congenital heart disease
Cranial nerve involvement
Developmental delay
External traumas
Failure to thrive or protein energy malnutrition
Gastroesophageal reflux disease
History of tube feeding
Internal traumas
Laryngeal abnormalities
Mechanical obstruction (eg, edema, tracheostomy tube, tumor)
Nasal or nasopharyngeal cavity defects
Neuromuscular impairment (eg, decreased or absent gag reflex,
    decreased strength or excursion of muscles involved in masti-
    cation, perceptual impairment, facial paralysis)
Oral cavity or oropharynx abnormalities
Premature infants
Respiratory disorders
Self-injurious behavior
Tracheal, laryngeal, or esophageal defects
Traumatic head injury
Upper airway anomalies

Suggestions for Use

Impaired swallowing may be associated with a variety of medical conditions (eg, cerebral palsy, CVA, Parkinson's disease, malignancies affecting the brain, reconstructive surgery of the head and neck, and decreased consciousness from anesthesia or other causes). It may also be related to *Fatigue*.

Suggested Alternative Diagnoses

Aspiration, risk for
Infant feeding pattern, ineffective

NOC Suggested Outcomes

Muscle Function: Adequacy of muscle contraction needed for movement
Neurologic Status: Consciousness: Extent to which an individual arouses, orients, and attends to the environment
Neurologic Status: Cranial Sensory/Motor Function: Extent to which cranial nerves convey sensory and motor information
Self-Care: Eating: Ability to prepare and ingest food

Goals/Evaluation Criteria

Examples Using NOC Language

- Demonstrates **Neurologic Status: Consciousness**, as evidenced by the following indicators (specify 1–5: extremely, substantially, moderately, mildly, or not compromised):
    Cognitive orientation
    Attends to environmental stimuli

Other Examples

Patient will:
- Identify emotional/psychologic factors that interfere with swallowing
- Tolerate food ingestion without choking or aspiration
- Have no impairment of facial and throat muscles, swallowing, tongue movement, or gag reflex

NIC Priority Interventions

Aspiration Precautions: Prevention or minimization of risk factors in the patient at risk for aspiration
Swallowing Therapy: Facilitating swallowing and preventing complications of impaired swallowing

Nursing Activities

Assessments

- Evaluate family's comfort level
- *(NIC) Aspiration Precautions:*
  Monitor level of consciousness, cough reflex, gag reflex, and swallowing ability
  Monitor for signs and symptoms of aspiration
- *(NIC) Swallowing Therapy:*
  Monitor patient's tongue movements while eating
  Monitor for sealing of lips during eating, drinking, and swallowing
  Check mouth for pocketing of food after eating
  Monitor body hydration (eg, intake, output, skin turgor, and mucous membranes)

Patient/Family Teaching

- *(NIC) Swallowing Therapy:*
  Instruct patient to reach for particles of food on lips or chin with tongue
  Instruct patient/caregiver on emergency measures for choking

Collaborative Activities

- Consult dietitian for food that can be easily swallowed
- *(NIC) Aspiration Precautions:* Request medication in elixir form
- *(NIC) Swallowing Therapy:*
  Collaborate with other members of health care team (eg, occupational therapist, speech pathologist, and dietitian) to provide continuity in patient's rehabilitative plan
  Collaborate with speech therapist to instruct patient's family about swallowing exercise regimen

Other

- Reassure patient during episodes of choking
- *(NIC) Aspiration Precautions:*
  Position upright 90 degrees or as far as possible
  Keep tracheal cuff inflated
  Keep suction setup available
  Feed in small amounts
  Avoid liquids or use thickening agent
  Cut food into small pieces
  Break or crush pills before administration

- *(NIC) Swallowing Therapy:*
  Provide mouth care, as needed
  Provide/use assistive devices, as appropriate
  Avoid use of drinking straws
  Assist patient to position head in forward flexion in preparation for swallowing ("chin tuck")
  Acknowledge patient's embarrassment regarding impaired swallowing
  Involve family during ingestion of food/medications to provide support and reassurance
  Assist patient to place food at back of mouth and on unaffected side

Thermoregulation, Ineffective
(1.2.2.4) (1986)

Definition: The state in which an individual's temperature fluctuates between hypothermia and hyperthermia

Defining Characteristics

Objective
Cyanotic nail beds
Cool skin
Fluctuations in body temperature above or below normal range
Flushed skin
Hypertension
Increased respiratory rate
Pallor (moderate)
Piloerection
Reduction in body temperature below normal range
Seizures/convulsions
Shivering (mild)
Slow capillary refill
Tachycardia
Warm to touch

Related Factors

Aging
Fluctuating environmental temperature
Immaturity
Trauma or illness

Suggestions for Use

This label is most appropriate for patients who are especially vulnerable to environmental conditions (eg, newborns and the elderly).

Suggested Alternative Diagnoses

Body temperature, risk for altered
Hyperthermia
Hypothermia

NOC Suggested Outcomes

Thermoregulation: Balance among heat production, heat gain, and heat loss

Thermoregulation: Neonate: Balance among heat production, heat gain, and heat loss during the neonatal period

Goals/Evaluation Criteria

For specific patient outcomes and evaluation criteria, refer to "Goals/Evaluation Criteria" for "Hyperthermia," p. 203, "Hypothermia," pp. 206–207, and *Risk for Altered Body Temperature*," p. 35.

NIC Priority Interventions

Temperature Regulation: Attaining and/or maintaining body temperature within a normal range

Temperature Regulation: Intraoperative: Attaining and/or maintaining desired intraoperative body temperature

Nursing Activities

Nursing interventions focus on teaching for prevention of ineffective thermoregulation and on maintaining a normal body temperature by manipulating external factors, such as clothing and room temperature. Refer to "Nursing Activities" for "Risk for Altered Body Temperature," pp. 36–37, "Hyperthermia," pp. 204–205, and "Hypothermia," pp. 207–208.

Thought Processes, Altered
(8.3) (1976, 1996)

Definition: A state in which an individual experiences a disruption in cognitive operations and activities [eg, conscious thought, reality orientation, problem solving, and judgment]

Defining Characteristics

Subjective
Cognitive dissonance
Inaccurate interpretation of environment
Inappropriate nonreality-based thinking
Objective
Distractibility
Egocentricity
Hyper- or hypovigilance
Memory deficit/problems

Related Factors

To be developed

Non-NANDA Related Factors
Mental disorders (specify)
Organic mental disorders (specify)
Personality disorders (specify)
Substance abuse

Suggestions for Use

This diagnosis is a result of mental/personality or chronic organic disorders that may be exacerbated by situational crises. It may be the etiology of other problems, such as *Self-care deficit, Impaired home maintenance management, Risk for injury, Ineffective management of therapeutic regimen.*

Suggested Alternative Diagnoses

Communication, impaired verbal
Confusion, acute/chronic
Environmental interpretation syndrome, impaired
Sensory/perceptual alterations: auditory, gustatory, kinesthetic, olfactory, tactile, visual

NOC Suggested Outcomes

Cognitive Ability: Ability to execute complex mental processes

Cognitive Orientation: Ability to identify person, place, and time

Concentration: Ability to focus on a specific stimulus

Decision Making: Ability to choose between two or more alternatives

Distorted Thought Control: Ability to self-restrain disruption in perception, thought processes, and thought content

Identity: Ability to distinguish between self and non-self and to characterize one's essence

Information Processing: Ability to acquire, organize, and use information

Memory: Ability to cognitively retrieve and report previously stored information

Neurologic Status: Consciousness: Extent to which an individual arouses, orients, and attends to the environment

Goals/Evaluation Criteria

Examples Using NOC Language

- Demonstrates **Cognitive Orientation**, as evidenced by the following indicators (specify 1–5: never, rarely, sometimes, often, or consistently demonstrated): Identifies self; significant other; current place; and correct day, month, year, and season

- Demonstrates appropriate **Decision Making** (specify 1–5: never, rarely, sometimes, often, or consistently demonstrated)

- Demonstrates **Identity**, as evidenced by the following indicators (specify 1–5: never, rarely, sometimes, often, or consistently demonstrated):

    Verbalizes clear sense of personal identity

    Differentiates self from environment and other human beings

    Recognizes interpersonal versus intrapersonal conflicts

- Demonstrates **Neurologic Status: Consciousness**, as evidenced by the following indicators (specify 1–5: extremely, substantially, moderately, mildly, or not compromised):

    Opens eyes to external stimuli

    Obeys commands

    Attends to environmental stimuli

Other Examples

Patient/family will:

- Accurately recall immediate, recent, and remote information
- Correctly identify familiar people and objects
- Demonstrate logical, organized thought processes

- Compare and contrast two items
- Not be easily distracted
- Perform serial subtractions from 100 by 7s or 3s
- Spell simple words backwards
- Respond appropriately to environmental and communication cues (eg, auditory, written)
- Not act on hallucinations or delusions

NIC Priority Interventions

Delusion Management: Promoting the comfort, safety, and reality orientation of a patient experiencing false, fixed beliefs that have little or no basis in reality

Dementia Management: Provision of a modified environment for the patient who is experiencing a chronic confusional state

Nursing Activities

Assessments

- Assess and document patient's orientation to person, place, time, and situation q _____
- *(NIC) Delusion Management:*
  Monitor self-care ability
  Monitor physical status of patient
  Monitor delusions for presence of content that is self-harmful or violent
  Monitor cognitive functioning, using a standardized assessment tool
  Monitor carefully for physiologic causes of increased confusion that may be acute and reversible
  Monitor patient for medication side effects and desired therapeutic effects

Patient/Family Teaching

- *(NIC) Delusion Management:*
  Educate family and significant others about ways to deal with patient who is experiencing delusions
  Provide illness teaching to patient/significant others if delusions are illness-based (eg, delirium, schizophrenia, or depression)

Collaborative Activities

- Identify community resources
- Involve social services for additional support

- *(NIC) Delusion Management:* Administer antipsychotic and anti-anxiety medications on a routine and as-needed basis

Other
- Post schedule of activities in room
- Call patient by preferred name
- Refer to calendar and clock often
- Use familiar items from home provided by family
- Provide positive feedback and reinforcement of appropriate behavior
- Provide support to patient/family during patient's periods of disorientation
- *(NIC) Delusion Management:*

  Avoid arguing about false beliefs; state doubt matter-of-factly

  Focus discussion on the underlying feelings, rather than the content of the delusion ("It appears as if you may be feeling frightened")

  Encourage patient to verbalize delusions to caregivers before acting on them

  Provide recreational, diversional activities that require attention or skill

  Decrease excessive environmental stimuli, as needed

  Assign consistent caregivers on a daily basis

- *(NIC) Dementia Management:*

  Provide a low-stimulation environment (eg, quiet, soothing music; nonvivid and simple, familiar patterns in décor; performance expectations that do not exceed cognitive-processing ability; and dining in small groups)

  Identify and remove potential dangers in environment for patient

  Prepare for interaction with eye contact and touch, as appropriate

  Give one simple direction at a time

  Speak in a clear, low, warm, respectful tone of voice

  Provide unconditional positive regard

  Use distraction, rather than confrontation, to manage behavior

  Provide cues—such as current events, seasons, location, and names—to assist orientation

  Label familiar photos with names of the individuals in the photos

  Assist family to understand it may be impossible for patient to learn new material

  Limit number of choices patient has to make, so not to cause anxiety

Tissue Integrity, Impaired
(1.6.2.1) (1986, 1998)

Definition: A state in which an individual experiences damage to mucous membrane, corneal, integumentary, or subcutaneous tissues. It is a state in which an individual has altered body tissue.

Defining Characteristics

Objective

Damaged or destroyed tissue (eg, corneal, mucous membrane, integumentary, or subcutaneous)

Related Factors

Altered circulation
Chemical irritants (eg, body excretions and secretions, medications)
Fluid deficit/excess
Impaired physical mobility
Knowledge deficit
Mechanical factors (eg, pressure, shear, friction)
Nutritional deficit or excess
Radiation (including therapeutic radiation)
Thermal factors (eg, temperature extremes)

Suggestions for Use

1. If tissue integrity is at risk because of immobility and if other systems are also at risk, consider using *Risk for disuse syndrome.*
2. If the necessary defining characteristics are present, use the more specific problems of *Altered oral mucous membrane* or *Impaired skin integrity. Impaired tissue integrity* should be used only when the damage is to tissue *other* than the skin and mucous membranes.
3. Do not use *Impaired tissue integrity* to rename a surgical incision or ostomy.

Suggested Alternative Diagnoses

Disuse syndrome, risk for
Oral mucous membrane, altered
Skin integrity, impaired
Surgical recovery, delayed

NOC Suggested Outcomes

Tissue Integrity: Skin and Mucous Membranes: Structural intactness and normal physiologic function of skin and mucous membranes

Wound Healing: Primary Intention: The extent to which cells and tissues have regenerated following intentional closure

Wound Healing: Secondary Intention: The extent to which cells and tissues in an open wound have regenerated

Goals/Evaluation Criteria

Also refer to "Goals/Evaluation Criteria" for "Impaired Skin Integrity," p. 421

Examples Using NOC Language

- Demonstrates **Tissue Integrity**, as evidenced by the following indicators (specify 1–5: extremely, substantially, moderately, mildly, or not compromised):

     Tissue texture and thickness in expected range

     Tissue perfusion

NIC Priority Interventions

Wound Care: Prevention of wound complications and promotion of wound healing

Nursing Activities

For specific nursing activities, refer to the following nursing diagnoses:

Infection, risk for (pp. 240–243)

Oral mucous membrane, altered (pp. 308–309)

Sensory/perceptual alterations (visual) (pp. 411–413)

Skin integrity, impaired (pp. 422–423)

Skin integrity, risk for impaired (pp. 426–428)

Tissue perfusion, altered (peripheral) (pp. 491–492)

Tissue Perfusion, Altered (Specify: Cardio-pulmonary, Cerebral, Gastrointestinal, and Renal) (1.4.1.1) (1980, 1998)

Definition: A decrease in oxygen resulting in the failure to nourish the tissues at the capillary level

Defining Characteristics

Cardiopulmonary

Subjective

Chest pain

Dyspnea

Sense of "impending doom"

Objective

Abnormal arterial blood gases

Altered respiratory rate outside of acceptable parameters

Arrhythmias

Bronchospasms

Capillary refill greater than 3 seconds

Chest retraction

Nasal flaring

Use of accessory muscles

Cerebral

Objective

Altered mental status

Behavioral changes

Changes in motor response

Changes in pupillary reactions

Difficulty in swallowing

Extremity weakness or paralysis

Speech abnormalities

Gastrointestinal

Subjective

Abdominal pain or tenderness

Nausea

Objective

Abdominal distention

Hypoactive or absent bowel sounds

Renal

Objective

Altered blood pressure outside of acceptable parameters

Diminished arterial pulsations

Elevation in BUN [blood urea nitrogen]/creatinine ratio

Hematuria

Oliguria or anuria

Skin color pale on elevation

Related Factors

Altered affinity of hemoglobin for oxygen

Decreased hemoglobin concentration in blood

Enzyme poisoning

Exchange problems

Hypervolemia

Hypoventilation

Impaired transport of the oxygen across alveolar and/or capillary membrane

Interruption of flow, arterial

Interruption of flow, venous

Mechanical reduction of venous and/or arterial blood flow

Mismatch of ventilation with blow flow

Suggestions for Use

With the exception of *Altered peripheral tissue perfusion*, I do not recommend use of this diagnosis. The following Suggested Alternative Diagnoses offer alternative labels that specifically address responses to impaired perfusion of renal, cerebral, cardiopulmonary, and gastrointestinal tissue. *Altered tissue perfusion* can be used appropriately as an etiology for other diagnoses (eg, *Acute confusion related to Altered cerebral tissue perfusion*).

Altered cardiopulmonary, cerebral, gastrointestinal, and renal tissue perfusion actually represent medical diagnoses/conditions. The outcomes and interventions for altered tissue perfusion are medical/surgical treatments; the nurse's role is to monitor and detect changes in the patient's condition. Therefore, nursing care may be better directed by the use of other nursing diagnoses or collaborative problems. However, because NOC and NIC have linked outcomes and interventions to this diagnosis, this text also includes them.

Suggested Alternative Diagnoses

Cardiopulmonary

Activity intolerance
Activity intolerance, risk for
Breathing pattern, ineffective
Cardiac output, decreased
Dysfunctional ventilatory weaning response (DVWR)
Fatigue
Gas exchange, impaired
Spontaneous ventilation, inability to sustain

Cerebral

Communication, impaired: verbal
Confusion, acute/chronic
Injury, risk for
Sensory/perceptual alterations: (auditory, gustatory, kinesthetic, olfactory, visual)

Gastrointestinal

Infection; risk for
Pain

Renal

Fluid volume excess
Fluid volume imbalance, risk for

NOC Suggested Outcomes

Cardiopulmonary Tissue Perfusion

Cardiac Pump Effectiveness: Extent to which blood is ejected from the left ventricle per minute to support systemic perfusion pressure

Circulation Status: Extent to which blood flows unobstructed, unidirectionally, and at an appropriate pressure through large vessels of the systemic and pulmonary circuits

Tissue Perfusion: Cardiac: Extent to which blood flows through the coronary vasculature and maintains heart function

Tissue Perfusion: Peripheral: Extent to which blood flows through the small vessels of the extremities and maintains tissue perfusion

Vital Signs Status: Temperature, pulse, respiration, and blood pressure within expected range for the individual

Cerebral Tissue Perfusion

Circulation Status: Extent to which blood flows unobstructed, unidirectionally, and at an appropriate pressure through large vessels of the systemic and pulmonary circuits

Cognitive Ability: Ability to execute complex mental processes

Neurologic Status: Extent to which the peripheral and central nervous systems receive, process, and respond to internal and external stimuli

Tissue Perfusion: Peripheral: Extent to which blood flows through the small vessels of the extremities and maintains tissue function

Gastrointestinal Tissue Perfusion

Bowel Elimination: Ability of the gastrointestinal tract to form and evacuate stool effectively

Circulation Status: Extent to which blood flows unobstructed, unidirectionally, and at an appropriate pressure through large vessels of the systemic and pulmonary circuits

Electrolyte and Acid-Base Balance: Balance of electrolytes and nonelectrolytes in the intracellular and extracellular compartments of the body

Fluid Balance: Balance of water in the intracellular and extracellular compartments of the body

Hydration: Amount of water in the intracellular and extracellular compartments of the body

Nutritional Status: Extent to which nutrients are available to meet metabolic needs

Renal Tissue Perfusion

Circulation Status: Extent to which blood flows unobstructed, unidirectionally, and at an appropriate pressure through the large vessels of the systemic and pulmonary circuits

Electrolyte & Acid-Base Balance: Balance of electrolytes and nonelectrolytes in the intracellular and extracellular compartments of the body

Fluid Balance: Balance of water in the intracellular and extracellular compartments of the body

Hydration: Amount of water in the intracellular and extracellular compartment of the body

Urinary Elimination: Ability of the urinary system to filter wastes, conserve solutes, and collect and discharge urine in a healthy pattern

Goals/Evaluation Criteria

Cardiopulmonary

Examples Using NOC Language

- Demonstrates Cardiac Pump Effectiveness, Cardiac Tissue Perfusion, and Peripheral Tissue Perfusion
- Demonstrates **Circulation Status,** as evidenced by the following indicators (specify 1–5: extremely, substantially, moderately, mildly, or not compromised):

  Systolic BP [blood pressure], diastolic BP, pulse pressure, mean BP, central venous pressure, and pulmonary wedge pressure in expected ranges

  Peripheral pulses strong and symmetrical.

  Peripheral edema and ascites not present

  Heart rate, cardiac index, blood gases, and ejection fraction in expected ranges

  Abnormal heart sounds not present

  Angina not present

  No adventitious breath sounds, neck vein distention, pulmonary edema, or large vessel bruits

  Extreme fatigue not present

  Orthostatic hypotension not present

Cerebral

Examples Using NOC Language

- Demonstrates **Circulation Status,** as evidenced by the following indicators (specify 1–5: extremely, substantially, moderately, mildly, or not compromised):

  Systolic and diastolic BP in expected ranges

  Orthostatic hypotension not present

  Large-vessel bruits not present

- Demonstrates **Cognitive Ability,** as evidenced by the following indicators (specify 1–5: extremely, substantially, moderately, mildly, or not compromised):

  Communicates clearly and appropriately for age and ability

  Demonstrates attentiveness, concentration, and orientation

  Demonstrates recent and remote memory

  Processes information

  Makes appropriate decisions

Other Examples

  Patient will:

- Have intact central and peripheral nervous systems

- Demonstrate intact cranial sensorimotor function
- Exhibit intact autonomic functioning
- Have pupils equal and reactive
- Be free from seizure activity
- Not experience headache

Gastrointestinal

Examples Using NOC Language

- Demonstrates **Bowel Elimination**, as evidenced by the following indicators (specify 1–5: extremely, substantially, moderately, mildly, or not compromised):

    Stool color, amount, odor, and consistency within normal limits
    Visible peristalsis, painful cramps, and bloating not present
    Bowel sounds not compromised

- Demonstrates **Circulation Status**, as evidenced by the following indicators (specify 1–5: extremely, substantially, moderately, mildly, or not compromised):

    Systolic and diastolic BP in expected ranges
    Peripheral tissue perfusion not compromised
    Neck vein distention not present

- Demonstrates **Electrolyte and Acid-Base Balance**, as evidenced by the following indicators (specify 1–5: extremely, substantially, moderately, mildly, or not compromised):

    Mental alertness, cognitive orientation, and muscle strength not compromised
    Lab tests in expected range (eg, serum Na^+, K^+, Cl^-, Ca^+, Mg^+, bicarbonate)

- Demonstrates **Fluid Balance**, as evidenced by the following indicators (specify 1–5: extremely, substantially, moderately, mildly, or not compromised):

    Neck vein distention not present
    Adventitious breath sounds not present
    24-hour intake and output balanced

- Demonstrates **Hydration**, as evidenced by the following indicators (specify 1–5: extremely, substantially, moderately, mildly, or not compromised):

    Ascites and peripheral edema not present
    Abnormal thirst not present
    Moist mucous membranes
    Fever not present
    Urine output within normal limits
    Hematocrit within normal limits

Other Examples

- Demonstrates adequate food, fluid, and nutrient intake
- Reports sufficient energy
- Displays body mass and weight in expected range

Renal

Examples Using NOC Language

- Demonstrates **Circulation Status**, as evidenced by the following indicators (specify 1–5: extremely, substantially, moderately, mildly, or not compromised):

    Systolic and diastolic BP in expected ranges

    Peripheral tissue perfusion not compromised

- Demonstrates **Electrolyte and Acid-Base Balance,** as evidenced by the following indicators (specify 1–5: extremely, substantially, moderately, mildly, or not compromised):

    Mental alertness, cognitive orientation, and muscle strength not compromised

    Lab tests in expected range (eg, serum Na^+, K^+, Cl^-, Ca^+, Mg^+, bicarbonate, BUN, creatinine)

- Demonstrates **Fluid Balance**, as evidenced by the following indicators (specify 1–5: extremely, substantially, moderately, mildly, or not compromised):

    Neck vein distention not present

    Adventitious breath sounds not present

    24-hour intake and output balanced

- Demonstrates **Hydration**, as evidenced by the following indicators (specify 1–5: extremely, substantially, moderately, mildly, or not compromised):

    Ascites and peripheral edema not present

    Abnormal thirst not present

    Moist mucous membranes

    Fever not present

    Urine output within normal limits

    Hematocrit within normal limits

Other Examples

- Urine odor and color in expected range
- Urine clear
- Laboratory tests within normal limits (eg, urine specific gravity, glucose, ketone, pH, and protein levels and microscopic results)
- Arterial PCO_2 within normal limits

NIC Priority Interventions

Cardiopulmonary

Cardiac Care: Acute: Limitation of complications for a patient recently experiencing an episode of an imbalance between myocardial oxygen supply and demand, resulting in impaired cardiac function

Circulatory Care: Promotion of arterial and venous circulation

Respiratory Monitoring: Collection and analysis of patient data to ensure airway patency and adequate gas exchange

Shock Management: Cardiac: Promotion of adequate tissue perfusion for a patient with severely compromised pumping function of the heart

Cerebral

Cerebral Perfusion Promotion: Promotion of adequate perfusion and limitation of complications for a patient experiencing or at risk for inadequate cerebral perfusion

Circulatory Care: Promotion of arterial and venous circulation

Intracranial Pressure (ICP) Monitoring: Measurement and interpretation of patient data to regulate intracranial pressure

Neurologic Monitoring: Collection and analysis of patient data to prevent or minimize neurologic complications

Peripheral Sensation Management: Prevention or minimization of injury or discomfort in the patient with altered sensation

Gastrointestinal

Fluid/Electrolyte Management: Regulation and prevention of complications from altered fluid and/or electrolyte levels

Gastrointestinal Intubation: Insertion of a tube into the gastrointestinal tract

Nutrition Management: Assisting with or providing a balanced dietary intake of foods and fluids

Renal

Fluid/Electrolyte Management: Regulation and prevention of complications from altered fluid and/or electrolyte levels

Fluid Management: Promotion of fluid balance and prevention of complications resulting from abnormal or undesired fluid levels

Hemodialysis Therapy: Management of extracorporeal passage of the patient's blood through a dialyzer

Peritoneal Dialysis Therapy: Administration and monitoring of dialysis solution into and out of the peritoneal cavity

Nursing Activities

Cardiopulmonary

Assessments

- Monitor chest pain (eg, intensity, duration, and precipitating factors)
- Observe for S-T changes on ECG
- Monitor cardiac rate and rhythm
- Auscultate heart and lung sounds
- Monitor coagulation studies (eg, prothrombin time [PT], partial thromboplastin time [PTT], and platelet counts)
- Weigh patient daily
- Monitor electrolyte values associated with dysrhythmias (eg, serum potassium and magnesium)
- *(NIC) Circulatory Care:*

  Perform a comprehensive appraisal of peripheral circulation (eg, check peripheral pulses, edema, capillary refill, color and temperature of extremity)

  Apply antiembolism stockings (eg, elastic or pneumatic stockings), if appropriate

  Monitor fluid status, including intake and output

  Evaluate peripheral edema and pulses
- *(NIC) Respiratory Monitoring:*

  Monitor for increased restlessness, anxiety, and air hunger

  Note changes in SaO_2, SvO_2, and changes in ABG values, as appropriate

Patient/Family Teaching

- Instruct the patient to avoid performing Valsalva's maneuver (eg, do not strain during bowel movement)
- Explain restrictions on caffeine, sodium, cholesterol, and fat intake
- Explain rationale for eating small, frequent meals

Collaborative Activities

- Administer medications according to order or protocols (eg, analgesics, anticoagulants, nitroglycerin, vasodilators, diuretics, and positive inotropic/contractility medications)

Other

- Reassure patient and family that call bells, lights, and pages will be answered promptly
- Promote rest (eg, limit visitors, control environmental stimuli)
- Do not take rectal temperatures

Cerebral

Assessments

Monitor the following:

- Vital signs: temperature, blood pressure, pulse, and respirations
- PO_2, PCO_2, pH, and bicarbonate levels
- $PaCO_2$, SaO_2, and hemoglobin levels to determine delivery of oxygen to tissues
- Pupil size, shape, symmetry, and reactivity
- Diplopia, nystagmus, blurred vision, and visual acuity
- Headache
- Level of consciousness and orientation
- Memory, mood, and affect
- Cardiac output
- Corneal, cough, and gag reflexes
- Muscle tone, motor movement, gait, and proprioception
- *(NIC) Intracranial Pressure (ICP) Monitoring:*
  Monitor patient's ICP and neurological response to care activities
  Monitor cerebral perfusion pressure
  Note patient's change in response to stimuli
- *(NIC) Peripheral Sensation Management:*
  Monitor for paresthesia: numbness and tingling
  Monitor fluid status, including intake and output

Collaborative Activities

- Maintain hemodynamic parameters (eg, systemic arterial pressure) within prescribed range
- Administer medications to expand intravascular volume, as ordered
- Induce hypertension to maintain cerebral perfusion pressure, as ordered
- Administer osmotic and loop diuretics, as ordered
- Elevate head of bed from 0 to 45 degrees, depending on patient's condition and medical orders

Other

- *(NIC) Circulatory Care:* Apply antiembolism stockings (eg, elastic or pneumatic stockings), if appropriate

Gastrointestinal

Assessments

- Monitor vital signs
- Monitor serum electrolyte levels
- Monitor for manifestations (eg, neuromuscular) of electrolyte imbalance

- Monitor cardiac rhythm
- Keep accurate record of fluid intake and output
- Assess for signs of altered fluid and electrolyte balance (eg, dry mucous membranes, cyanosis, and jaundice)
- *(NIC) Nutrition Management:*
  Monitor recorded intake for nutritional content and calories
  Weigh patient at appropriate intervals

Collaborative Activities

- Administer supplemental electrolytes, as ordered
- *(NIC) Nutrition Management:*
  Determine—in collaboration with dietitian, as appropriate—number of calories and type of nutrients needed to meet nutrition requirements
  Insert gastrointestinal tube, if needed. (Consult agency procedure manual or fundamentals text.)
  Monitor gastric output and administer nasogastric replacement, per order
  Restrict food or fluid intake, if appropriate.

Renal

Assessments

- *(NIC) Fluid Management:*
  Observe hydration status (eg, moist mucous membranes, adequacy of pulses, and orthostatic blood pressure)
  Monitor lab results relevant for fluid balance (eg, hematocrit, BUN, albumin, total protein, serum osmolality, and urine specific gravity)
  Monitor lab results for fluid retention (eg, increased specific gravity, increased BUN, decreased hematocrit, and increased urine osmolality)
  Observe for signs of fluid overload/retention (eg, crackles, elevated CVP or pulmonary capillary wedge pressure, edema, neck vein distention, and ascites)
  Maintain accurate intake and output record
  Monitor vital signs
  Monitor patient's response to prescribed electrolyte therapy
  Weigh daily and monitor trends

  For hemodialysis patients:
- Monitor serum electrolyte levels
- Monitor blood pressure
- Weigh patient before and after procedure

- Monitor BUN, serum creatinine, serum electrolytes, and hematocrit levels between dialysis treatments
- Assess for signs of dialysis disequilibrium syndrome (eg, headache, nausea and vomiting, hypertension, and altered level of consciousness)
- Observe for dehydration, muscle cramps, or seizure activity
- Assess for bleeding at the dialysis access site or elsewhere
- Observe for transfusion reaction, if appropriate
- Assess patency of arteriovenous fistula (eg, palpate for pulse, auscultate for bruit)
- Assess mental status (eg, consciousness, orientation)
- Monitor clotting times

For peritoneal dialysis patients:
- Assess temperature, orthostatic blood pressure, apical pulse, respirations, and lung sounds before dialysis
- Weigh patient daily
- Measure and record abdominal girth
- Note BUN, serum electrolyte, creatinine, pH, and hematocrit levels prior to dialysis and periodically during the procedure
- During instillation and dwell periods, observe for respiratory distress
- Record amount and type of dialysate instilled, dwell time, and amount and appearance of the drainage
- Monitor for signs of infection at exit site and in peritoneum

Patient/Family Teaching
- Explain all procedures and expected sensations to patient
- Explain the need for fluid restrictions, as needed

For dialysis patients:
- Teach patient signs and symptoms that indicate the need to contact a physician (eg, fever, bleeding)
- Teach procedure to patients having home dialysis

Collaborative Activities
- Administer diuretics, as ordered
- Notify physician if signs and symptoms of fluid volume excess worsen

For hemodialysis patients:
- Administer heparin according to protocol and adjust dosage

Other
- Distribute prescribed fluid intake appropriately over 24-hour period

- Maintain fluid and diet restrictions (eg, low sodium, no salt), as ordered

  For hemodialysis patients:
- Do not perform venipunctures or take blood pressures on the arm with a fistula

  For peritoneal dialysis patients:
- Use strict aseptic technique at all times
- Warm dialysate to body temperature before dialysis
- Place in semi-Fowler position and slow instillation rate if respiratory distress occurs

Tissue Perfusion, Altered (Peripheral)
(1.4.1.1) (1980, 1998)

Definition: A decrease in oxygen resulting in the failure to nourish the tissues at the capillary level

[**NOTE:** NANDA includes *Altered peripheral tissue perfusion* with *Altered tissue perfusion (cardiopulmonary/cerebral/gastrointestinal/renal).*]

Defining Characteristics

Altered sensations
Altered skin characteristics (eg, hair, nails, moisture)
Bruits
Blood pressure changes in extremities
Claudication
Delayed healing
Diminished arterial pulsations
Edema
Positive Homan's sign
Skin color pale on elevation; does not return on lowering the leg
Skin discolorations
Skin temperature changes
Weak or absent pulses

Related Factors

Altered affinity of hemoglobin for oxygen
Decreased hemoglobin concentration in blood
Enzyme poisoning
Exchange problems
Hypervolemia

Hypoventilation

Hypovolemia

Impaired transport of the oxygen across alveolar and/or capillary
  membrane

Interruption of arterial flow

Interruption of venous flow

Mechanical reduction of venous and/or arterial blood flow

Mismatch of ventilation with blow flow

The following table provides help in identifying *Altered tissue
perfusion (peripheral)*

Table 10

Objective Data	Chances that characteristics will be present in given diagnosis	Chances that characteristics will not be explained by any other diagnosis
Skin temperature: cold extremities	High	Low
Skin color: dependent blue or purple	Moderate	Low
Pale on elevation, color does not return on lowering of leg	High	High
Diminished arterial pulsations	High	High
Skin quality: shining	High	Low
Lack of lanugo; round scars covered with atrophied skin	High	Moderate
Gangrene	Low	High
Slow-growing, dry brittle nails	High	Moderate
Claudication	Moderate	High
Blood pressure changes in extremities	Moderate	Moderate
Bruits	Moderate	Moderate
Slow healing of lesions	High	Low

Suggestions for Use

Because some of the nursing interventions are different, it is
usually important to determine whether *Altered peripheral tissue
perfusion* is of arterial or venous origin.

Suggested Alternative Diagnoses

Injury, risk for
Peripheral neurovascular dysfunction, risk for
Skin integrity, risk for impaired
Tissue integrity, impaired

NOC Suggested Outcomes

Fluid Balance: Balance of water in the intracellular and extracellular compartments of the body

Muscle Function: Adequacy of muscle contraction for movement

Tissue Integrity: Skin and Mucous Membranes: Structural intactness and normal physiologic function of skin and mucous membranes

Tissue Perfusion: Peripheral: Extent to which blood flows through the small vessels of the extremities and maintains tissue function

Goals/Evaluation Criteria

Examples Using NOC Language

- Demonstrates **Fluid Balance**, as evidenced by the following indicators (specify 1–5: extremely, substantially, moderately, mildly, or not compromised):
    Blood pressure in expected range
    Peripheral pulses palpable
    Peripheral edema not present
    Skin hydration
- Demonstrates **Tissue Integrity: Skin and Mucous Membranes**, as evidenced by the following indicators (specify 1–5: extremely, substantially, moderately, mildly, or not compromised):
    Tissue temperature, sensation, elasticity, hydration, pigmentation, color, and thickness
    Tissue lesion-free
- Demonstrates **Tissue Perfusion: Peripheral**, as evidenced by the following indicators (specify 1–5: extremely, substantially, moderately, mildly, or not compromised):
    Proximal and distal peripheral pulses strong and symmetrical
    Sensation level normal
    Muscle function intact
    Skin intact, color normal
    Extremity temperature warm
    Localized extremity pain not present

Other Examples

Patient will:

• Be able to describe plan for care at home

NIC Priority Interventions

Circulatory Care: Promotion of arterial and venous circulation

Intracranial Pressure (ICP) Monitoring: Measurement and interpretation of patient data to regulate intracranial pressure. [**NOTE:** This nursing diagnosis is directly concerned only with *peripheral* tissue perfusion.]

Neurologic Monitoring: Collection and analysis of patient data to prevent or minimize neurologic complications

Peripheral Sensation Management: Prevention or minimization of injury or discomfort in the patient with altered sensation

Nursing Activities

Assessments

• *(NIC) Circulatory Care:*

Perform a comprehensive appraisal of peripheral circulation (eg, check peripheral pulses, edema, capillary refill, color, and temperature of extremity)

Assess degree of discomfort or pain

Monitor fluid status, including intake and output

• *(NIC) Peripheral Sensation Management:*

Monitor [peripherally] sharp/dull and/or hot/cold discrimination

Monitor for paresthesia: numbness, tingling, hyperesthesia, and hypoesthesia

Monitor for thrombophlebitis and deep vein thrombosis

Monitor fit of bracing devices, prosthesis, shoes, and clothing

Monitor position of body parts while bathing, sitting, lying, or changing position

Examine skin daily for alteration in skin integrity

Patient/Family Teaching

Instruct patient/family about:

• Avoiding extremes of temperature to extremities

• The importance of adhering to diet and medication regimen

• Reportable signs and symptoms that may require notification of physician

• *(NIC) Circulatory Care:*

Proper foot care

The importance of prevention of venous stasis (eg, not crossing legs, elevating feet without bending knees, and exercise)

Collaborative Activities

- Give pain medications. Notify physician if pain is unrelieved.
- *(NIC) Circulatory Care:* Administer antiplatelet or anticoagulant medications, as appropriate

Other

- Avoid chemical, mechanical, or thermal trauma to involved extremity
- Discourage smoking and use of stimulants
- *(NIC) Circulatory Care:*

  Lower extremity to improve arterial circulation, as appropriate

  Apply antiembolism stockings (eg, elastic or pneumatic stockings), if appropriate

  Elevate affected limb 20 degrees or greater above the level of the heart to improve venous return, as appropriate

  Encourage passive or active range-of-motion exercises during bed rest, as appropriate

- *(NIC) Peripheral Sensation Management:*

  Avoid or carefully monitor use of heat or cold, such as heating pads, hot-water bottles, and ice packs

  Place cradle over affected body parts to keep bedclothes off affected areas

  Discuss or identify causes of abnormal sensations or sensation changes

Transfer Ability, Impaired
(6.1.1.1.5) (1998)

Definition: Limitation of independent movement between two nearby surfaces. [Specify level.]

Defining Characteristics

Objective

Impaired ability to transfer:

    From bed to chair and chair to bed

    On or off a toilet or commode

    Between uneven levels

    From chair to car or car to chair

    From chair to floor or floor to chair

    From standing to floor or floor to standing

Other Defining Characteristics (Non-NANDA)

Cognitive impairment

Decreased muscle strength, control, and/or mass

Depressive mood state or anxiety

Developmental delay

Intolerance to activity, decreased strength and endurance

Joint stiffness or contractures

Lack of physical or social environmental supports

Limited cardiovascular endurance

Loss of integrity of bone structures

Medications

Musculoskeletal impairment

Neuromuscular impairment

Pain

Prescribed movement restrictions

Reluctance to initiate movement

Sedentary lifestyle or disuse or deconditioning

Selective or generalized malnutrition

Sensoriperceptual impairments

Related Factors

To be developed

Suggestions for Use

(1) Use *Impaired transfer ability* to describe individuals with limited ability for independent physical movement, such as decreased ability to move arms or legs or generalized muscle weakness, or when nursing interventions will focus on restoring mobility and function or preventing further deterioration. Do not use this label to describe temporary conditions that cannot be changed by the nurse (eg, traction, prescribed bedrest, or permanent paralysis). When the patient's transfer ability cannot be improved, this label should be used as a related or risk factor for other nursing diagnoses, such as *Risk for injury: falls.* (2) Specify level of mobility, using the same criteria as for *Impaired physical mobility.*

Level 0: Is completely independent

Level 1: Requires use of equipment or device

Level 2: Requires help from another person for assistance, supervision, or teaching

Level 3: Requires help from another person and equipment/device

Level 4: Is dependent; does not participate in activity

(3) See "Suggestions for Use" for "Impaired Physical Mobility" on p. 279.

Suggested Alternative Diagnoses

Disuse syndrome, risk for
Injury, risk for
Mobility: bed, impaired
Mobility: physical, impaired
Mobility: wheelchair, impaired
Self-care deficit
Walking, impaired

NOC Suggested Outcomes

NOTE: Because this is a new NANDA label, NOC has not yet published suggested outcomes for it. However, the following seem to be appropriate choices

Joint Movement: Active: Range of motion of joints with self-initiated movement
Mobility Level: Ability to move purposefully
Transfer Performance: Ability to change body locations

Goals/Evaluation Criteria

• The patient will perform full range of motion of all joints
• The patient will transfer:
> From bed to chair or bed to standing
> To and from a toilet or commode
> From wheelchair to car or car to wheelchair
> From standing to floor or floor to standing

NIC Priority Interventions

NOTE: NIC has not yet published priority interventions for *Impaired transfer ability.* The following are the priority interventions presently linked to the NOC outcome Transfer Performance.
Exercise Therapy: Balance: Use of specific activities, postures, and movements to maintain, enhance, or restore balance
Exercise Therapy: Muscle Control: Use of specific activity or exercise protocols to enhance or restore controlled body movement
Teaching: Psychomotor Skill: Preparing a patient to perform a psychomotor skill

Nursing Activities

Assessments

- Perform ongoing assessment of patient's transfer ability
- Assess need for assistance from home health agency or other placement service and assess need for durable medical equipment
- Assess vision, hearing, and proprioception
- *(NIC) Exercise Therapy: Muscle Control:*
  Determine patient's readiness to engage in activity or exercise protocol
  Determine accuracy of body image
  Monitor patient's emotional, cardiovascular, and functional responses to exercise protocol
  Monitor patient's self-exercise for correct performance

Patient/Family Teaching

- Instruct in active/passive range-of-motion exercises
- Give step-by-step directions
- Provide written information/diagrams
- Give frequent feedback to prevent formation of bad habits
- Provide information about assistive devices that may help with transfers
- Teach home caregivers how to incorporate balance and strength exercises into ADLs
- *(NIC) Exercise Therapy: Muscle Control:*
  Provide step-by-step cuing for each motor activity during exercise or ADLs
  Instruct patient to "recite" each movement as it is being performed

Collaborative Activities

- Use occupational and physical therapy as resources in developing plan to maintain/increase transfer mobility. Plan should include balance and muscle-strengthening exercises

Other

- Position call light/button within easy reach
- Provide positive reinforcement during activities
- Implement pain control measures before beginning exercises or physical therapy
- Be sure care plan includes number of personnel needed to transfer patient
- Assist patient to transfer, as needed

- *(NIC) Exercise Therapy: Muscle Control:*
  Dress patient in nonrestrictive clothing
  Assist to maintain trunk and/or proximal joint stability during
  motor activity
  Reorient patient to movement functions of the body
  Incorporate ADLs into exercise protocol, if appropriate
  Assist patient to prepare and maintain a progress graph/chart to
  motivate adherence with exercise protocol

Trauma, Risk for
(1.6.1.3) (1980)

Definition: Accentuated risk of accidental tissue injury (eg,
wound, burn, fracture)

Risk Factors

External (Environmental)

High-crime neighborhood and vulnerable clients; pot handles
facing toward front of stove; use of thin or worn pot holders;
knives stored uncovered; inappropriate call-for-aid mechanisms
for bed-resting client; inadequately stored combustibles or corro-
sives (eg, matches, oily rags, lye); highly flammable children's toys
or clothing; obstructed passageways; high beds; large icicles hang-
ing from the roof; snow or ice collected on stairs, walkways; over-
exposure to sun, sunlamps, radiotherapy; overloaded electrical
outlets; overloaded fuse boxes; play or work near vehicle pathways (eg, driveways, laneways, railroad tracks); playing with fire-
works or gunpowder; guns or ammunition stored unlocked; contact with rapidly moving machinery, industrial belts, or pulleys;
litter or liquid spills on floors or stairways; defective appliances;
bathing in very hot water (eg, unsupervised bathing of young children); bathtub without handgrip or antislip equipment; children
playing with matches, candles, cigarettes, sharp-edged toys; children playing without gates at the top of the stairs; delayed lighting
of gas burner or oven; contact with intense cold; grease waste collected on stoves; children riding in the front seat in car; driving a
mechanically unsafe vehicle; driving after partaking of alcoholic
beverages or drugs; nonuse or misuse of seat restraints; driving at
excessive speeds; driving without necessary visual aids; entering
unlighted rooms; experimenting with chemical or gasoline; exposure to dangerous machinery; faulty electrical plugs; frayed wires;

unanchored electric wires; contact with acids or alkalis; unsturdy or absent stair rails; use of unsteady ladders or chairs; use of cracked dishware or glasses; wearing plastic apron or flowing clothes around open flame; unscreened fires or heaters; unsafe window protection in homes with young children; sliding on coarse bed linen or struggling within bed restraints; misuse of necessary headgear for motorized cyclists or young children carried on adult bicycles; potential igniting gas leaks; unsafe road or road-crossing conditions; slippery floors (eg, wet or highly waxed); smoking in bed or near oxygen; unanchored rugs

Internal (Individual)

Weakness, poor vision, balancing difficulties, reduced temperature or tactile sensation, reduced large or small muscle coordination, reduced hand-eye coordination, lack of safety education, lack of safety precautions, insufficient finances to purchase safety equipment or effect repairs, cognitive or emotional difficulties, history of previous trauma

Suggestions for Use

Use a more specific diagnosis when possible.

Suggested Alternative Diagnoses

Aspiration, risk for
Home maintenance management, impaired
Injury, risk for
Perioperative positioning injury, risk for
Poisoning, risk for

NOC Suggested Outcomes

Risk Control: Actions to eliminate or reduce actual, personal, and modifiable health threats

Safety Behavior: Fall Prevention: Individual or caregiver actions to minimize risk factors that might precipitate falls

Goals/Evaluation Criteria

Examples Using NOC Language

• Demonstrates **Risk Control,** as evidenced by the following indicators (specify 1–5: never, rarely, sometimes, often, or consistently demonstrated):

    Monitors environmental and personal behavior risk factors
    Follows selected risk-control strategies
    Modifies lifestyle to reduce risk

Participates in screening for identified risks

Uses personal support systems and community resources to control risk

- Practices **Safety Behavior: Fall Prevention**, as evidenced by the following indicators (specify 1–5: not, slightly, moderately, substantially, or totally adequate):

Correct use of assistive devices

Placement of barriers to prevent falls

Placement of handrailings, as needed

Elimination of clutter, spills, glare from floors

Taking down rugs

Arrangement for removal of snow and ice from walking surfaces

Use of rubber mats and grab bars in tub/shower

Use of precautions when taking medications that increase risk for falls

Use of vision-correcting devices

Other Examples

- Patient will avoid physical injury

NIC Priority Interventions

Environmental Management: Safety: Monitoring and manipulation of the physical environment to promote safety

Skin Surveillance: Collection and analysis of patient data to maintain skin and mucous membrane integrity

Nursing Activities

Assessments

- *(NIC) Environmental Management: Safety:*

Identify the safety needs of the patient based on level of physical and cognitive function and past history of behavior

Identify safety hazards in the environment (ie, physical, biological, and chemical)

Patient/Family Teaching

- Instruct patient/family in safety measures specific to risk area
- Provide educational materials related to strategies for prevention of trauma
- Provide information on environmental hazards and characteristics (eg, stairs, windows, cupboard locks, swimming pools, streets, or gates)

Collaborative Activities

- Refer to educational classes in the community (eg, CPR, first-aid, or swimming classes)
- *(NIC) Environmental Management: Safety:* Assist patient in relocating to safer environment (eg, referral for housing assistance)

Other

- *(NIC) Environmental Management: Safety:*

  Modify the environment to minimize hazards and risk

  Provide adaptive devices (eg, step stools and handrails) to increase the safety of the environment

  Use protective devices (eg, restraints, side rails, locked doors, fences, and gates) to physically limit mobility or access to harmful situations

Unilateral Neglect
(7.2.1.1) (1986)

Definition: The state in which an individual is perceptually unaware of and inattentive to one side of the body

Defining Characteristics

Objective

Consistent inattention to stimuli on affected side

Does not look toward affected side

Inadequate self-care

Leaves food on plate on affected side

Positioning and/or safety precautions in regard to the affected side

Related Factors

Effects of disturbed perceptual abilities (eg, hemianopsia)

Neurologic illness or trauma

One-sided blindness

Other Related Factors (Non-NANDA)

Anesthesia of one side of the body (ie, hemianesthesia)

Blindness in half of the field of vision in one or both eyes (ie, hemianopia)

Paralysis of one side of body (ie, hemiplegia)

Real or pretended ignorance of presence of paralysis (ie, anosognosia)

Weakness of one side of body (ie, hemiparesis)

Suggestions for Use

Unilateral neglect may occur with medical conditions such as brain injuries, cerebral aneurysms or tumors, and cerebrovascular accidents. There are usually other nursing diagnoses associated with the pathophysiology of *Unilateral neglect*, for example, those in the following section, "Suggested Alternative Diagnoses."

Suggested Alternative Diagnoses

Anxiety
Injury, risk for
Self-care deficit
Sensory/perceptual alterations

NOC Suggested Outcomes

Body Image: Positive perception of own appearance and body functions

Body Positioning: Self-Initiated: Ability to change own body positions

Self-Care: Activities of Daily Living (ADLs): Ability to perform the most basic physical tasks and personal care activities

Goals/Evaluation Criteria

Examples Using NOC Language

- Demonstrates **Body Image,** as evidenced by the following indicators (specify 1–5: never, rarely, sometimes, often, or consistently positive):

    Positive internal picture of self

    Congruence between body reality, body ideal, and body presentation

    Adjustment to changes in body function

- Performs **Self-Care: Activities of Daily Living (ADLs),** as evidenced by the following indicators (specify 1–5: dependent, does not participate, requires assistive person and device, requires assistive person—independent with assistive device; or completely independent): eating, dressing, toileting, bathing, grooming, hygiene, ambulation, and transfer

Other Examples

Patient will:

- Be able to change own body positions (specify: lying to sitting, sitting to lying, kneeling to standing, and so forth)
- Acknowledge extent of deficit

- Modify behavior/environment to accommodate deficit
- Demonstrate improving perception of environment
- Not experience falls or other accidents

NIC Priority Interventions

Unilateral Neglect Management: Protecting and safely reintegrating the affected part of the body while helping the patient adapt to disturbed perceptual abilities

Nursing Activities

Assessments

- Assess the nature and extent of deficit
- *(NIC) Unilateral Neglect Management:* Monitor for abnormal responses to three primary types of stimuli: sensory, visual, and auditory

Patient/Family Teaching

- Explain and reinforce nature and extent of deficit to patient/ family
- Provide information about community resources
- *(NIC) Unilateral Neglect Management:* Instruct caregivers on the cause, mechanisms, and treatment of unilateral neglect

Collaborative Activities

- *(NIC) Unilateral Neglect Management:* Consult with occupational and physical therapists concerning timing and strategies to facilitate reintegration of neglected body parts and function

Other

- Provide visual, olfactory, and tactile stimulation
- *(NIC) Unilateral Neglect Management:*
  Provide realistic feedback about patient's perceptual deficit
  Touch unaffected shoulder when initiating conversation
  Place food and beverages within field of vision and turn plate, as necessary
  Rearrange the environment to use the right or left visual field, such as positioning personal items, television, or reading materials within view on unaffected side
  Gradually move personal items and activity to affected side as patient demonstrates an ability to compensate for neglect
  Assist patient to bathe and groom affected side first as patient demonstrates an ability to compensate for neglect
  Keep side rail up on affected side, as appropriate

Ensure that affected extremities are properly and safely positioned

Include family in rehabilitation process to support the patient's efforts and assist with care, as appropriate

Urinary Elimination, Altered
(1.3.2) (1973)

Definition: The state in which the individual experiences a disturbance in urine elimination

Defining Characteristics

Subjective
Dysuria
Urgency

Objective
Frequency
Hesitancy
Incontinence
Nocturia
Retention

Related Factors

Multiple causality, including anatomic obstruction, sensory or motor impairment, urinary tract infection

Suggestions for Use

Use a more specific label when possible. For specific patient outcomes, evaluation criteria, and nursing interventions, refer to the following suggested alternative diagnoses.

Suggested Alternative Diagnoses

Incontinence, urinary, functional
Incontinence, urinary reflex
Incontinence, urinary, stress
Incontinence, urinary, total
Incontinence, urinary, urge
Incontinence: urinary, urge, risk for
Urinary retention

NOC Suggested Outcomes

Knowledge: Medication: Extent of understanding conveyed about the safe use of medication

Urinary Continence: Control of the elimination of urine

Urinary Elimination: Ability of the urinary system to filter wastes, conserve solutes, and to collect and discharge urine in a healthy pattern

Goals/Evaluation Criteria

Examples Using NOC Language

- Demonstrates **Urinary Continence,** as evidenced by the following indicators (specify 1–5: never, rarely, sometimes, often, or consistently positive):

    Able to toilet independently

    Absence of urinary tract infection (<100,000 WBC [white blood cells])

    Voids >150 cc each time

    Predictable pattern to passage of urine

Other Examples

Patient will:

- Be continent of urine
- Demonstrate adequate knowledge of medications that affect urinary function
- Urinary elimination will not be compromised:

    Urine odor, amount, and color in expected range

    No hematuria

    Passes urine without pain, hesitancy, or urgency

    BUN, serum creatinine, and specific gravity within normal limits

    Urine proteins, glucose, ketones, pH, and electrolytes within normal limits

NIC Priority Interventions

Urinary Elimination Management: Maintenance of an optimum urinary elimination pattern

Nursing Activities

Also refer to "Nursing Activities" for the preceding "Suggested Alternative Diagnoses."

Assessments

- *(NIC) Urinary Elimination Management:*

  Monitor urinary elimination, including frequency, consistency, odor, volume, and color, as appropriate

  Obtain midstream voided specimen for urinalysis, as appropriate

Patient/Family Teaching

- *(NIC) Urinary Elimination Management:*

  Teach patient signs and symptoms of urinary tract infection

  Instruct patient/family to record urinary output, as appropriate

  Instruct patient to respond immediately to urge to void

  Teach patient to drink 8 oz of liquid with meals, between meals, and in early evening

Collaborative Activities

- *(NIC) Urinary Elimination Management:* Refer to physician if signs and symptoms of urinary tract infection occur

Urinary Retention
(1.3.2.2) (1986)

Definition: The state in which an individual experiences incomplete emptying of the bladder

Defining Characteristics

Subjective

Dysuria

Sensation of bladder fullness

Objective

Bladder distention

Dribbling

Overflow incontinence

Residual urine

Small, frequent voiding or absence of urine output

Related Factors

Blockage

High urethral pressure caused by weak detrusor

Inhibition of reflex arc

Strong sphincter

Suggestions for Use

None

Suggested Alternative Diagnoses

Incontinence, urinary, functional
Incontinence, urinary, stress
Incontinence, urinary, urge
Urinary elimination, altered

NOC Suggested Outcomes

Urinary Continence: Control of the elimination of urine
Urinary Elimination: Ability of the urinary system to filter wastes, conserve solutes, and to collect and discharge urine in a healthy pattern

Goals/Evaluation Criteria

Examples Using NOC Language

• Demonstrates **Urinary Continence,** as evidenced by the following indicators (specify 1–5: never, rarely, sometimes, often, or consistently positive):

    Free of urine leakage between voidings
    Empties bladder completely
    Absence of postvoid residual >100–200 cc
    Fluid intake in expected range

Other Examples

Patient will:

• Demonstrate bladder evacuation by clean intermittent self-catheterization procedure
• Describe plan of care at home
• Remain free of urinary tract infection
• Report a decrease in bladder spasms
• Have a balanced 24-hour intake and output

NIC Priority Interventions

Urinary Catheterization: Insertion of a catheter into the bladder for temporary or permanent drainage of urine
Urinary Retention Care: Assistance in relieving bladder distention

Nursing Activities

Assessments

- Identify and document patient's bladder evacuation pattern
- *(NIC) Urinary Retention Care:*

  Monitor use of nonprescription agents with anticholinergic or alpha agonist properties

  Monitor effects of prescribed pharmaceuticals, such as calcium channel blockers and anticholinergics

  Monitor intake and output

  Monitor degree of bladder distention by palpation and percussion

Patient/Family Teaching

- Instruct patient in reportable signs/symptoms of urinary tract infection (eg, fever, chills, flank pain, hematuria, change in consistency and odor of urine)
- *(NIC) Urinary Retention Care:* Instruct patient/family to record urinary output, as appropriate

Collaborative Activities

- Refer to enterostomal therapy nurse for instruction in clean intermittent self-catheterization q4–6 hours while awake.
- *(NIC) Urinary Retention Care:* Refer to urinary continence specialist, as appropriate

Other

- Establish a bladder-evacuation training program
- Space fluids throughout the day to ensure adequate intake without bladder overdistention
- Encourage oral intake of fluids: ____ cc for day; ____ cc for evening; ____ cc for nights
- *(NIC) Urinary Retention Care:*

  Provide privacy for elimination

  Use the power of suggestion by running water or flushing the toilet

  Stimulate the reflex bladder by applying cold to the abdomen, stroking the inner thigh, or running water

  Provide enough time for bladder emptying (10 minutes)

  Use spirits of wintergreen in bedpan or urinal

  Provide Credé's maneuver, as necessary

  Catheterize for residual, as appropriate

  Insert urinary catheter, as appropriate

Ventilatory Weaning Response, Dysfunctional (DVWR) (1.5.1.3.2) (1992)

Definition: A state in which a patient cannot adjust to lowered levels of mechanical ventilator support, which interrupts and prolongs the weaning process

Defining Characteristics

Nurses have defined three levels of DVWR in which these defining characteristics occur in response to weaning (Logan and Jenny 1991).

Mild DVWR

Subjective

Breathing discomfort
Expressed feelings of increased need for oxygen
Fatigue
Queries about possible machine malfunction
Warmth

Objective

Increased concentration on breathing
Restlessness
Slight increase in respiratory rate from baseline
Warmth

Moderate DVWR

Subjective

Apprehension

Objective

Color changes; pale, slight cyanosis
Decreased air entry on auscultation
Diaphoresis
Eye widening ("wide-eyed" look)
Hypervigilance to activities
Inability to cooperate
Inability to respond to coaching
Baseline increase in respiratory rate < 5 breaths/minute
Slight increase from baseline blood pressure < 20mm Hg
Slight increase from baseline heart rate < 20 beats/minute
Slight respiratory accessory muscle use

Severe DVWR

Objective

Adventitious breath sounds, audible airway secretions

Agitation

Cyanosis

Decreased level of consciousness

Deterioration in arterial blood gases from current baseline data

Discoordinated breathing with the ventilator

Full respiratory accessory muscle use

Increase from baseline blood pressure > 20 mm Hg

Increase from baseline heart rate > 20 beats/minute

Paradoxical abdominal breathing

Profuse diaphoresis

Respiratory rate increases significantly from baseline

Shallow, gasping breaths

Related Factors

Physiologic

Inadequate nutrition

Ineffective airway clearance

Sleep pattern disturbance

Uncontrolled pain or discomfort

Situational

Adverse environment (eg, noisy, active environment, negative events in the room, low nurse-patient ratio, extended nurse absence from bedside, unfamiliar nursing staff)

History of multiple unsuccessful weaning attempts

History of ventilator dependence > one week

Inadequate social support

Inappropriate pacing of diminished ventilator support

Uncontrolled episodic energy demands or problems

Psychologic

Anxiety: moderate, severe

Decreased motivation

Decreased self-esteem

Fear

Hopelessness

Insufficient trust in the nurse

Knowledge deficit of the weaning process

Patient perceived inefficacy about the ability to wean

Patient role

Powerlessness

Suggestions for Use

DVWR is concerned specifically with patient responses to separation from the mechanical ventilator. Other respiratory diagnoses may also occur during weaning, for example, *Ineffective airway clearance, Ineffective breathing pattern,* and *Impaired gas exchange.* This diagnostic label does not include the reasons for the weaning problems. If you do not know the etiology of the DVWR, use "unknown etiology."

Suggested Alternative Diagnoses

Airway clearance, ineffective
Breathing pattern, ineffective
Gas exchange, impaired

NOC Suggested Outcomes

Respiratory Status: Gas Exchange: Alveolar exchange of CO_2 or O_2 to maintain arterial blood gas concentrations

Respiratory Status: Ventilation: Movement of air in and out of the lungs

Vital Signs Status: Temperature, pulse, respiration, and blood pressure within expected range for the individual

Goals/Evaluation Criteria

Examples Using NOC Language

- Demonstrates **Vital Signs Status,** as evidenced by the following indicators (specify 1–5: extreme, substantial, moderate, mild, or no deviation from expected range): temperature, apical and radial pulse rate, respiration rate, and systolic and diastolic BP
- Demonstrates **Respiratory Status: Gas Exchange**, as evidenced by the following indicators (specify 1–5: extremely, substantially, moderately, mildly, or not compromised):
    Neurologic status in expected range
    Chest x-ray findings in expected range
    PaO_2, $PaCO_2$, arterial pH, and O_2 saturation within normal limits
- Demonstrates **Respiratory Status: Ventilation,** as evidenced by the following indicators (specify 1–5: extremely, substantially, moderately, mildly, or not compromised):
    Restlessness, cyanosis, and fatigue not present
    Accessory muscle use not present
    Chest retraction not present
    Shortness of breath and dyspnea not present

Other Examples

Patient will:

- Achieve established weaning goals
- Be physiologically stable for weaning process
- Be psychologically and emotionally ready for weaning process

NIC Priority Interventions

Mechanical Ventilation: Use of an artificial device to assist a patient to breathe

Mechanical Ventilatory Weaning: Assisting the patient to breathe without the aid of a mechanical ventilator

Nursing Activities

Assessments

- Assess patient's readiness to wean by considering the following respiratory indicators:

    Arterial blood gases stable with $PaO_2 > 60$ on 40- to 60-percent oxygen

    Maximum inspiratory force > -20 cm H_2O so independent respiration can be initiated

    Unassisted tidal volume > 5 mL/Kg ideal body weight

    Vital capacity > 13 mL/Kg ideal body weight

    Stable spontaneous respiratory rate < 30 breaths/minute

    Cough effective enough to handle secretions

    Length of time on ventilator

- Assess patient's readiness to wean by considering the following nonrespiratory indicators:

    Absence of constipation, diarrhea, or ileus

    Absence of fever and/or infection

    Adequate nutritional status as evidenced by acceptable serum albumin and transferrin and midarm muscle circumference > 15th percentile

    Adequate rest and sleep

    Hemoglobin and hematocrit within normal limits for patient

    Improvements in body strength and endurance

    Normal blood pressure for patient

    Psychologic/emotional readiness

    Satisfactory fluid and electrolyte balance

    Stable heart rate and rhythm

    Tolerable pain or discomfort level

- Determine why previous weaning attempts were unsuccessful, if applicable
- Monitor patient's response to current medications and correlate response with weaning goals
- *(NIC) Mechanical Ventilatory Weaning:*
  Monitor degree of shunt, vital capacity, V_d/V_t, MVV, inspiratory force, and FEV_1 for readiness to wean from mechanical ventilation, based on agency protocol
  Monitor for signs of respiratory muscle fatigue (eg, abrupt rise in $PaCO_2$ level; rapid, shallow ventilation; and paradoxical abdominal wall motion), hypoxemia, and tissue hypoxia while weaning is in process

Patient/Family Teaching

- Instruct patient/family in weaning process and goals, which should include:
  How patient may feel as process evolves
  Participation of family
  Participation required by patient
  What patient can expect from nurse
  Reasons why weaning is necessary
- *(NIC) Mechanical Ventilatory Weaning:* Assist the patient to distinguish spontaneous breaths from mechanically-delivered breaths

Collaborative Activities

- Discuss weaning process and goals with physician and respiratory care practitioner, including patient's present and preexisting medical conditions
- *(NIC) Mechanical Ventilatory Weaning:* Collaborate with other health team members to optimize patient's nutritional status, ensuring that 50 percent of the diet's nonprotein calorie source is fat, rather than carbohydrate

Other

- Encourage self-care to increase sense of control and participation in own care
- Normalize ADLs to patient's tolerance level
- Establish a trusting relationship that instills patient's confidence in nurse to assist patient with weaning process
- Establish effective methods of communication between patient and others (eg, writing, blinking eyes, squeezing hand)

- Initiate weaning process by:

  Checking equipment to make sure it is attached to oxygen and that settings are correct

  Checking for presence of bilateral breath sounds

  Checking tubing for kinks and excessive moisture

  Checking vital signs and patient for indicators of nontolerance or fatigue q5–15 minutes

  Documenting weaning process and patient's tolerance

  Explaining procedure to patient and family

  Measuring and recording baseline respiratory rate, heart rate, blood pressure, ECG rhythm, lung sounds, vital capacity, tidal volume, inspiratory force, and saturated oxygen via pulse oximeter

  Preoxygenating, hyperinflating, suctioning, and reoxygenating patient prior to weaning

  Providing a quiet environment during weaning time

  Providing diversions such as television or radio

  Sitting patient in an upright position to decrease abdominal pressure on the diaphragm and allow for better lung expansion

  Starting the weaning time when patient has rested and is awake and alert

  Staying with patient during weaning time to provide coaching and reassurance

  Understanding the rationale for weaning orders (eg, use of continuous positive airway pressure [CPAP], synchronized intermittent mandatory ventilation [SIMV], pressure support ventilation [PSV], and mandatory minute ventilation [MMV], or T-piece)

- Reconnect patient to ventilator at preweaning settings if indicators of nontolerance occur

- Document in nursing care plan those strategies that promote success with weaning process to ensure consistency (eg, communication method with patient, family participation, and coaching methods)

- *(NIC) Mechanical Ventilatory Weaning:*

  Alternate periods of weaning trials with sufficient periods of rest and sleep

  Avoid delaying return of patient with fatigued respiratory muscles to mechanical ventilation

  Set a schedule to coordinate other patient care activities with weaning trials

  Use relaxation techniques, as appropriate

Violence: Directed at Others, Risk for
(9.2.2) (1980, 1996)

Definition: Behaviors in which an individual demonstrates that he/she can be physically, emotionally, and/or sexually harmful to others

Risk Factors

Objective

Availability and/or possession of weapon(s)

Body language: rigid posture, clenching of fists and jaw, hyperactivity, pacing, breathlessness, threatening stances

Cognitive impairment (eg, learning disabilities, attention-deficit disorder, decreased intellectual functioning)

Cruelty to animals

Fire setting

History of childhood abuse

History of drug/alcohol abuse

History of violence against others (eg, hitting someone, kicking someone, spitting at someone, scratching someone, throwing objects at someone, biting someone, attempted rape, rape, sexual molestation, urinating/defecating on a person)

History of violence of threats (eg, verbal threats against property, verbal threats against person, social threats, cursing, threatening notes/letters, threatening gestures, sexual threats)

History of violence, indirect (eg, tearing off clothes, ripping objects off walls, writing on walls, urinating on floor, defecating on floor, stamping feet, temper tantrum, running in corridors, yelling, throwing objects, breaking a window, slamming doors, sexual advances)

History of violent antisocial behavior (eg, stealing, insistent borrowing, insistent demand for privileges, insistent interruption of meetings, refusal to eat, refusal to take medication, ignoring instructions)

History of witnessing family violence

Impulsivity

Motor vehicle offenses (eg, frequent traffic violations, use of a motor vehicle to release anger)

Neurologic impairment (eg, positive EEG, CAT or MRI, head trauma, positive neurologic findings, seizure disorders)

Pathological intoxication

Prenatal and perinatal complications/abnormalities

Psychotic symptomatology (eg, auditory, visual, command hallucinations; paranoid delusions; loose, rambling, or illogical thought processes)

Suicidal behavior

Other Risk Factors (Non-NANDA)

Arrest/conviction pattern

Catatonic excitement

History of abuse by spouse

Manic excitement

Toxic reactions to medications

Suggestions for Use

Use this diagnosis for patients who need nursing interventions for the purpose of protecting others and preventing/decreasing violent episodes. The diagnosis *Ineffective family coping: disabling* may be more useful for situations in which there is domestic violence. If the need is to focus on anxiety or poor self-esteem, consider using those suggested alternative diagnoses.

Suggested Alternative Diagnoses

Anxiety

Coping: family, ineffective

Coping: individual, ineffective

Self-esteem, chronic low

Self-esteem disturbance

Self-esteem, situational low

NOC Suggested Outcomes

Abusive Behavior Self-Control: Management of own behaviors to avoid abuse and neglect of dependents or significant others

Aggression Control: Ability to restrain assaultive, combative, or destructive behavior toward others

Impulse Control: Ability to restrain compulsive or impulsive behavior

Goals/Evaluation Criteria

Examples Using NOC Language

• Demonstrates **Aggression Control,** as evidenced by the following indicators (specify 1–5: never, rarely, sometimes, often, or consistently demonstrated):

Refrains from:
> Verbal outbursts
> Striking others
> Violating others' personal space
> Harming others; harming animals
> Destroying property

Identifies when angry, frustrated, or feeling aggressive

Vents negative feelings [eg, anger, frustration] appropriately

- Demonstrates **Impulse Control,** as evidenced by the following indicators (specify 1–5: never, rarely, sometimes, often, or consistently demonstrated):
> Identifies feelings or behaviors that lead to impulsive actions
> Identifies consequences of impulsive actions to self or others
> Avoids high-risk environments and situations
> Verbalizes control of impulses

Other Examples

Patient will:
- Identify factors that precipitate violent behaviors
- Identify alternative ways to cope with problems
- Identify support systems in the community
- Not abuse others physically, emotionally, or sexually

NIC Priority Interventions

Anger Control Assistance: Facilitation of the expression of anger in an adaptive nonviolent manner

Environmental Management: Violence Prevention: Monitoring and manipulation of the physical environment to decrease the potential for violent behavior directed toward self, others, or environment

Nursing Activities

Assessments

- Identify behaviors that signal impending violence against others. Specify behaviors.
- *(NIC) Anger Control Assistance:* Monitor potential for inappropriate aggression and intervene before its expression
- *(NIC) Environmental Management: Violence Prevention:*
  Monitor the safety of items being brought to the environment by visitors
  Monitor patient during use of potential weapons (eg, razor)

Patient/Family Teaching

- *(NIC) Anger Control Assistance:* Instruct on use of calming measures (eg, time-outs and deep breaths)

Collaborative Activities

- Clarify use of 72-hour hold for evaluation and treatment in psychiatric unit in the event of abuse against others
- Confer with physician on use of appropriate restraining measures when necessary to prevent injury to others
- Follow hospital/agency policy regarding legal responsibility for reporting abuse to authorities
- Initiate a multidisciplinary patient care conference to develop a plan of care

Other

- Encourage patient to verbalize anger
- Identify situations that provoke violence. Specify situations.
- Provide positive feedback when patient adheres to behavior limits
- *(NIC) Anger Control Assistance:*
  Use a calm, reassuring approach
  Limit access to frustrating situations until patient is able to express anger in an adaptive manner
  Encourage patient to seek assistance of nursing staff or responsible others during periods of increasing tension
  Prevent physical harm if anger is directed at self or others (eg, restrain and remove potential weapons)
  Provide physical outlets for expression of anger or tension (eg, punching bag, sports, clay, and writing in a journal)
  Identify consequences of inappropriate expression of anger
  Establish expectation that patient can control his/her behavior
  Assist in developing appropriate methods of expressing anger to others (eg, assertiveness and use of feeling statements)
- *(NIC) Environmental Management: Violence Prevention:*
  Assign single room to patient with potential for violence toward others
  Place patient in a room near nursing station
  Limit access to windows, unless locked and shatterproof, as appropriate
  Place patient in least restrictive environment that allows for necessary level of observation
  Maintain a designated safe area (eg, seclusion room) for patient to be placed when violent

Provide plastic, rather than metal, clothes hangers, as appropriate

Provide paper dishes and plastic utensils at meals

Violence: Self-Directed, Risk for
(9.2.2.2) (1994)

Definition: Behaviors in which an individual demonstrates that he/she can be physically, emotionally, and/or sexually harmful to self

Risk Factors

Age 15–19

Age over 45

Behavioral clues (eg, writing forlorn love notes, directing angry messages at a significant other who has rejected the person, giving away personal items, taking out a large life insurance policy)

Conflictual interpersonal relationships

Emotional status (eg, hopelessness, despair, increased anxiety, panic, anger, hostility)

Employment (eg, unemployed, recent job loss/failure)

Family background (eg, chaotic or conflictual, history of suicide)

History of multiple suicide attempts

Marital status (eg, single, widowed, divorced)

Mental health (eg, severe depression, psychosis, severe personality disorder, alcoholism, or drug abuse)

Occupation (eg, executive, administrator/owner of business, professional semiskilled worker)

People who engage in autoerotic sexual acts

Personal resources (eg, poor achievement, poor insight, affect unavailable and poorly controlled)

Physical health (eg, is hypochondriac, chronic or terminal illness)

Sexual orientation (eg, bisexual [active], homosexual [inactive])

Social resources (eg, poor rapport, socially isolated, unresponsive family)

Suicidal ideation (frequent, intense, prolonged)

Suicidal plan (clear and specific, lethality, method and availability of destructive means)

Verbal clues (eg, talking about death, better off without me, asking questions about lethal dosages and drugs)

Suggestions for Use

If the specific risk factors for *Risk for self-mutilation* are present, that more specific nursing diagnosis should be used instead of *Risk for violence: self-directed*

Suggested Alternative Diagnoses

Self-mutilation, risk for

NOC Suggested Outcomes

Because this is a new nursing diagnosis, NOC outcomes have not yet been linked to it. The following seem to be appropriate choices:
Impulse Control: Ability to restrain compulsive or impulsive behavior
Suicide Self-Restraint: Ability to refrain from gestures and attempts at killing self

Goals/Evaluation Criteria

Examples Using NOC Language

* Demonstrates **Impulse Control,** as evidenced by the following indicators:
    Vents negative feelings appropriately
    Identifies feelings or behaviors that lead to impulsive actions
    Identifies consequences of impulsive actions to self or others
    Avoids high-risk environments and situations
    Verbalizes control of impulses

Other Examples

Patient will:
* Identify alternative ways to cope with problems
* Identify support systems in the community
* Report a decrease in suicidal thoughts
* Not attempt suicide

NIC Priority Interventions

Anger Control Assistance: Facilitation of the expression of anger in an adaptive nonviolent manner
Environmental Management: Violence Prevention: Monitoring and manipulation of the physical environment to decrease the potential for violent behavior directed toward self, others, or environment

Nursing Activities

Assessments

- Assess and document patient's potential for suicide q _____
- Identify behaviors that signal impending violence against self. Specify behaviors.
- *(NIC) Environmental Management: Violence Prevention:*
  Monitor the safety of items being brought to the environment by visitors
  Monitor patient during use of potential weapons (eg, razor)

Patient/Family Teaching

- *(NIC) Anger Control Assistance:* Instruct on use of calming measures (eg, time-outs and deep breaths)

Collaborative Activities

- Clarify use of 72-hour hold for evaluation and treatment in psychiatric unit in the event of abuse against self
- Confer with physician on use of appropriate restraining measures when necessary to prevent injury to self
- Initiate a multidisciplinary patient care conference to develop a plan of care

Other

- Institute suicide precautions, as needed (eg, 24-hour attendant)
- Reassure patient that you will protect him/her against own suicidal impulses until able to regain control by: (1) constantly observing patient, (2) frequently checking patient, and (3) taking patient's suicidal ideation seriously
- Discuss with patient/family the role of anger in self-harm
- Encourage patient to verbalize anger
- *(NIC) Anger Control Assistance:*
  Use a calm, reassuring approach
  Limit access to frustrating situations until patient is able to express anger in an adaptive manner
  Encourage patient to seek assistance of nursing staff or responsible others during periods of increasing tension
  Prevent physical harm if anger is directed at self (eg, restrain and remove potential weapons)
  Provide physical outlets for expression of anger or tension (eg, punching bag, sports, clay, and writing in a journal)
  Establish expectation that patient can control his/her behavior

- *(NIC) Environmental Management: Violence Prevention:*
  Place patient with potential for self-harm with a roommate to decrease isolation and opportunity to act on self-harm thoughts, as appropriate
  Place patient in a room near nursing station
  Limit access to windows, unless locked and shatterproof, as appropriate
  Place patient in least restrictive environment that allows for necessary level of observation
  Apply mitts, splints, helmets, or restraints to limit mobility and ability to initiate self-harm, as appropriate
  Provide plastic, rather than metal, clothes hangers, as appropriate
  Provide paper dishes and plastic utensils at meals

Walking, Impaired
(6.1.1.1.3) (1998)

Definition: Limitation of independent movement within the environment on foot. [Specify level.]

Defining Characteristics
Impaired ability to:
  Climb stairs
  Navigate curbs
  Walk on an incline or decline
  Walk on uneven surfaces
  Walk required distances

Related Factors
  To be developed

Non-NANDA Related Factors
Altered cellular metabolism
Cognitive impairment
Cultural beliefs regarding age-appropriate activity
Decreased muscle strength, control, and/or mass
Depressive mood state or anxiety
Developmental delay
Intolerance to activity, decreased strength and endurance
Joint stiffness or contractures
Lack of knowledge regarding value of physical activity

Lack of physical or social environmental supports
Limited cardiovascular endurance
Loss of integrity of bone structures
Medications
Musculoskeletal impairment
Neuromuscular impairment
Pain
Reluctance to initiate movement
Sedentary lifestyle, disuse, or deconditioning
Selective or generalized malnutrition
Sensoriperceptual impairments

Suggestions for Use

As with other mobility diagnoses, the author recommends specifying the patient's functional level, as follows:

Level 0: Completely independent
Level 1: Requires use of equipment or device
Level 2: Requires help from another person for assistance, supervision, or teaching
Level 3: Requires help from another person and equipment/device
Level 4: Dependent; does not participate in activity

Use *Impaired walking* to describe individuals with limited ability for independent physical movement or generalized muscle weakness or when nursing interventions will focus on restoring mobility and function or preventing further deterioration. An example of an appropriate diagnosis would be *Impaired walking related to ineffective management of chronic pain secondary to rheumatoid arthritis.*

Do not use this label to describe temporary immobility that cannot be changed by the nurse (eg, traction, prescribed bed rest) or permanent paralysis. *Impaired walking* may be used effectively as the etiology of a nursing diagnosis, for example, *Self-care deficit: toileting related to impaired walking +4.*

Suggested Alternative Diagnoses

Disuse syndrome, risk for
Injury, risk for
Self-care deficit
Transfer ability, impaired

NOC Suggested Outcomes

Because this is a new diagnosis, NOC outcomes have not yet been specified. However, the following seem to be appropriate choices:

Ambulation: Walking: Ability to walk from place to place

Joint Movement: Active: Range of motion of joints with self-initiated movement

Mobility Level: Ability to move purposefully

Transfer Performance: Ability to change body locations

Goals/Evaluation Criteria

Examples Using NOC Language

- Demonstrates **Mobility Level,** as evidenced by the following indicators (specify 1–5: dependent, does not participate, requires assistive person and device, requires assistive person, is independent with assistive device, or is completely independent):

    Balance performance
    Body positioning performance
    Muscle and joint movement
    Transfer performance
    Ambulation: walking

Other Examples

Patient will:

- Bear weight and walk with adequate gait
- Walk a distance appropriate to his/her overall condition
- Demonstrate correct use of assistive devices (eg, crutches, cane) with supervision
- Request assistance with mobilization activities, as needed
- Perform activities of daily living independently with assistive devices (specify activity and device)

NIC Priority Interventions

Because this is a new diagnosis, NIC has not yet published the priority interventions for it. However, the following seem to be logical possibilities:

Exercise Therapy, Ambulation: Promotion and assistance with walking to maintain or restore autonomic and voluntary body functions during treatment and recovery from illness or injury

Exercise Therapy, Joint Mobility: Use of active or passive body movement to maintain or restore joint flexibility

Nursing Activities

Assessments

Assessment is an ongoing process to determine the performance level at which the patient's mobility is impaired.

Level 1 Nursing Activities

- Provide positive reinforcement during activities
- Collaborate with physical therapist in developing strength, balance, and flexibility exercises
- Assess need for assistance from home health agency and need for durable medical equipment
- *(NIC) Exercise Therapy: Ambulation:*
  Monitor patient's use of crutches or other walking aids
  Instruct patient how to position self throughout the transfer process
  Apply/provide assistive device (eg, cane, walker, or wheelchair) for ambulation if the patient is unsteady
  Assist patient to use footwear that facilitates walking and prevents injury
  Encourage independent ambulation within safe limits

Level 2 Nursing Activities

- Assess patient's learning needs regarding _____ (specify)
- Assess need for assistance from home health agency and need for durable medical equipment
- Instruct and encourage patient in active/passive range-of-motion exercises
- Instruct patient regarding weight-bearing status
- Instruct patient regarding correct body alignment
- Instruct and encourage patient to use a trapeze and/or weights to enhance and maintain strength of upper extremities
- Use occupational and physical therapy as resources in developing a plan for maintaining/increasing mobility
- Provide positive reinforcement during activities
- Supervise all mobilization attempts
- *(NIC) Exercise Therapy: Ambulation:*
  Instruct patient/caregiver about safe transfer and ambulation techniques
  Assist patient to stand and ambulate specified distance with specified number of staff

Levels 3 and 4 Nursing Activities

- Use occupational and physical therapy as resources in planning patient care activities

- Encourage patient/family to view limitations realistically
- Provide positive reinforcement during activities
- Develop a plan to include the following:
  Perform passive range-of-motion (PROM) or assisted range-of-motion (AROM) exercises, as indicated
  Type of assistive device
  Number of personnel needed to mobilize patient
  Schedule of activities
  Maximization of patient's mobility, given necessary constraints
- Assess patient motivation level for overcoming limitations
- Administer analgesics before beginning exercises/walking, as needed
- *(NIC) Exercise Therapy: Ambulation:*
  Use a gait belt to assist with transfer and ambulation, as needed

Clinical Conditions Guide to Nursing Diagnoses and Collaborative Problems

Medical Conditions
Surgical Conditions
Psychiatric Conditions
Antepartum and Postpartum Conditions
Newborn Conditions
Pediatric Conditions

This section contains lists of potential complications (also called multidisciplinary problems and collaborative problems) and nursing diagnoses associated with selected conditions (eg, medical, surgical, childbearing). However, because nursing diagnoses represent *human responses*, and because human beings respond in infinite ways, *any* nursing diagnosis could occur with *any* disease process or condition. In a sense, then, all nursing diagnoses on these lists are *potential* diagnoses. When using these lists, keep in mind that for each condition (eg, congestive heart failure) (1) every patient with that condition must be monitored for the associated complications, (2) a patient may have nursing diagnoses that are not included in the list, and (3) the list may include many nursing diagnoses that the patient does not have.

For the nursing diagnoses in this section, the etiologies (which follow "related to") are stated in broad, general terms. Etiologies, like problems, are highly individual. Therefore, when writing a nursing diagnosis, use the list as a starting point and expand the etiology to fully describe that patient's pathophysiology, disease process, situation, or other related factors. The format used for collaborative problems is adapted from Carpenito (1997b, pp. 28–29), for example, Potential Complication (PC) of burns: Hypovolemic shock.

Some patient teaching is required for every patient. Therefore, the nursing diagnosis *Knowledge deficit* is not listed for any of the clinical conditions in this section. It is assumed that all clients, regardless of disease or medical diagnosis, will be assessed for *Knowledge deficit*.

Also note that almost every patient is at risk for the nursing diagnosis *Ineffective individual management of therapeutic regimen related to lack of knowledge of disease process, therapies, and self-care.* This text includes that diagnosis only in situations where the processes, therapies, and so forth are complex, or where the patient could be expected to lack the abilities to manage for other reasons (eg, memory loss, confusion).

Medical Conditions

Acquired immune deficiency syndrome (AIDS)
Arthritis
Autoimmune disorders
Blood disorders
Burns
Cancer
Cardiac disorders (angina, coronary insufficiency, myocardial infarction, congestive heart failure, pericarditis/endocarditis)
Chest trauma
Dying patient
Endocrine disorders (Cushing's disease, diabetes mellitus, hypoglycemia, hyperthyroidism, hypothyroidism)
Gastrointestinal disorders (inflammation, bleeding, ulcers, abdominal pain)
Immobilized patient
Liver disease
Neurologic disorders (cerebrovascular accident, other)
Obesity
Pancreatitis
Renal failure, acute
Renal failure, chronic
Respiratory disorders, acute (pneumonia, pulmonary edema, pulmonary embolism)
Respiratory disorders, chronic
Urologic disorders
Vascular disease

Acquired Immune Deficiency Syndrome (AIDS)

Potential Complications (Collaborative Problems)

PC of AIDS: Human immunodeficiency virus [HIV] wasting syndrome, malignancies (eg, Kaposi's sarcoma [KS], lymphoma), meningitis, opportunistic infections (eg, candidiasis, cytomegalovirus [CMV], herpes, *Pneumocystis carinii* pneumonia)

Nursing Diagnoses

Activity intolerance Related factors: Fatigue, weakness, medication side effects, fever, malnutrition, *Impaired gas exchange* (secondary to lung infections or malignancy)

Airway clearance, ineffective Related factors: Decreased energy/ fatigue, respiratory infections, tracheobronchial secretions, pulmonary malignancy, pneumothorax

Anxiety Related factors: Uncertain future, perception of effects of disease and treatments on lifestyle

Body image disturbance Related factors: Chronic illness, lesions of KS, alopecia, weight loss, changes in sexuality

Caregiver role strain (actual/risk for) Related/risk factors: Illness severity of the care receiver, unpredictable illness course or instability in the care receiver's health, duration of caregiving required, inadequate physical environment for providing care, lack of respite and recreation for caregiver, complexity/number of caregiving tasks

Confusion, acute/chronic Related factors: Infection of central nervous system (CNS) (eg, toxoplasmosis), CMV infection, KS, lymphoma, progress of HIV

Coping: family, ineffective, compromised/disabling (also consider *Family processes, altered*) Related factors: Inadequate or incorrect information or understanding by family member/close friend, chronic illness, chronically unresolved feelings

Coping: individual, ineffective Related factor: Personal vulnerability in a situational crisis (eg, terminal illness)

Diarrhea Related factors: Medication, diet, infections

Diversional activity deficit Related factors: Frequent/lengthy medical treatments, long-term hospitalization, prolonged bed rest

Fatigue Related factors: Disease process, overwhelming psychologic or emotional demands

Fear Related factors: Powerlessness, real threat to own well-being, possibility of disclosure, possibility of death

Fluid volume deficit Related factors: Inadequate fluid intake secondary to oral lesions, *Diarrhea*

Grieving, anticipatory/dysfunctional Related factors: Impending death or impending changes in lifestyle, loss of body function, changes in appearance, abandonment by significant others

Home maintenance management, impaired Related factors: Inadequate support systems, lack of knowledge, lack of familiarity with community resources

Hopelessness Related factors: Deteriorating physical condition, poor prognosis

Infection, risk for Risk factor: Cellular immunodeficiency

Infection transmission, risk for (non-NANDA) Risk factor: Contagious nature of body fluids

Injury (falls), risk for Related factors: *Fatigue*, weakness, cognitive changes, encephalopathy, neuromuscular changes

Management of therapeutic regimen: individual, ineffective Related factors: Complexity of medication regimen; *Knowledge deficit* of disease, medications, and community resources; depression; illness/malaise

Nutrition: less than body requirements, altered Related factors: Difficulty in swallowing, loss of appetite, oral/esophageal lesions, gastrointestinal malabsorption, increased metabolic rate, *Nausea*

Oral mucous membrane, altered Risk factors: Compromised immune system, opportunistic infections (eg candidiasis, herpes)

Pain, [acute] Related factors: Progression of disease process, medication side effects, lymphedema secondary to KS, headaches secondary to CNS infection, peripheral neuropathy, severe myalgias

Powerlessness Related factors: Terminal illness, treatment regimen, unpredictable nature of disease

Self-care deficit: (specify) Related factors: Decreased strength and endurance; *Activity intolerance; Confusion, acute/chronic*

Self-esteem disturbance Related factors: Chronic illness, situational crisis

Sensory/perceptual alterations (auditory/visual) Related factors: Hearing loss secondary to medications, visual loss related to CMV infection

Sexuality patterns, altered Related factors: Safer sex practices, fear of HIV transmission, abstinence, impotence secondary to medications

Skin integrity, impaired Related factors: Tissue and muscle wasting secondary to altered nutritional state, perineal excoriation secondary to *Diarrhea* and lesions (eg, candidiasis, herpes), *Impaired physical mobility*, KS lesions

Sleep pattern disturbance Related factors: *Pain*, night sweats, medication regimen, medication side effects, *Anxiety*, depression, drug withdrawal (eg, heroin, cocaine)

Social isolation Related factors: Stigma, others' fear of contracting disease, own fear of HIV transmission, cultural and religious mores, physical appearance, *Self-esteem* and *Body image disturbances*

Spiritual distress Related factors: Challenged belief and value system, test of spiritual beliefs

Violence: directed at self, risk for Risk factor: Suicidal ideation, *Hopelessness*

Arthritis

Includes but is not limited to rheumatoid arthritis, osteoarthritis, juvenile rheumatoid arthritis, gouty arthritis, and septic arthritis.

Potential Complications (Collaborative Problems)

PC of arthritis: Fibrous and/or bony ankylosis, joint contractures, neuropathy

PC of corticosteroids (intraarticular injections): Intraarticular infection, joint degeneration

PC of corticosteroids (systemic administration): Cushing's syndrome, hyperglycemia, delayed wound healing, osteoporosis, muscle wasting, hypertension, edema, congestive heart failure, hypokalemia, depressed immune response, peptic ulcers, renal failure, growth retardation (children), psychotic reactions, cataract formation, atherosclerosis, thrombophlebitis

PC of nonsteroidal anti-inflammatory medications: Gastric ulceration/bleeding, nephropathy

Nursing Diagnoses

Body image disturbance Related factors: Chronic illness, joint deformities, *Impaired mobility*

Coping: individual, ineffective Related factors: Personal vulnerability in a situational crisis (eg, new diagnosis of illness, declining health), unpredictable exacerbations

Family processes, altered Related factors: Change in family roles, disability of family member, lack of support system

Fatigue Related factors: Pain, overwhelming psychologic or emotional demands, systemic inflammation, anemia

Home maintenance management, impaired Related factors: *Impaired physical mobility, Fatigue, Pain*

Management of therapeutic regimen: individual, ineffective Related factors: *Knowledge deficit* of medication and therapies, forgetful about taking medications because of *Impaired memory*, reliance on quackery

Pain, acute/chronic Related factors: Progression of joint abnormalities, inflammation

Mobility: physical, impaired Related factors: Stiffness, pain, joint ankylosis, contractures, decreased muscle strength

Powerlessness Related factors: Incurable nature of the disease, not feeling better even when following therapeutic regimen

Self-care deficit: (specify) Related factors: Musculoskeletal impairment, *Pain, Impaired physical mobility, Fatigue*

Sexuality patterns, altered Related factors: *Fatigue, Pain, Impaired physical mobility*

Sleep pattern disturbance Related factor: *Pain*

Social interaction, impaired Related factors: *Fatigue,* difficulty ambulating

Autoimmune Disorders

Includes but is not limited to systemic lupus erythematosus (SLE), scleroderma, rheumatic fever, glomerulonephritis, and multiple sclerosis.

Potential Complications (Collaborative Problems)

PC of lupus erythematosus: Vasculitis, pericarditis, pleuritis, cerebral infarction, hemolytic anemia, glomerulonephritis

PC of glomerulonephritis or renal failure: Ascites, anasarca, sepsis

PC of corticosteroid therapy: Cushing's syndrome, hyperglycemia, delayed wound healing, osteoporosis, muscle wasting, hypertension, edema, congestive heart failure, hypokalemia, depressed immune response, peptic ulcers, renal failure, growth retardation (children), psychotic reactions, cataract formation, atherosclerosis, thrombophlebitis

Nursing Diagnoses

Activity intolerance Related factors: *Anxiety, Acute/chronic pain,* weakness, *Fatigue*

Adjustment, impaired Related factors: Necessity for major lifestyle/behavior change

Body image disturbance Related factors: Chronic illness, *Chronic pain*, rash, lesions, ulcers, purpura, mottling of hands, alopecia, and altered body function

Caregiver role strain Related/risk factors: Illness severity of care receiver, duration of caregiving required, lack of respite and recreation for caregiver, complexity/number of caregiving tasks

Coping: family, ineffective, compromised See *Family processes*

Coping: individual, ineffective Related factors: Personal vulnerability in a situational crisis (eg, declining health), unpredictable course of disease, exacerbations

Diversional activity deficit Related factors: Long-term hospitalization, frequent/lengthy treatments, forced inactivity

Family processes, altered Related factors: Chronic illness/disability, complex therapies, change in family roles, hospitalization/change in environment, disability of family member

Fatigue Related factors: Increased energy needs secondary to chronic inflammation, altered body chemistry, effects of medication therapy

Fear Related factors: Environmental stressors/hospitalization, *Powerlessness*, real or imagined threat to own well-being

Fluid volume excess Related factor: Decreased urine output secondary to sodium retention or glomerulonephritis

Grieving, anticipatory/dysfunctional Related factors: Potential loss of body function, potential loss of social role, terminal illness, chronic illness

Home maintenance management, impaired Related factors: *Pain, Impaired physical mobility*

Hopelessness Related factors: Failing or deteriorating physical condition, long-term stress

Incontinence, functional, urinary Related factor: *Impaired physical mobility*

Infection, risk for Risk factors: Immunosuppression, chronic disease, pharmaceutical agents, secondary to glomerulonephritis

Management of therapeutic regimen: individual, ineffective Related factors: *Knowledge deficit* (disease process, balanced rest and exercise, symptoms of exacerbations and complications, medications and treatment, community resources)

Mobility: physical, impaired Related factors: *Pain*, medically prescribed limitations, (joint) changes, neuromuscular impairment

Noncompliance Related factors: Denial of illness, negative perception or consequences of treatment regimen, perceived benefits of continued illness

Nutrition: less than body requirements, altered Related factors: Difficulty in chewing, *Impaired swallowing*, loss of appetite, *Nausea*, and vomiting

Oral mucous membrane, altered Related factors: Pathophysiology of the disease, medication side effects

Pain Related factors: Inflammation of connective tissues, blood vessels, and mucous membranes

Powerlessness Related factors: Unpredictability of chronic, terminal disease; complex treatment regimen; physical and psychologic changes associated with the disease

Protection, altered Related factor: Corticosteroid therapy

Role performance, altered Related factors: Chronic illness, *Chronic pain*

Self-care deficit: (specify) Related factors: Decreased strength and endurance, *Pain, Activity intolerance*, stiffness, *Fatigue*

Self-esteem disturbance Related factors: Chronic illness, *Chronic pain, Altered role performance*, inability to achieve developmental tasks because of disabling condition

Sensory/perceptual alterations (visual, kinesthetic, tactile) Related factor: Disease process

Sexuality patterns, altered Related factors: *Fatigue, Pain, Impaired physical mobility*

Skin integrity, impaired (actual/risk for) Related/risk factors: Rashes, lesions, medications, altered circulation, *Impaired physical mobility*, photosensitivity, edema

Sleep pattern disturbance Related factors: *Pain*/discomfort, *Anxiety*, inactivity

Social interaction, impaired Related factors: *Self-esteem disturbance,* limited physical mobility, *Fatigue*, embarrassment over appearance

Social isolation Related factor: Others' response to appearance

Blood Disorders

Includes but is not limited to anemias, polycythemia, and coagulation disorders.

Potential Complications (Collaborative Problems)

PC of anemias: Cardiac failure, iron overload, bleeding, infection

PC of coagulation disorders: Hemorrhage, thrombus formation, renal failure, congestive heart failure

Nursing Diagnoses

Activity intolerance Related factors: Insufficient oxygen transport secondary to low red blood cell count, pulmonary congestion, tissue hypoxia, *Acute pain, Fatigue*, decreased strength and endurance

Anxiety Related factors: Lack of knowledge of disease and treatments, uncertainty of outcome

Constipation Related factors: Atrophy of gastrointestinal mucosa, medication (iron) side effects

Diarrhea Related factors: Atrophy of gastrointestinal mucosa

Family processes, altered Related factors: Hospitalization/change in environment, illness/disability of family member

Fear Related factors: Environmental stressors/hospitalization, treatments

Injury (bleeding), risk for Risk factors: Abnormal blood profile, sickle cells, decreased hemoglobin, thrombocytopenia, splenomegaly

Infection, risk for Risk factors: Decreased resistance secondary to abnormal white blood cells

Nutrition: less than body requirements, altered Related factors: Loss of appetite secondary to sore mouth, *Nausea*

Oral mucous membrane, altered Related factors: Atrophy of gastrointestinal mucosa, tissue hypoxia, papillary atrophy, and inflammatory changes (pernicious anemia)

Pain Related factor: Altered body function (eg, bleeding in joint spaces)

Protection, altered See *Injury, risk for*

Tissue perfusion, altered (peripheral) Related factors: Deficit or malfunction of RBCs, hyperviscosity (in polycythemia)

Burns

Potential Complications (Collaborative Problems)

PC of burns: Hypovolemic shock, hypervolemia, paralytic ileus, renal failure, sepsis, stress ulcers

Nursing Diagnoses

Airway clearance, ineffective Related factors: Tracheal edema, decreased pulmonary ciliary action

Anxiety Related factors: Suddenness of injury, pain from injury and treatments, uncertainty of prognosis, immobility

Aspiration, risk for Risk factors: Presence of tracheostomy or endotracheal tube, tube feeding, *Impaired swallowing*, hindered elevation of upper body

Body image disturbance Related factors: Physical impairment, scarring, contractures

Body temperature, risk for altered Risk factor: Dehydration secondary to *Impaired skin integrity*

Breathing pattern, ineffective Related factor: *Pain*

Caregiver role strain Related factors: Illness severity of care receiver, duration of caregiving required, lack of respite and recreation for caregiver, complexity/number of caregiving tasks

Constipation Related factors: Decreased activity, medications (eg, narcotic analgesics)

Coping: family, ineffective Related factors: See *Family processes, altered*

Disuse syndrome, risk for Risk factor: Severe *Pain*

Diversional activity deficit Related factors: Monotony of long-term hospitalization, separation from family, *Social isolation*

Family processes, altered Related factors: Long-term, complex therapies; long-term hospitalization; change in environment; separation from family members; critical nature of injury

Fatigue Related factors: *Pain*, overwhelming psychologic or emotional demands

Fear Related factors: Environmental stressors/hospitalization, painful procedures, threat of dying, projected effects of injury on lifestyle and relationships

Fluid volume deficit Related factor: Abnormal fluid loss (eg, intravascular to interstitial fluid shift)

Gas exchange, impaired Related factors: Smoke inhalation, heat damage to lungs, carbon monoxide poisoning

Hypothermia Related factor: Loss of epithelial tissue

Infection, risk for Risk factors: Tissue destruction (loss of skin barrier), impaired immune response, invasive procedures, and other increased environmental exposures

Management of therapeutic regimen: individual/family, ineffective Related factors: *Knowledge deficit* of wound care, exercise and other therapies, nutrition, pain management, and signs and symptoms of complications

Mobility: physical, impaired Related factors: *Pain*, edema, dressings, splints, wound contractures

Nutrition: less than body requirements, altered Related factors: Difficulty swallowing, high metabolic rate needed for wound healing

Pain Related factors: Burn injury, exposed nerve endings, treatments

Powerlessness Related factor: Inability to control situation (eg, due to treatment regimen, health care environment, *Pain*)

Self-care deficit: (specify) Related factors: *Pain*, dressings, splints, enforced immobility, *Activity intolerance*, decreased strength and endurance, limited range of motion

Self-esteem disturbance Related factors: *Body image disturbance*, loss of role responsibilities, loss of functional abilities, delay in achieving developmental tasks secondary to effects of injury

Sensory/perceptual alterations: auditory, gustatory, kinesthetic, olfactory, tactile, visual (specify) Related factors: Sensory deficit, sensory overload (environmental), stress, *Sleep deprivation*, protective isolation, enforced immobility

Sleep pattern disturbance (or sleep deprivation) Related factors: *Pain*, *Anxiety*, dressings, splints, invasive lines

Social isolation Related factors: Separation from family, infection control measures, embarrassment over appearance, response of others to appearance

Tissue perfusion, altered (peripheral): Related factor: Constriction from circumferential burns

Cancer

NOTE: Nursing diagnoses depend greatly upon the location, type, and stage of the cancer.

Potential Complications (Collaborative Problems)

PC of cancer: Cachexia, electrolyte imbalance, pathological fractures, hemorrhage, malnutrition (negative nitrogen balance), metastasis to vital organs (eg, brain, bones, kidneys, lungs, liver), spinal cord compression, superior vena cava syndrome

PC of chemotherapy: Anaphylactic reaction, anemia, CNS toxicity, congestive heart failure, electrolyte imbalance, hemorrhagic cystitis, leukopenia, necrosis at IV site, renal failure, thrombocytopenia

PC of narcotic medications: Depressed respiration, consciousness and blood pressure; cardiovascular collapse; profound brain damage; biliary spasm

PC of radiation therapy: Increased intracranial pressure, myelosuppression, inflammation, fluid/electrolyte imbalances

Nursing Diagnoses

Activity intolerance Related factors: See *Fatigue*

Adjustment, impaired Related factors: Necessity for major lifestyle changes, incomplete grieving

Airway clearance, ineffective Related factors: Tracheobronchial obstruction; ineffective cough secondary to decreased energy, *Fatigue*, and *Pain*; increased viscosity of secretions

Anxiety Related factors: Unfamiliar hospital environment, uncertainty of prognosis, lack of knowledge about cancer and treatment, threat of death, threat of or change in role functioning, inadequate pain relief

Body image disturbance Related factors: Hair loss, edema, blebs and blisters, petechiae, erythema

Bowel incontinence Related factors: Decreased awareness of need to defecate, disease process, loss of rectal sphincter control

Breathing pattern, ineffective Related factors: Medications, *Chronic pain, Fatigue,* anemia

Caregiver role strain Related factors: Illness severity of care receiver, duration of caregiving required, lack of respite and recreation for caregiver, complexity/number of caregiving tasks

Constipation Related factors: Decreased activity, dietary changes, medications (eg, narcotic analgesics, chemotherapy), radiation therapy, painful defecation

Coping: individual, ineffective Related factors: Personal vulnerability in a maturational crisis (eg, terminal illness in childhood) or in a situational crisis (eg, terminal illness)

Decisional conflict Related factors: Lack of relevant information, multiple or divergent sources of information, multiple treatment choices, lack of support system

Diarrhea Related factors: Dietary changes, impaction, radiation, chemotherapy (specify), antibiotics, stress

Disuse syndrome, risk for Risk factors: Severe *Pain,* altered level of consciousness

Family processes, altered Related factors: Change in family roles, complex therapies, hospitalization/change in environment, illness/disability of family member, separation of family members, fears associated with the diagnosis, financial effects of illness

Fatigue Related factors: *Pain,* disease process, overwhelming psychologic or emotional demands, malnutrition, hypoxia/*Impaired gas exchange*

Fear Related factors: Real or imagined threat to own well-being, environmental stressors/hospitalization, impending death, fear of pain

Fluid volume deficit Related factors: Inadequate fluid intake (eg, altered ability to obtain fluids, weakness, fatigue, anorexia, *Nausea,* depression), abnormal fluid loss (eg, vomiting, diarrhea)

Grieving, anticipatory/dysfunctional Related factors: Terminal illness, impending loss of body function, effects of cancer on lifestyle, withdrawal from/of others

Home maintenance management, impaired Related factors: Lack of support system, inadequate finances, *Knowledge deficit* regarding community and other supports, *Acute/chronic confusion, Altered thought processes, Sensory/perceptual alterations*

Hopelessness Related factors: Failing or deteriorating physical condition, long-term stress, lost spiritual belief, overwhelming functional losses, impending death

Infection, risk for Risk factors: Immunosuppression, neutropenia, pharmaceutical agents

Injury (falls), risk for Risk factors: Weakness, *Sensory/perceptual alterations, Altered thought processes, Confusion*

Mobility: physical, impaired Related factors: Decreased strength and endurance, musculoskeletal impairment, neuromuscular impairment, *Pain,* sedation, *Fatigue,* edema, enforced immobility (eg, for chemotherapy infusions)

Nausea Related factors: Side effects of chemotherapy and other medications, stress, *Pain,* difficulty swallowing

Nutrition: less than body requirements, altered Related factors: Difficulty in swallowing, *Nausea,* vomiting, loss of appetite, changes in taste, isolation, *Anxiety,* stress, *Altered oral mucous membrane, Fatigue,* increased metabolic demands of the tumor

Oral mucous membrane, altered Related factors: Chemotherapy, radiation to head and neck, *Altered nutrition: less than body requirements,* inadequate hydration, immunosuppression

Pain, acute/chronic Related factors: Ongoing tissue destruction (ie, localizations), infection, stomatitis, chemotherapy

Powerlessness Related factor: Terminal illness, feelings of inability to change the progression of events, uncertainty about prognosis and treatments

Role performance, altered Related factors: *Chronic pain,* treatment side effects

Self-care deficit: (specify) Related factors: Developmental disability, maturational age, *Pain, Activity intolerance, Fatigue,* depression

Sexual dysfunction/Sexuality patterns, altered Related factors: *Pain,* change in body image, *Fear* (patient and/or partner), *Fatigue* from treatments or disease, lack of privacy

Skin integrity, impaired Related factors: Radiation, chemotherapy, allergic reactions to medications, loss of muscle and subcutaneous tissue secondary to poor nutritional status, immunologic deficit, *Impaired physical mobility* secondary to weakness

Sleep pattern disturbance/Sleep deprivation Related factors: *Anxiety,* emotional state, medical treatment regimen, *Pain,* pruritus

Social interaction, impaired Related factors: *Fear* of rejection, actual rejection by others, *Self-esteem disturbance,* therapeutic isolation (eg, secondary to radiation or protective isolation)

Spiritual distress Related factors: Test of spiritual beliefs, challenged belief and value system, unresolved conflicts, *Dysfunctional grieving*

Swallowing, impaired Related factors: Irritated oropharyngeal cavity, mechanical obstruction, head and neck radiation

Thought processes, altered Related factors: Chemotherapy, toxicity, cerebellar localization

Cardiac Disorders

Potential Complications (Collaborative Problems)

PC of angina/coronary insufficiency: Myocardial infarction

PC of congestive heart failure: Cardiogenic shock, deep vein thrombosis, hepatic failure, acute pulmonary edema, renal failure

PC of digitalis administration: Toxicity

PC of dysrhythmias: Decreased cardiac output, causing decreased myocardial perfusion, causing heart failure; severe atrioventricular conduction blocks; thromboemboli formation; ventricular fibrillation

PC of myocardial infarction (chest pain, arrhythmias): Cardiogenic shock, dysrhythmia, thromboembolism, pulmonary edema, pulmonary embolism, pericarditis

PC of pericarditis/endocarditis: Congestive heart failure, emboli (eg, pulmonary, cerebral, renal, spleen, coronary), cardiac tamponade, valvular stenosis

Nursing Diagnoses

Angina/Coronary Insufficiency

Activity intolerance Related factors: Anxiety, arrhythmias, *Pain*, lack of exercise/conditioning due to fear of pain

Anxiety Related factors: Chest pain, threat to self-concept, change in role functioning

Breathing pattern, ineffective Related factors: Acute *Pain, Anxiety*

Denial, ineffective Related factors: Fear of effects of diagnosis on lifestyle, *Fear* of "heart attack"

Family processes, altered Related factors: Change in family roles, hospitalization, inability of family member to perform usual roles

Fear Related factors: Environmental stressors/hospitalization, unknown future

Injury (falls), risk for Risk factors: Dizziness and hypotension secondary to vasodilator, calcium channel blockers, and opiate analgesic medications

Nausea Related factors: Side effects of calcium channel blockers and opiate analgesics, *Pain*

Noncompliance Related factors: Denial of illness, negative side effects of medications, negative perception of treatment regimen, perceived benefits of continued illness, dysfunctional patient/provider relationship

Pain Related factors: Myocardial ischemia, headache secondary to vasodilators

Role performance, altered Related factors: Chronic illness, treatment side effects, *Fear* of "heart attack"

Sexual dysfunction/Sexuality patterns, altered Related factors: *Pain, Fear* of pain, *Self-esteem disturbance*

Sleep pattern disturbance Related factors: *Pain*/discomfort, *Anxiety*

Myocardial Infarction (Chest Pain, Arrhythmias)

Activity intolerance Related factors: Acute *Pain*, weakness/*Fatigue* because of insufficient oxygen secondary to cardiac ischemia

Anxiety Related factors: Severe *Pain*, threat to or change in health status, anticipated change in role functioning, unknown outcome, unfamiliar environment

Cardiac output, decreased Related factors: Dysfunctional electrical conduction, increased ventricular workload, ventricular ischemia, ventricular damage

Constipation Related factors: Decreased peristalsis secondary to medications (eg, opiate analgesics), decreased activity, nothing by mouth (NPO) or soft diet

Coping: individual, ineffective Related factors: Personal vulnerability to situational crisis (eg, new diagnosis of illness, declining health)

Denial, ineffective Related factors: Fear of consequences of disease on roles, lifestyle, and so forth

Family processes, altered Related factors: Inability of patient to assume family roles, hospitalization, separation of family members

Fear Related factors: *Pain*, unknown future, real or imagined threat to own well-being, strange (eg, hospital) environment, *Fear* of death

Fluid volume excess Related factor: Decreased kidney perfusion secondary to heart failure

Gas exchange, impaired Related factor: *Decreased cardiac output*, decreased pulmonary blood supply secondary to pulmonary hypertension/congestive heart failure

Grieving, dysfunctional Related factors: Actual or perceived losses resulting from illness

Home maintenance management, impaired Related factors: *Pain, Fear* of pain, *Activity intolerance, Fear* of another "heart attack"

Nausea Related factors: Severe chest pain, side effect of medications

Pain Related factor: Myocardial ischemia

Powerlessness Related factors: Treatment regimen, hospital environment, anticipated lifestyle changes

Role performance, altered Related factors: Situational crisis, treatment side effects, *Pain, Fear* of pain, *Activity intolerance*

Self-care deficit: (specify) Related factors: *Pain, Activity intolerance*

Self-esteem disturbance Related factors: Treatment side effects, perceived or actual role changes

Sexual dysfunction/Sexuality patterns, altered Related factors: *Fear* of pain, *Activity intolerance, Self-esteem disturbance,* disease-related role changes

Sleep deprivation/Sleep pattern disturbance Related factors: Strange (eg, hospital) environment, *Pain*, treatments

Congestive Heart Failure

Activity intolerance Related factors: Weakness due to prolonged bed rest/sedentary lifestyle, *Fatigue*, insufficient oxygenation secondary to decreased cardiac output

Anxiety Related factors: Shortness of breath, dyspnea, progressive nature of disease

Anxiety, death Related factor: Possibility of dying

Family processes, altered Related factors: Hospitalization/change in environment, illness/disability of family member

Fatigue Related factors: Inadequate oxygenation secondary to decreased cardiac output, difficulty sleeping

Fear See *Anxiety*

Fluid volume excess Related factors: Decreased cardiac output; reduced glomerular filtration; increased antidiuretic hormone (ADH) production, causing sodium/water retention

Gas exchange, impaired Related factors: Alveolar capillary membrane changes, fluid in alveoli, decreased pulmonary blood supply

Home maintenance management, impaired Related factors: *Fatigue,* shortness of breath, clouded sensorium secondary to insufficient oxygen

Hopelessness Related factors: Failing or deteriorating physical condition, lack of energy for coping

Management of therapeutic regimen: individual, ineffective Related factors: *Knowledge deficit* (cardiac function/disease process, diet, activity exercise, medications, signs/symptoms of complications, and self-care), *Impaired memory, Fatigue*

Nutrition: less than body requirements, altered Related factors: *Nausea,* anorexia secondary to venous congestion of gastrointestinal tract, *Fatigue*

Powerlessness Related factors: Chronic illness, progressive nature of illness

Self-care deficit: (specify) Related factors: *Fatigue,* dyspnea

Skin integrity, impaired Related factors: *Decreased peripheral tissue perfusion, Impaired physical mobility,* edema

Sleep deprivation/Sleep pattern disturbance Related factors: *Anxiety,* nocturia, inability to assume preferred sleep position because of nocturnal dyspnea

Pericarditis/Endocarditis

Activity intolerance Related factors: Inadequate oxygenation secondary to restriction of cardiac filling, causing reduced cardiac output

Anxiety Related factors: *Pain,* change in health status, threat of death

Breathing pattern, ineffective Related factors: Acute *Pain* secondary to inflammation

Cardiac output, decreased Related factors: Restriction of cardiac filling/ventricular contractility, effusion, dysrhythmias, increased ventricular workload

Fear See *Anxiety*

Pain Related factors: Effusion, tissue inflammation

Chest Trauma

Includes but is not limited to hemothorax and pneumothorax.

Potential Complications (Collaborative Problems)

PC of chest trauma: Flail chest, hemothorax, pneumothorax, tension pneumothorax and mediastinal shift

Nursing Diagnoses

Breathing pattern, ineffective Related factors: Acute *Pain, Anxiety*

Dysfunctional ventilatory weaning response (DVWR) Related factors: *Anxiety,* history of ventilator dependence > one week, inappropriate pacing of diminished ventilatory support, uncontrolled episodic energy demands or problems

Fear Related factors: Real or imagined threat to own well-being, sudden injury, unknown extent of or prognosis for injury

Mobility: physical, impaired Related factors: *Pain*/discomfort, presence of chest tubes, intravenous lines

Pain Related factor: Chest injury

Self-care deficit: (specify) Related factors: *Pain*/discomfort, presence of tubes and lines

Sleep deprivation/Sleep pattern disturbance Related factors: *Pain*/discomfort, medical regimen

Spontaneous ventilation, inability to sustain Related factors: Injury to thoracic cage and/or lung tissue, flail chest

Dying Patient

Nursing Diagnoses

Activity intolerance Related factors: *Chronic pain*, weakness, *Fatigue* secondary to disease process, medications, and/or inadequate intake of calories

Adjustment, impaired Related factor: Incomplete grieving over loss of physical and/or role function

Airway clearance, ineffective Related factors: Decreased energy, *Fatigue*, *Pain*, tracheobronchial obstruction

Anxiety, death Related factors: Imminence of death, lack of resolution

Bowel incontinence Related factors: Loss of sphincter control, decreased awareness of need to defecate

Caregiver role strain Related factors: Illness severity of the care receiver, inability to change outcome for the patient, inadequate physical environment for providing care, lack of respite and recreation for caregiver, complexity/amount of caregiving tasks

Communication, impaired verbal Related factors: Inability to speak, inability to speak clearly

Coping: family, ineffective, compromised Related factor: Family member's temporary preoccupation with own emotional conflicts and personal suffering

Coping: individual, ineffective Related factor: Personal vulnerability to situational crisis (terminal illness)

Denial, ineffective Related factors: *Fear* of dying, *Fear* of effect on others

Family processes, altered Related factors: Change in family roles, hospitalization/change in environment, illness/disability of family member, separation of family members

Fatigue Related factors: Disease process, overwhelming psychologic or emotional demands, decreased intake of nutrients for energy

Fear Related factors: *Powerlessness*, environmental stressors/hospitalization, *Fear* of pain, *Fear* of the unknown, *Fear* of dying

Grieving, anticipatory Related factor: Impending death of self

Grieving, dysfunctional Related factors: *Ineffective denial*, unresolved family issues, loss of faith (eg, *Spiritual distress*), lack of support system

Hopelessness Related factors: Failing or deteriorating physical condition, lack of social/family support, loss of spiritual belief

Incontinence, urinary, functional/total Related factors: Disorientation, *Impaired mobility*, neurologic dysfunction

Nutrition: less than body requirements, altered Related factors: *Impaired swallowing*, loss of appetite, *Nausea*/vomiting

Oral mucous membrane, altered Related factors: Chemotherapy, inability to perform oral hygiene or obtain fluids, radiation to head and neck

Pain Related factors: Specific to patient's cause of death

Powerlessness Related factors: Inability to change outcome of terminal illness, loss of independence, overwhelming treatment regimen

Self-care deficit: (specify) Related factors: *Pain*/discomfort, *Activity intolerance*, decreased strength and endurance

Skin integrity, impaired Related factors: *Impaired physical mobility*, *Urinary/Bowel incontinence*, radiation therapy, poor nutritional status, dehydration

Sleep pattern disturbance Related factors: *Pain*/discomfort, *Anxiety*
Social isolation Related factors: Medical condition, alteration in physical appearance
Sorrow, chronic Related factors: See *Grieving*
Spiritual distress Related factors: Challenged belief and value system, separation from religious/cultural ties, test of spiritual beliefs

Endocrine Disorders

Include but are not limited to Cushing's disease, diabetes mellitus, hyperthyroidism, hypothyroidism, hypoglycemia, and pancreatic tumors.

Potential Complications (Collaborative Problems)

PC of Cushing's disease: Hypertension, congestive heart failure, potassium and sodium imbalance, psychosis, hyperglycemia, osteoporosis

PC of diabetes mellitus: Ketoacidosis, coma, hypoglycemia, infections, coronary artery disease, peripheral vascular disease, retinopathy, neuropathy, nephropathy

PC of hyperthyroidism: Thyroid storm, heart disease, exophthalmos

PC of hypothyroidism: Arteriosclerotic heart disease, myxedema coma, psychosis

PC of repeated or prolonged hypoglycemia: Neuropathy, retinal hemorrhage, cerebrovascular accidents, personality changes, intellectual damage

Nursing Diagnoses

Cushing's Disease

Activity intolerance Related factors: Muscle weakness secondary to protein wasting, hyperglycemia, and potassium depletion; congestive heart failure

Body image disturbance Related factors: Change in appearance (eg, moon face, virilism in women, acne) secondary to disease process and medication therapy, changes in social involvement

Infection, risk for Risk factors: Skin and capillary fragility, negative nitrogen balance, compromised immune response, hyperglycemia, lowered resistance to stress, poor wound healing

Injury, risk for Risk factors: Fractures secondary to osteoporosis, hypertension secondary to sodium and water retention

Management of therapeutic regimen: individual, ineffective Related factors: *Knowledge deficit* (disease process, therapeutic diet, diagnostic tests, surgical treatment, self-administration of steroids, indications of need to call physician)

Nutrition: less than body requirements, altered Related factors: Disturbance of carbohydrate metabolism, increased resistance to insulin

Skin integrity, impaired Related factors: Decreased connective tissue, edema secondary to sodium and water retention, thinning and dryness of the skin

Self-care deficit: (specify) Related factors: *Fatigue*, generalized weakness, demineralization of bones

Sexuality patterns, altered Related factors: Impotence, cessation of menses, loss of libido secondary to excessive adrenocorticotropic hormone (ACTH) production

Thought processes, altered Related factors: Increased levels of glucocorticoids and ACTH

Diabetes Mellitus/Hypoglycemia

Coping: family, ineffective, compromised/disabling Related factors: Complex self-care regimen, chronic disease, inability to predict future, inadequate or incomplete information/understanding, changes required in family functioning

Fear Related factors: Effects on lifestyle, need for self-injections, diabetes complications

Infection, risk for Risk factors: Decreased leukocyte function, delayed healing, impaired circulation

Injury, risk for Risk factors: Impaired vision, hypoglycemia, impaired tactile sensation

Management of therapeutic regimen: individual, ineffective Related factors: *Knowledge deficit* (disease process, diet and exercise balance, self-monitoring and self-medication, foot care, signs and symptoms of complications, community resources)

Noncompliance Related factors: Complexity of self-care and medical regimen, chronicity of disease, denial

Nutrition: less than body requirements, altered Related factors: Inability to utilize glucose, resulting in weight loss, muscle weakness, and thirst

Powerlessness Related factors: Perceived inability to prevent complications such as blindness and amputations

Sensory/perceptual alterations (tactile, visual) Related factors: Glucose/insulin or electrolyte imbalance, peripheral neurovascular changes

Sexual dysfunction/Sexuality patterns, altered Related factors: Impotence secondary to peripheral neuropathy, psychologic conflicts (male), psychologic stressors, frequent genitourinary problems (female)

Hyperthyroidism

Anxiety Related factor: Central nervous system irritability

Comfort, altered (heat intolerance) (non-NANDA) Related factor: Increased metabolic rate

Diarrhea Related factor: Increased peristalsis secondary to increased metabolic rate

Fatigue Related factors: Increased energy requirements, central nervous system irritability

Hyperthermia, risk for: Risk factor: Inability to compensate for excess thyroid activity

Nutrition: less than body requirements, altered Related factors: Hypermetabolic rate, constant activity, inability to ingest enough calories, vomiting, *Diarrhea*

Tissue integrity, impaired [corneal] Related factors: Periorbital edema, reduced ability to blink, eye dryness, corneal abrasions/ulcerations

Hypothyroidism

Activity intolerance Related factors: Apathy, weakness, inadequate oxygen and decreased energy secondary to decreased metabolic rate

[Comfort, altered (cold intolerance)] Related factor: Slowed metabolic rate

Constipation Related factors: Decreased activity and decreased peristalsis secondary to decreased metabolic rate

Fatigue Related factors: See *Activity intolerance*

Hypothermia Related factor: Decreased metabolic rate

Injury, risk for Related factors: Hypersensitivity to sedatives, narcotics, and anesthetics secondary to decreased metabolic rate

Mobility: physical, impaired Related factors: *Fatigue*, weakness, mucin deposits in joints and interstitial spaces, changes in reflexes and coordination

Nutrition: more than body requirements, altered Related factor: Intake greater than body needs secondary to decreased metabolic rate

Skin integrity, impaired Related factors: Dryness and edema secondary to movement of fluid into interstitial spaces

Social interaction, impaired Related factors: Weakness, apathy, changes in appearance, depression

Gastrointestinal Disorders

Potential Complications (Collaborative Problems)

PC of GI inflammatory diseases (eg, diverticulitis): GI bleeding, anal fissure, fluid/electrolyte imbalances, anemia, intestinal obstruction, fistula, abscess, perforation

PC of GI bleeding: Hypovolemic shock, anemia

PC of peptic ulcers: Perforation, pyloric obstruction, hemorrhage

Nursing Diagnoses

GI Inflammation (eg, Diverticulitis, Inflammatory Bowel Disease)

Constipation Related factors: Inadequate ingestion of dietary fiber, narrowing of intestinal lumen secondary to scar tissue

Coping: individual, ineffective Related factors: Chronic condition, no definitive treatment, *Chronic pain, Sleep pattern disturbance*, ostomy

Diarrhea Related factors: Inflammation of GI tract, malabsorption

Fluid volume deficit Related factors: *Diarrhea*, vomiting, decreased fluid intake

Nutrition: less than body requirements, altered Related factors: *Diarrhea*, nausea and abdominal cramping associated with eating, ulcers of the mucous membrane, decreased absorption of nutrients

Pain, chronic Related factors: Inflammation or obstruction of GI tract, hyperperistalsis

GI Bleeding

Activity intolerance Related factor: Weakness/*Fatigue* secondary to anemia or blood loss

Coping: individual, ineffective Related factor: Personal vulnerability to situational crisis (eg, acute illness)

Fatigue Related factors: Disease process, low hemoglobin level

Fear Related factor: Real or imagined threat to own well-being

Fluid volume deficit Related factor: Abnormal fluid loss (eg, emesis, diarrhea)

Nutrition: less than body requirements, altered Related factors: Loss of appetite, *Nausea*/vomiting

Ulcers

Constipation Related factors: Effects of antacids and anticholinergics
Diarrhea Related factor: Effects of magnesium-containing antacids
Pain, acute/chronic Related factors: Lesions secondary to increased gastric secretions

Abdominal Pain/Irritable Bowel Syndrome

Anxiety Related factors: Necessity for frequent bowel movements, *Diarrhea*, *Pain*, chronicity of the condition
Constipation Related factors: Decreased activity, decreased fluid intake, dietary changes, medications (specify)
Diarrhea Related factors: Dietary changes, increased intestinal motility, medications (specify), alcohol intake, smoking, *Fatigue*, cold drinks
Fluid volume deficit Related factors: Abnormal fluid loss (specify), inadequate fluid intake, abnormal blood loss (specify), excessive continuous consumption of alcohol
Nutrition: less than body requirements, altered Related factors: Loss of appetite, *Nausea*, vomiting, food intolerance, fear of precipitating *Diarrhea*
Pain, acute Related factors: Injury, noxious stimulus (eg, fruits, alcohol)
Pain, chronic Related factors: Specific to patient
Sleep deprivation/Sleep pattern disturbance Related factors: *Pain*/discomfort, *Anxiety, Diarrhea*

Immobilized Patient

Potential Complications (Collaborative Problems)

PC of immobility: Contractures; joint ankylosis; osteoporosis; thrombophlebitis, embolus; hypostatic pneumonia; renal calculi

Nursing Diagnoses

Activity intolerance Related factors: Generalized weakness, *Fatigue*, compromised circulatory and/or respiratory system
Constipation Related factors: Decreased activity, decreased colon motility secondary to increased adrenaline production
Coping: individual, ineffective Related factor: Personal vulnerability to a situational crisis (specify), inability to perform usual role functions, dependence on others, *Self-esteem disturbance*
Disuse syndrome, risk for Risk factors: Paralysis, mechanical immobilization, prescribed immobility, severe *Pain*, altered level of consciousness
Diversional activity deficit Related factor: Prolonged bed rest
Dysreflexia Related factor: Spinal cord injury T7 or above
Incontinence, urinary functional/total Related factor: Neurologic impairment
Mobility: physical, impaired Related factors: Decreased strength and endurance; *Activity Intolerance; Pain*; neuromuscular, musculoskeletal, and cognitive impairment; depression, severe *Anxiety*
Self-care deficit: (specify) Related factors: *Pain, Activity intolerance*, decreased strength and endurance, prescribed immobility
Skin integrity, impaired Related factors: *Impaired physical mobility*, atrophy of dermis and subcutaneous tissues, loss of skin turgor, impaired circulation

Sleep pattern disturbance Related factors: Lack of physical activity, *Pain*/discomfort, inability to change positions independently or assume usual sleep position

Urinary Retention Related factors: Decreased muscle tone of bladder, inability to relax the perineal muscles, embarrassment of using bedpan, lack of privacy, unnatural position for urination

Liver Disease

Includes but is not limited to cirrhosis and hepatitis.

Potential Complications (Collaborative Problems)

PC of liver disease: Anemia; hepatic encephalopathy; glomerulonephritis, renal failure; esophageal varices; gastrointestinal bleeding, hemorrhage; hypokalemia; negative nitrogen balance; disseminated intravascular coagulation (DIC)

Nursing Diagnoses

Activity intolerance Related factors: Weakness, extreme *Fatigue* secondary to bed rest, impaired respiratory function secondary to ascites

Anxiety Related factors: Unknown prognosis of the disease, uncertainty of the future, alcohol withdrawal

Body image disturbance Related factors: Change in appearance (eg, jaundice, ascites), chronic illness

Breathing patterns, ineffective Related factor: Pressure on diaphragm secondary to ascites

Confusion, acute Related factors: Alcohol abuse, inability of liver to detoxify certain substances, increased serum ammonia level

Coping: individual, ineffective Related factor: Personal vulnerability to situational crisis (eg, new diagnosis of illness, declining health)

Diarrhea Related factors: Dietary changes, inability to metabolize fats, stress

Family processes, altered Related factors: Change in family roles, illness/disability of family member

Fatigue Related factors: Disease process, malnutrition

Fear Related factor: Real or imagined threat to own well-being

Fluid volume excess Related factors: Malnutrition, portal hypertension, sodium retention

Infection, risk for Related factors: Hypoproteinemia, enlarged spleen, leukopenia

Injury, risk for Related factors: Continued intake of hepatotoxins (eg, alcohol), decreased prothrombin and coagulation factors

Management of therapeutic regimen: individual, ineffective Related factors: *Knowledge deficit* (eg, disease process, nutritional needs, symptoms of complications, effects of alcohol), lack of motivation to stop drinking

Mobility: physical, impaired Related factor: Weakness secondary to prolonged bed rest

Nutrition: less than body requirements, altered Related factors: Loss of appetite; *Nausea*; vomiting; bile stasis; decreased absorption and storage of fat-soluble vitamins; impaired fat, glucose, and protein metabolism; *Diarrhea*

Pain, acute/chronic Related factors: Ascites, liver enlargement

Self-care deficit: (specify) Related factors: *Pain, Fatigue, Activity intolerance*

Self-esteem disturbance Related factors: Chronic illness, situational crisis, *Body image disturbance*, inability to stop drinking alcohol

Skin integrity, impaired Related factors: Physical immobility; itching secondary to jaundice, edema, and ascites

Thought processes, altered Related factors: See *Confusion*

Neurologic Disorders

Includes but is not limited to cerebrovascular accident (CVA, stroke), multiple sclerosis, amyotrophic lateral sclerosis, brain tumors, Guillain-Barré syndrome, myasthenia gravis, seizure disorders, Alzheimer's disease, coma, head injury, cerebral thrombosis, and transient ischemic attack. Associated psychiatric diagnoses include central nervous system infections (eg, tertiary neurosyphilis, viral encephalitis, Jakob-Creutzfeldt disease), brain trauma, Huntington's chorea, Parkinson's disease, and meningitis.

Potential Complications (Collaborative Problems)

PC of cerebrovascular accident (stroke): Increased intracranial pressure, respiratory infection, brain stem failure, cardiac dysrhythmias

PC of brain tumor: Increased intracranial pressure, paralysis, hyperthermia, sensory-motor changes

PC of other neurologic disorders (eg, multiple sclerosis): Pneumonia, respiratory failure, renal failure

Nursing Diagnoses

Cerebrovascular Accident (Stroke)

NOTE: Nursing diagnoses for CVA will vary depending upon the location and severity of the lesion. CVA can have mild to severe effects.

Activity intolerance Related factors: *Anxiety, Fatigue*, weakness, deconditioning secondary to immobility, neuromuscular deficits

Airway clearance, ineffective Related factors: Decreased energy, *Fatigue*, decreased cough and gag reflexes, muscle paralysis

Aspiration, risk for. Risk factors: Reduced level of consciousness, *Impaired swallowing*, depressed cough and gag reflexes

Body image disturbance Related factors: Chronic illness, diminished physical function, loss of control over body

Caregiver role strain Related factors: Illness severity of care receiver, duration of caregiving required, lack of respite and recreation for caregiver, complexity/number of caregiving tasks, elderly caregiver

Communication, impaired verbal Related factors: Aphasia, dysarthria, inability to speak, inability to speak clearly

Constipation Related factors: Decreased activity, medications (specify), weak abdominal muscles

Disuse syndrome, risk for Risk factors: Altered level of consciousness, paralysis

Family processes, altered Related factors: Hospitalization/change in environment, separation of family members, illness/disability of family member, change in family roles

Fluid volume deficit Risk factors: Decreased access to, intake of, or absorption of fluids secondary to weakness, impaired motor functions (eg, swallowing), impaired cognition and level of consciousness

Grieving, dysfunctional Related factors: Actual loss (eg, of function), chronic illness, inability to fulfill usual roles

Home maintenance management, impaired Related factors: Home environment obstacles; inadequate support system; lack of familiarity with community resources; sensorimotor/cognitive deficits; caregiver's lack of knowledge of reality orientation, skin care, and so forth

Hopelessness Related factor: Failing or deteriorating physical condition

Incontinence, urinary, functional Related factors: Cognitive impairment, inability to reach toilet secondary to *Impaired physical mobility*

Incontinence, urinary, total Related factors: Loss of bladder tone and/or sphincter control; inability to perceive need to void, secondary to neurologic dysfunction

Injury (falls), risk for Risk factors: *Impaired physical mobility, Sensory/perceptual alterations*

Memory, impaired Related factor: Residual effects of CVA

Mobility: physical, impaired Related factors: Neuromuscular impairment (eg, weakness, paresthesia, flaccid paralysis, spastic paralysis) secondary to damage of upper motor neurons, perceptual impairment, cognitive impairment

Nutrition: less than body requirements, altered Related factors: Difficulty chewing, *Impaired swallowing*, inability to prepare food secondary to mobility deficits

Powerlessness Related factors: Treatment regimen, chronic disease

Relocation stress syndrome Related factors: Change in environment/location (eg, transfer to long-term care facility), *Anxiety*, depression

Self-care deficit: (specify) Related factors: Neuromuscular impairment, decreased strength and endurance, *Activity intolerance*, decreased range of motion, weakness secondary to disease and immobility

Sensory/perceptual alterations: (specify: auditory, gustatory, kinesthetic, olfactory, tactile, visual) Related factors: Altered sensory reception, transmission, and/or integration, secondary to hypoxia and compression or displacement of brain tissue

Skin integrity, impaired Related factors: Altered sensation, *Impaired mobility*, incontinence of stool or urine, poor nutritional status

Social interaction, impaired Related factors: *Impaired verbal communication, Impaired physical mobility*, embarrassment about disabilities

Swallowing, impaired Related factors: Muscle paralysis secondary to damaged upper motor neurons, impaired perception/level of consciousness

Unilateral neglect (specify side) Related factors: *Sensory/perceptual alterations* (visual) with perceptual loss of corresponding body segment

Other Neurologic Disorders

Activity intolerance Related factors: *Acute/Chronic pain*, weakness/*Fatigue*

Airway clearance, ineffective Related factor: Decreased energy/*Fatigue*, neuromuscular weakness

Anxiety Related factors: Change in health status, threat to or change in role functioning, change in interaction patterns, seriousness of condition, threat to self-concept, separation from support system

Aspiration, risk for Risk factors: *Impaired swallowing*, presence of tracheostomy or endotracheal tube, reduced level of consciousness, depressed cough and gag reflexes, tube feedings, hindered elevation of upper body

Breathing pattern, ineffective Related factors: Neuromuscular paralysis/weakness, decreased energy/*Fatigue*

Caregiver role strain Related factors: Complex, long-term needs of patient

Communication, impaired verbal Related factors: Psychologic impairment, aphasia, inability to speak, inability to speak clearly, tracheostomy, muscle weakness

Constipation Related factors: Decreased activity, inability to ingest adequate fiber

Coping: individual, ineffective Related factor: Personal vulnerability to situational crisis (eg, new diagnosis of illness, declining health, terminal illness)

Disuse syndrome, risk for Risk factors: Paralysis, altered level of consciousness

Diversional activity deficit Related factors: Forced inactivity, long-term hospitalization

Family processes, altered Related factors: Change in family roles; change in family structure; cognitive and emotional changes of family member; hospitalization/change in environment; *Impaired verbal communication*, secondary to central nervous system changes

Fatigue Related factors: Disease process, immobility

Fear Related factor: Real threat to well-being (see *Anxiety*)

Fluid volume deficit Related factors: Inadequate fluid intake, vomiting secondary to increased intracranial pressure

Grieving, anticipatory or dysfunctional Related factors: Functional losses, role changes, uncertain prognosis, inability to change outcome of disease process

Home maintenance management, impaired Related factors: *Activity intolerance*, effects of debilitating disease, home environment obstacles, inadequate support system, insufficient family organization or planning, psychologic impairment, lack of familiarity with community resources

Hopelessness Related factors: Failing or deteriorating physical condition, perception of having no way to improve situation

Incontinence, urinary, functional Related factors: Cognitive impairment; *Impaired physical mobility; Confusion acute/chronic;* disorientation; lack of sphincter control; spastic bladder

Incontinence, urinary, total Related factor: Neurologic dysfunction (see *Functional urinary incontinence*)

Injury (eg, falls), risk for Risk factors: Sensory dysfunction (eg, visual disturbances), cognitive, and psychomotor deficits secondary to compression/displacement of brain tissue, muscular weakness, unsteady gait

Mobility: physical, impaired Related factors: Neuromuscular impairment, decreased strength and endurance, *Pain*/discomfort, medically prescribed treatment, muscle rigidity, tremors

Nutrition: less than body requirements, altered Related factors: Difficulty chewing secondary to cranial nerve involvement, *Impaired swallowing*, psychologic impairment, loss of appetite, *Fatigue*

Pain, acute/chronic Related factors: Neurologic injury, headache secondary to displaced brain tissue or increased intracranial pressure

Powerlessness See *Hopelessness*

Role performance, altered Related factors: Chronic illness, treatment side effects, brain changes

Self-care deficit: (specify) Related factors: *Pain* (eg, headache, joint pain), decreased strength and endurance, sensory-motor impairments, cognitive deficits, *Fatigue*, paralysis

Sexual dysfunction/Sexuality patterns, altered Related factors: Loss of perineal sensation, *Fatigue*, decreased libido, *Self-esteem disturbance, Impaired physical mobility*

Skin integrity, impaired Related factors: Physical immobilization, impaired circulation

Social interaction, impaired Related factors: Communication barriers, Self-esteem disturbance, extended hospitalization, *Impaired physical mobility*, embarrassment

Spontaneous ventilation, inability to sustain Related factors: Impaired neuromuscular function, pressure on brain stem

Swallowing, impaired Related factors: Impairment of laryngeal/pharyngeal neuromuscular function; impaired sensory transmission, reception, and/or integration secondary to cerebellar lesions

Thought processes, altered Related factors: Chronic organic disorder, pressure on brain tissue

Urinary retention Related factor: Sensory/motor impairment

Violence: self-directed or directed at others, risk for Risk factor: Organic mental disorder

Obesity

Nursing Diagnoses

Activity intolerance Related factors: Sedentary lifestyle, exertional discomfort (eg, shortness of breath)

Coping: individual, ineffective Related factors: Personal vulnerability in situational crisis, use of food to cope with stressors

Family processes, altered Related factor: Effects of weight-loss therapy on family relationships

Health maintenance, altered Related factor: Lack of ability to make deliberate and thoughtful judgments about exercise, nutrition, and so forth

Health seeking behaviors (specify) Related factors: Specific to patient

Mobility: physical, impaired Related factor: Decreased strength and endurance

Nutrition: more than body requirements, altered Related factors: Eating disorder, lack of physical exercise, decreased metabolic requirements, lack of basic nutritional knowledge

Self-esteem disturbance Related factors: Responses of peers and family to obesity, negative view of self as compared to societal ideal, *Body image disturbance*

Sexuality patterns, altered Related factors: *Body image disturbance*, difficulty assuming sexual positions, rejection by partner

Social interaction, impaired Related factors: Self-concept disturbance, feelings of embarrassment, actual rejection by others because of appearance

Pancreatitis

Potential Complications (Collaborative Problems)

PC of pancreatitis: Coma, delirium tremens, hemorrhage, hypovolemic shock, hypocalcemia, hyperglycemia/hypoglycemia, psychosis, pleural effusion/respiratory failure

Nursing Diagnoses

Activity intolerance Related factors: Acute *Pain*, weakness/*Fatigue*, malnutrition

Anxiety Related factors: Change in health status, unfamiliar environment, fear of reoccurrence of *Pain*

Breathing patterns, ineffective Related factors: Abdominal distention, ascites, *Pain*, pleural effusion, respiratory failure

Coping: individual, ineffective Related factors: Alcohol abuse, severity of illness, chronicity of illness

Denial, ineffective Related factors: Failure to acknowledge alcohol abuse or dependency (see *Coping: individual, ineffective*)

Diarrhea Related factor: Excessive fats in stools secondary to insufficient pancreatic enzymes

Family processes: alcoholism, altered Related factors: Hospitalization/ change in environment, change in family roles, alcohol abuse by family member/patient

Fear Related factor: Real or imagined threat to own well-being (see *Anxiety*)

Fluid volume deficit Related factors: Abnormal fluid loss (eg, nasogastric suctioning, vomiting, fever, diaphoresis), inadequate fluid intake (eg, NPO status), fluid shifts (eg, into retroperitoneal space), bleeding

Infection, risk for Related factors: Stasis and shifts of body fluids (eg, retroperitoneal effusion), change in pH of fluids, immunosuppression, chronicity of disease, impaired nutritional status

Management of therapeutic regimen: individual, ineffective Related factors: *Knowledge deficit* (eg, related to disease process, treatments, therapeutic diet, follow-up care, alcohol treatment programs, signs/symptoms of addiction), impaired judgment secondary to alcohol abuse

Noncompliance Related factors: Negative perception of treatment regimen, dysfunctional relationship between patient and provider, poor judgment secondary to alcohol abuse

Nutrition: less than body requirements, altered Related factors: Loss of appetite, *Nausea*/vomiting, decreased ability to digest foods secondary to loss of insulin and digestive enzymes, chemical dependence, NPO status, nasogastric suctioning

Pain Related factors: Inflammation of pancreas and surrounding tissue, pancreatic duct obstruction, interruption of blood supply, pleural effusion, pancreatic enzymes in peritoneal tissues, nasogastric suctioning

Self-care deficit: (specify) Related factors: *Pain*/discomfort, *Activity intolerance, Confusion*

Renal Failure, Acute

Potential Complications (Collaborative Problems)

PC of renal failure: Electrolyte imbalance, fluid overload, metabolic acidosis, pericarditis, platelet dysfunction, secondary infections

Nursing Diagnoses

Activity intolerance Related factors: Increased energy requirements (eg, fever, inflammation), decreased energy production, inadequate nutrition, anemia

Anxiety Related factors: Unknown prognosis, severity of illness

Cardiac output, decreased Related factor: Increased ventricular workload secondary to volume overload

Confusion See *Thought processes, altered*

Environmental interpretation syndrome, impaired See *Thought processes, altered*

Fear Related factors: Environmental stressors/hospitalization, *Powerlessness*, threat to own well-being, threat to child's well-being, severity of illness, multisystem effects

Fluid volume excess Related factors: Changes in renal vascular supply resulting in ischemia, tubular necrosis, decreased glomerular filtration rate

Infection, risk for Risk factors: Invasive procedures, disease process, lowered resistance, malnutrition

Nutrition: less than body requirements, altered Related factors: Anorexia, *Nausea*/vomiting, dietary restrictions, change in taste, loss of smell, stomatitis, increased metabolic needs

Oral mucous membrane, altered Related factors: Extracellular fluid depletion, stomatitis

Skin integrity, impaired Related factors: Poor skin turgor secondary to extracellular fluid, *Diarrhea*

Thought processes, altered Related factors: Decreased cerebral perfusion, accumulation of toxic wastes

Renal Failure, Chronic

Potential Complications (Collaborative Problems)

PC chronic renal failure: Anemia, congestive heart failure, fluid and electrolyte imbalance, fluid overload, hyperparathyroidism, infections, medication toxicity, metabolic acidosis, gastrointestinal bleeding, pericarditis, cardiac tamponade, pleural effusion, pulmonary edema, uremia

Nursing Diagnoses

Activity intolerance Related factors: Weakness/fatigue secondary to anemia, inadequate oxygenation secondary to cardiac and/or pulmonary complications

Body image disturbance Related factors: *Altered growth and development*, treatment side effects, chronic illness, surgery (eg, insertion of hemodialysis blood access or peritoneal catheter, amputations), kidney transplant

Breathing pattern, ineffective Related factors: Anemia, volume overload, pressure of dialysate on diaphragm

Caregiver role strain Related factors: Complexity, amount, and duration of caregiving tasks; illness severity; situational stressors within the family; caregiver's health, knowledge, skills, experience, competing role commitments, and coping styles; isolation, lack of opportunity for respite and recreation

Comfort, altered (non-NANDA) Related factors: Pruritus, fluid retention, vomiting, urate or calcium phosphate crystals on skin

Confusion, acute/chronic Related factors: Uremic encephalopathy, inadequate oxygenation secondary to cardiac and/or respiratory complications, anemia

Constipation Related factors: Restriction of fluids and fiber-rich foods, decreased activity, presence of phosphate-binding agents, medications

Coping: family, ineffective, disabling Related factors: Chronically unresolved feelings, chronic illness and uncertain future of patient, complexity of home care (eg, home dialysis)

Coping: individual, ineffective Related factors: Personal vulnerability in situational crisis (eg, new diagnosis of chronic illness, declining health, terminal illness), inability to concentrate, short attention span, and impaired reasoning secondary to central nervous system involvement

Diversional activity deficit Related factor: Frequent/lengthy medical treatments, lack of energy and mobility to participate

Fatigue Related factors: Altered renal function, inactivity, inadequate nutrition (see *Activity Intolerance*).

Fear Related factors: Environmental stressors/hospitalization, *Powerlessness*, real or imagined threat to well-being

Fluid volume deficit Related factors: Abnormal fluid loss (eg, vomiting), abnormal blood loss secondary to hemodialysis procedure, inadequate fluid intake, compensatory diuresis of dilute urine secondary to decreased ability to concentrate urine, inability of tubules to reabsorb sodium, shifts between blood and dialysate

Fluid volume excess Related factors: Increased fluid intake secondary to excess sodium intake, sodium retention, hyperglycemia, *Noncompliance* with fluid restriction, shifts between blood and dialysate

Grieving, dysfunctional Related factors: Chronic illness, loss, terminal illness, separation from significant others, loss of role function

Hopelessness Related factors: Failing or deteriorating physical condition, lack of social supports, long-term stress, inability to change progression of disease

Infection, risk for Risk factors: Immunosuppression, malnutrition, invasive therapy (eg, dialysis)

Injury (falls), risk for Risk factors: Altered mobility, sensory impairment, hypotension, weakness

Management of therapeutic regimen: individual, ineffective Related factors: *Knowledge deficit* (eg, related to disease, dietary restrictions, medications, signs/symptoms of complications, community resources), complexity of regimen, *Acute/chronic confusion* and *Impaired memory* secondary to disease process

Memory, impaired Related factor: Neurologic changes

Mobility: physical, impaired Related factors: Decreased strength and endurance secondary to anemia, cardiac or respiratory complications, musculoskeletal impairment (eg, fractures secondary to osteoporosis), neuromuscular impairment

Noncompliance Related factors: Denial of illness, dysfunctional relationship between patient and provider, negative perception and/or consequence of treatment regimen, perceived benefits of continued illness

Nutrition: less than body requirements, altered Related factors: Loss of appetite, *Nausea*/vomiting, dietary restrictions, stomatitis, loss of taste/smell secondary to cranial nerve changes

Powerlessness Related factors: Treatment regimen, inability to change progressive course of the disease

Self-care deficit: (specify) Related factors: Depression, *Pain*/discomfort, *Activity intolerance*, neuromuscular impairment, musculoskeletal impairment

Self-esteem disturbance See *Body image disturbance*

Sexual dysfunction Related factors: *Self-esteem disturbance*, impotence, loss of libido, *Activity intolerance*

Skin integrity, impaired Related factors: Edema, dry skin, pruritus, impaired venous circulation secondary to surgical creation of hemodialysis blood access, impaired arterial circulation secondary to hypertension, hyperglycemia

Respiratory Disorders, Acute

Potential Complications (Collaborative Problems)

PC of pneumonia: Lung tissue necrosis

PC of pulmonary edema: Right-sided heart failure, anasarca, multiple organ system failure

PC of pulmonary embolism: pulmonary infarction with necrosis

Nursing Diagnoses

Pneumonia

Activity intolerance Related factor: Weakness/*Fatigue*

Anxiety Related factors: Threat to or change to health status, dyspnea

Fluid volume deficit Related factors: Factors affecting fluid needs (eg, fever)

Gas exchange, impaired Related factors: Decreased functional lung tissue secondary to consolidation, increased secretions

Nutrition: less than body requirements, altered Related factor: Loss of appetite

Pain Related factors: Injury, difficulty breathing

Self-care deficit: (specify) Related factors: *Pain*/discomfort, *Activity intolerance*

Sleep deprivation/Sleep pattern disturbance Related factors: Dyspnea, *Pain*

Pulmonary Edema

Activity intolerance Related factors: Imbalance between oxygen supply and demand, weakness/*Fatigue*

Cardiac output, decreased Related factors: Increased ventricular workload

Fatigue See *Activity intolerance*

Fear Related factors: Environmental stressors/hospitalization

Fluid volume excess Related factor: Decreased urine output secondary to pulmonary edema

Nutrition: less than body requirements, altered Related factor: Loss of appetite

Self-care deficit: (specify) Related factors: *Pain*/discomfort, *Activity intolerance*

Sleep deprivation/Sleep pattern disturbance Related factor: Dyspnea

Pulmonary Embolism

Activity intolerance Related factors: Acute *Pain*, imbalance between oxygen supply and demand

Fear Related factor: Real or imagined threat to own well-being

Gas exchange, impaired Related factor: Decreased pulmonary blood supply secondary to pulmonary embolus

Self-care deficit: (specify) Related factors: *Pain*/discomfort, *Activity intolerance*

Respiratory Disorders, Chronic

Includes but is not limited to asthma, chronic obstructive pulmonary disease, and chronic restrictive pulmonary disease.

Potential Complications (Collaborative Problems)

PC of chronic pulmonary disease: Hypoxemia, right-sided heart failure, respiratory infection, spontaneous pneumothorax

Nursing Diagnoses

Activity intolerance Related factors: Dyspnea, weakness/*Fatigue*, inadequate oxygenation, *Anxiety, Sleep pattern disturbance*

Airway clearance, ineffective Related factors: Tracheobronchial obstruction, excessive and tenacious secretions, ineffective cough secondary to decreased energy/*Fatigue*

Anxiety Related factors: Dyspnea, *Fear* of suffocation, smoking cessation

Caregiver role strain Related factors: Illness severity of the care receiver, unpredictable course of the illness, amount and duration of caregiving required, inadequate physical environment for providing care, lack of respite and recreation for caregiver

Communication, impaired verbal Related factor: Dyspnea

Coping: individual, ineffective Related factors: Personal vulnerability in situational crisis (eg, declining health), difficulty of smoking cessation

Family processes, altered Related factors: Change in family roles and/or structure, hospitalization/change in environment, chronic illness/disability of family member

Fear See *Anxiety*

Fluid volume deficit Related factors: Inadequate fluid intake secondary to difficulty in breathing, fluid loss secondary to fever and diaphoresis

Health maintenance, altered Related factors: Health beliefs, lack of social supports, difficulty with smoking cessation

Home maintenance management, impaired Related factors: *Fatigue, Activity intolerance*, lack of social support

Nutrition: less than body requirements, altered Related factors: Loss of appetite, *Nausea*/vomiting, decreased energy, dyspnea

Powerlessness Related factors: Treatment regimen, chronic illness, lifestyle changes, loss of control (eg, "too late" to improve lung function)

Self-care deficit: (specify) Related factors: Decreased strength and endurance, *Activity intolerance*

Sexual dysfunction/Sexuality patterns, altered Related factors: Dyspnea, lack of energy, relationship changes

Sleep pattern disturbance Related factors: *Anxiety*, medical regimen (eg, pulmonary treatments), inability to assume usual sleep position because of dyspnea, unfamiliar hospital environment, cough

Ventilatory weaning response, dysfunctional (DVWR) Related factors: *Ineffective airway clearance*, patient perceived inefficacy about the ability to wean, *Fear* of suffocation, lack of motivation, *Anxiety*, inappropriate pacing of diminished ventilator support, history of ventilator dependence > one week, history of multiple unsuccessful weaning attempts

Urologic Disorders

Includes but is not limited to cystitis, glomerulonephritis, pyelonephritis, and urolithiasis.

Potential Complications (Collaborative Problems)

PC of cystitis: Renal infection, ulceration of bladder
PC of urolithiasis: Pyelonephritis, renal insufficiency
PC of pyelonephritis: Chronic pyelonephritis, bacteremia, renal insufficiency

Nursing Diagnoses

Diarrhea Related factor: Stimulation of renal/intestinal reflexes
Fluid volume deficit Related factors: Fever, vomiting, *Diarrhea* secondary to stimulation of renal/intestinal reflexes
Hyperthermia Related factors: Inflammatory process, increased metabolic rate
Incontinence, urinary, urge Related factors: Bladder irritation, dysuria, pyuria, frequency
Nutrition: less than body requirements, altered Related factors: Anorexia secondary to fever, *Nausea*, vomiting, and *Pain*
Pain Related factors: Inflammation of bladder or renal tissues; headache; muscular pain; abdominal pain; distention, trauma, and smooth-muscle spasms; and edema in renal tissue (in urolithiasis)

Vascular Disease

Includes but is not limited to deep vein thrombosis, hypertension, stasis ulcers, varicosities, peripheral vascular disease, and thrombophlebitis.

Potential Complications (Collaborative Problems)

PC of varicose veins: Vascular rupture, hemorrhage, venous stasis ulcers, cellulitis
PC of peripheral arterial disease: Arterial thrombosis, cerebrovascular accident, hypertension, ischemic ulcers, cellulitis
PC of deep vein thrombosis: Chronic leg edema, stasis ulcers, pulmonary embolism

Nursing Diagnoses

Activity intolerance Related factors: *Pain*, claudication
Body image disturbance Related factors: Chronic illness, appearance of legs
Injury, risk for Risk factors: Sensory dysfunction, *Impaired physical mobility*

Pain Related factors: Tissue ischemia secondary to decreased peripheral circulation, engorgement/distention of veins

Role performance, altered Related factor: Chronic *Pain*

Self-esteem disturbance Related factor: Chronic illness (see *Body image disturbance*)

Skin integrity, impaired Related factors: Draining wound, tissue ischemia secondary to impaired circulation, physical immobilization, ankle/leg edema, decreased sensation secondary to chronic atherosclerosis

Tissue perfusion, altered (peripheral) Related factors: Impaired venous circulation, impaired arterial circulation

Surgical Conditions

Abdominal surgery

Breast surgery

Chest surgery

Craniotomy

Ear surgery

Eye surgery

Musculoskeletal surgery

Neck surgery

Rectal surgery

Skin graft

Spinal surgery

Urologic surgery

Vascular surgery

Abdominal Surgery

Includes but is not limited to appendectomy, cholecystectomy, colectomy, colon resection, colostomy, gastrectomy, gastric resection, gastroenterostomy, abdominal hysterectomy with or without salpingooophorectomy, ileostomy, laparotomy, lysis of adhesions, Marshall-Marchetti-Krantz operation, ovarian cystectomy, salpingotomy, small bowel resection, splenectomy, vagotomy, and hiatal hernia repair.

Potential Complications (Collaborative Problems)

PC of general anesthesia: Stasis pneumonia

PC of surgery: Dehiscence, evisceration, fistula formation, hemorrhage, paralytic ileus, peritonitis, pulmonary embolism, renal failure, surgical trauma (eg, to ureter, bladder, or rectum), thrombophlebitis, urinary retention

Nursing Diagnoses

Airway clearance, ineffective See *Breathing pattern, ineffective*

Anxiety Related factors: Surgical procedure, preoperative procedures (eg, intravenous insertion, Foley catheter, fluid restrictions), postoperative procedures (eg, coughing/deep breathing, NPO status)

Aspiration, risk for Risk factors: Decreased gastrointestinal motility and depressed cough and gag reflexes secondary to anesthesia and/or analgesics, presence of endotracheal tube, incomplete lower esophageal sphincter, gastrointestinal tubes, increased intragastric pressure, increased gastric residual, delayed gastric emptying, hindered elevation of upper body

Body image disturbance Related factors: Surgery (eg, ostomy), situational crisis, treatment side effects, cultural or spiritual factors

Breathing pattern, ineffective Related factors: *Pain*, immobility, postanesthesia state

Caregiver role strain Related factors: Illness severity of care receiver, discharge of family member with significant home care needs, past history of poor relationship between caregiver and care receiver

Constipation Related factors: Decreased activity, decreased fluid and fiber intake, lack of privacy, change in daily routine, decreased peristalsis secondary to anesthetic, narcotic analgesics

Fear Related factors: Environmental stressors/hospitalization, real or imagined threat to own well-being, unpredictable outcome of surgical procedure, general anesthesia, surgical outcome, *Pain.*

Fluid volume deficit Related factors: Abnormal blood loss, abnormal fluid loss (eg, vomiting), failure of regulatory mechanisms

Infection, risk for Risk factors: Stasis of body fluids, altered peristalsis, suppressed inflammatory response, invasive procedures and lines, surgical incision, urinary catheter

Nutrition: less than body requirements, altered Related factors: Loss of appetite, *Nausea*/vomiting, diet restrictions, increased protein/vitamin requirements for healing

Oral mucous membrane, altered Related factors: Mouth breathing and NPO status secondary to nasogastric tube

Pain Related factors: Incision, abdominal distention, immobility

Sexual dysfunction or Altered sexuality patterns Related factors: *Pain*, health-related transitions, *Body image disturbance*, altered body function or structure, reaction of partner (eg, to ostomy or hysterectomy), physiologic impotence or inadequate vaginal lubrication secondary to the surgery

Skin integrity, impaired Related factors: Mechanical factors, *Impaired physical mobility* secondary to pain and invasive lines, excretions/secretions, poor nutritional state, altered sensation

Social isolation Related factors: Embarrassment about odors, appearance, or appliance (eg, ostomy pouch); reaction of others to appearance and odors

Tissue perfusion, altered (gastrointestinal) Related factors: Interruption of arterial flow, exchange problems, hypervolemia, hypovolemia

Breast Surgery

Includes but is not limited to breast augmentation, mastectomy, reconstruction, lumpectomy, and biopsy.

Potential Complications (Collaborative Problems)

PC of breast surgery: Cellulitis, lymphedema, hematoma, seroma

Nursing Diagnoses

Anxiety Related factors: Threat to self-concept, threat to or change in health status, threat to or change in interaction patterns with significant others, situational/maturational crisis

Body image disturbance Related factors: Surgery, treatment side effects, cultural or spiritual factors pertaining to changes in breast and sexuality

Coping: individual, ineffective Related factors: Changes in appearance, concern over others' reaction, loss of function, diagnosis of cancer

Family processes, altered Related factors: Complex therapies (eg, radiation, chemotherapy), hospitalization/change in environment, reactions of significant others to disfigurement

Fear Related factors: Disease process/prognosis (eg, cancer), *Powerlessness*,

Grieving, anticipatory/dysfunctional Related factors: Loss of body part or function, change in appearance

Mobility: physical, impaired Related factors: Decreased range of motion of shoulder or arm secondary to lymphedema, nerve/muscle damage, and/or *Pain*

Pain Related factors: Surgical procedure, paresthesia

Self-care deficit: dressing/grooming Related factors: *Pain*/discomfort, neuromuscular impairment

Sexuality patterns, altered Related factors: *Pain*, altered body function or structure, illness/medical treatment, *Body image disturbance*, *Self-esteem disturbance*, reaction of significant other

Chest Surgery

Includes but is not limited to biopsy, cardiopulmonary bypass, coronary artery bypass, lobectomy, and thoracotomy.

Potential Complications (Collaborative Problems)

PC of coronary artery bypass graft: Cardiovascular insufficiency, respiratory insufficiency, renal insufficiency

PC of thoracotomy: Atelectasis, cardiac dysrhythmias, hemorrhage, pneumonia, pneumothorax, hemothorax, mediastinal shift, pulmonary edema, pulmonary embolus, subcutaneous emphysema, thrombophlebitis

PC of chest surgery: Myocardial infarction

Nursing Diagnoses

Activity intolerance Related factors: Imbalance between oxygen supply and demand, acute *Pain*, weakness/*Fatigue*, narcotic analgesics, loss of alveolar ventilation

Breathing pattern, ineffective Related factors: Ineffective cough secondary to decreased energy/*Fatigue*, acute *Pain*, increased tracheobronchial secretions

Cardiac output, decreased Related factors: Dysfunctional electrical conduction, ventricular ischemia, ventricular damage, diminished circulating volume, increased systemic vascular resistance

Communication, impaired verbal Related factor: Intubation

Coping: individual, ineffective Related factors: Personal vulnerability in situational crisis (specify), inability to perform usual roles, loss of body function (eg, respiratory), temporary dependence, need for changes in lifestyle

Family processes, altered Related factors: *Fear* of death/disability, disruption of family processes, stressful environment (eg, intensive care unit, hospital)

Fear Related factors: Environmental stressors/hospitalization, threat to own well-being, *Fear* of complications after being transferred out of intensive care unit

Gas exchange, impaired Related factors: Decreased functional lung tissue secondary to pneumonia or lung resection, respiratory distress syndrome, ventilation-perfusion imbalance

Infection, risk for Risk factor: Collection of fluid in thoracic cavity

Mobility, physical, impaired Related factors: Limited arm/shoulder movement secondary to muscle dissection and prescribed position restrictions, *Pain*

Noncompliance Related factors: Denial of illness, negative perception of treatment regimen, difficulty with smoking cessation

Pain Related factors: Surgical incisions, chest tubes, immobility

Role performance, altered Related factors: Surgery, treatment side effects, dependent role during recuperation, uncertain future

Self-care deficit: (specify) Related factors: *Pain*/discomfort, *Activity intolerance* secondary to inadequate oxygenation, *Impaired physical mobility* (arms, shoulders)

Self-esteem disturbance Related factors: Changes in lifestyle, symbolic meaning of the heart, inability to perform usual roles

Sleep deprivation/Sleep pattern disturbance Related factors: *Pain*/discomfort, unfamiliar surroundings, medically prescribed treatments (eg, nebulizer)

Ventilatory weaning response, dysfunctional (DVWR) Related factors: Uncontrolled *Pain*/discomfort, moderate/severe *Anxiety, Fear*, history of ventilatory dependence > one week

Craniotomy

Includes but is not limited to acoustic neuroma removal, cerebral aneurysm clipping, cerebral bleed, and cerebral trauma.

Potential Complications (Collaborative Problems)

PC of craniotomy: Cardiac dysrhythmias, cerebral/cerebellar dysfunction, cerebrospinal fluid leaks, cranial nerve impairment, fluid and electrolyte imbalance, gastrointestinal bleeding, hemorrhage, hematomas, hydrocephalus, hygromas, hyperthermia/hypothermia, hypoxemia, meningitis/encephalitis, seizures, residual neurologic defects

Nursing Diagnoses

Activity intolerance Related factors: Weakness/*Fatigue, Pain*, sleep deprivation, decreased level of consciousness

Airway clearance, ineffective Related factors: Tracheobronchial secretions, increased intracranial pressure

Aspiration, risk for Risk factor: Cranial nerve dysfunction

Body image disturbance Related factors: Surgery, treatment side effects (eg, difficulty speaking, appearance)

Breathing pattern, ineffective Related factors: Depression of respiratory center, neuromuscular paralysis/weakness, cranial nerve dysfunction, airway obstruction secondary to neck edema

Caregiver role strain Related factors: Illness severity of care receiver, discharge of family member with significant home care needs, unpredictable illness course, psychologic or cognitive problems in care receiver

Confusion, acute/chronic See *Thought processes, altered*

Communication, impaired verbal Related factors: Aphasia, dysarthria, *Acute confusion*, intubation

Disuse syndrome, risk for Risk factors: Paralysis, prescribed/mechanical immobilization, decreased level of consciousness

Environmental interpretation syndrome, impaired See *Thought processes, altered*

Fear Related factors: Environmental stressors/hospitalization, *Powerlessness*, threat to own well-being, seriousness of surgery, possibility of dying

Fluid volume excess Related factor: Decreased urine output secondary to renal dysfunction

Incontinence, bowel Related factor: Decreased level of consciousness

Incontinence, urinary, functional Related factors: Cognitive impairment, disorientation, *Impaired physical mobility*

Incontinence, urinary, total Related factors: Neuropathy preventing transmissions of reflex indicating bladder fullness, neurologic dysfunction causing triggering of micturition at unpredictable times, independent contraction of detrusor reflex due to surgery

Injury (contractures), risk for Risk factors: Sensory dysfunction, *Impaired physical mobility*

Management of therapeutic regimen: individual, ineffective Related factors: *Acute/chronic confusion; Impaired memory* and judgment secondary to residual effects on brain tissue; lack of social support

Memory, impaired Related factors: Brain tissue hypoxia or loss secondary to disease or surgery

Mobility, physical, impaired Related factors: Neuromuscular impairment, perceptual/cognitive impairment, depression, severe *Anxiety*

Nutrition: less than body requirements, altered Related factor: Inability to eat secondary to decreased level of consciousness

Pain Related factors: Surgical procedure, paresthesia

Role performance, altered Related factors: Surgery, psychologic impairment, treatment side effects, visual and speech disturbances, seizures, memory loss

Self-care deficit: (specify) Related factors: *Activity intolerance*, neuromuscular impairment, altered level of consciousness, *Sensory/perceptual alterations, Pain*, weakness

Sensory/perceptual alterations: (specify) Related factors: Altered sensory reception, transmission, and/or integration; sensory deficit; sensory overload

Swallowing, impaired Related factors: Cranial nerve dysfunction; altered sensory reception, transmission, and/or integration; neuromuscular impairment

Thought processes, altered Related factors: Increased intracranial pressure, sleep deprivation, brain tissue loss secondary to cerebral edema, hypoxia or surgical resection

Tissue perfusion, altered (cerebral) Related factors: Interruption of arterial blood flow, increased intracranial pressure

Ear Surgery

Ear surgery includes but is not limited to myringotomy, reconstruction, and stapedectomy.

Potential Complications (Collaborative Problems)

PC of ear surgery: Facial paralysis, hearing loss, infection

Nursing Diagnoses

Communication, impaired verbal Related factor: Hearing loss

Infection, risk for Risk factors: Exposure to upper respiratory infections, invasive procedures

Injury (falls), risk for Risk factors: Vertigo, nystagmus

Pain Related factors: Inflammation, tissue trauma, edema, presence of surgical packing

Self-care deficit: (specify) Related factor: *Activity intolerance* secondary to dizziness and loss of balance

Sensory/perceptual alterations (auditory) Related factors: Sensory deficit, sensory overload, surgical packing, edema, disturbance of middle-ear structures

Trauma, risk for Risk factor: Displacement of prosthesis secondary to increased middle-ear pressure

Eye Surgery

Includes but is not limited to blepharoplasty, cataract removal, cryosurgery for retinal detachment, iridectomy, iridotomy, and lens implant.

Potential Complications (Collaborative Problems)

PC of eye surgery: Bleeding, endophthalmus, hyphema (ie, blood in anterior chamber of the eye), increased intraocular pressure, infection, lens implant dislocation, macular edema, retinal detachment, secondary glaucoma

Nursing Diagnoses

Body image disturbance Related factor: Change in appearance (enucleation)

Fear Related factor: Real or imagined threat to own well-being (eg, permanent loss of vision)

Injury (falls), risk for Risk factors: Unsafe ambulation secondary to limited vision, eye patches, unfamiliar environment

Mobility: physical, impaired Related factors: Medically prescribed treatment and positioning, impaired vision

Self-care deficit: (specify) Related factors: Eye patches, impaired vision

Sensory/perceptual alterations (visual) Related factor: Sensory deficit secondary to eye patches or impaired vision

Musculoskeletal Surgery

Includes but is not limited to amputation, arthrotomy, bunionectomy, casts, hip pinning, hip prosthesis, open reduction/internal fixation of fracture, shoulder repair, total ankle replacement, total hip replacement, total knee replacement, and traction.

Potential Complications (Collaborative Problems)

PC of amputation: Edema of the stump

PC of fractures: Fat embolus, nonunion of bone, reflex sympathetic dystrophy

PC of fractures/casts: Compartment syndrome

PC of fractures and musculoskeletal surgery: Deep vein thrombosis, nerve damage

PC of joint replacement surgery: Joint dislocation/displacement of prosthesis

PC of musculoskeletal surgery: Flexion contractures, hematoma, hemorrhage, infection, pulmonary embolism, sepsis, stress fractures, synovial herniation,

PC of total hip replacement: Femoral head necrosis

Nursing Diagnoses

Activity intolerance Related factors: *Pain*, weakness, *Sleep deprivation*

Anxiety Related factors: Lack of knowledge of surgery and postoperative routines (eg, physical therapy, walking with crutches), threat to self-concept, threat to or change in role functioning

Body image disturbance Related factors: Surgery (eg, loss of limb), loss of functional abilities (eg, need to use wheelchair), fear of others' response to appearance

Confusion, acute Related factors: Hypoxemia, medications (eg, opiate analgesics), infection, impaction

Constipation Related factors: Decreased activity, dietary changes, medication (eg, opiates, anesthetics)

Coping: individual, ineffective Related factors: *Pain*, *Self-care deficits*, long-term and debilitating nature of disease

Disuse syndrome, risk for Risk factor: Prescribed immobilization

Diversional activity deficit Related factors: Prolonged bed rest, institutionalization

Grieving, anticipatory/dysfunctional Related factors: Loss of limb, changes in lifestyle, loss of ability to perform usual roles

Home maintenance management, impaired Related factors: Barriers (eg, stairs) and hazards (eg, throw rugs), *Activity intolerance*

Infection, risk for Risk factors: Inadequate primary defense secondary to exposure of joint, broken skin

Injury (contractures), risk for Risk factors: Immobility secondary to *Pain* and/or weakness

Injury (falls), risk for Risk factors: Unfamiliarity of assistive devices (eg, crutches), weakness secondary to surgery and immobility

Management of therapeutic regimen: individual, ineffective Related factors: Lack of knowledge of disease process, surgical treatment, self-care, complex rehabilitation regimen, alterations in lifestyle, insufficient energy to perform exercises

Mobility: physical, impaired Related factors: *Pain*, stiffness, decreased strength

Pain Related factors: Muscle cramps, paresthesia, inflammation, surgical procedure, joint destruction, phantom limb pain

Peripheral neurovascular dysfunction, risk for Related factors: Fractures, mechanical compression, orthopedic surgery, trauma, immobilization, casts and traction devices

Self-care deficit: (specify) Related factors: *Pain, Activity intolerance, Impaired physical mobility*, decreased strength and endurance

Skin integrity, impaired Related factors: Mechanical factors, prescribed physical immobilization, *Impaired physical mobility*, impaired circulation, altered sensation, casts and other appliances, edema (eg, of stump)

Sleep deprivation/Sleep pattern disturbance Related factors: *Pain*/discomfort, unfamiliar surroundings, medically induced regimen, inability to assume usual sleep position

Tissue perfusion, altered (peripheral) Related factors: Reduced arterial or venous blood flow, trauma to blood vessels, edema, dislocation of prosthesis

Neck Surgery

Includes but is not limited to carotid endarterectomy, laryngectomy, parathyroidectomy, radical neck dissection, thyroidectomy, tonsillectomy, and tracheostomy.

Potential Complications (Collaborative Problems)

PC of neck surgery: Airway obstruction, aspiration, cerebral infarction, cranial nerve damage (eg, facial, hypoglossal, glossopharyngeal, vagus), fistula formation (eg, between hypopharynx and skin), hemorrhage, hypertension, hypotension, infection, local nerve impairment, thyroid storm, tracheal stenosis, vocal cord paralysis,

PC radical neck dissection: Flap rejection

PC thyroidectomy/parathyroidectomy: Hypoparathyroidism, causing hypocalcemia and tetany

Nursing Diagnoses

Activity intolerance Related factors: Imbalance between oxygen supply and demand, *Anxiety, Pain*, weakness secondary to limited mobility, *Fatigue* secondary to accelerated metabolic rate (eg, thyroidectomy)

Airway clearance, ineffective Related factors: Decreased energy, edema, *Pain*, tracheobronchial obstruction, increased tracheobronchial secretions, edema of the glottis, tracheal compression secondary to hemorrhage, presence of tracheostomy tube

Anxiety See *Fear*

Aspiration, risk for Risk factors: Depressed cough or gag reflexes, presence of tracheostomy or endotracheal tube, *Impaired swallowing*, hindered elevation of upper body, removal of epiglottis (in partial laryngectomy), loss of normal reflexes and excessive secretions secondary to surgery

Body image disturbance Related factors: Changes in appearance secondary to surgery, depression, treatment side effects

Breathing pattern, ineffective Related factors: *Anxiety*, decreased energy, accidental decannulation

Communication, impaired verbal Related factors: *Acute confusion*, inability to speak, inability to speak clearly secondary to *Pain* and edema, tracheostomy, laryngectomy, weak or hoarse voice secondary to trauma to laryngeal nerve

Coping: individual, ineffective Related factors: Personal vulnerability in situational crisis (specify), inability to speak, disfigurement, inadequate support system (see *Body image disturbance*)

Fear Related factors: Real or imagined threat to own well-being (eg, fear of suffocation), unfamiliarity with environment and pre- and postoperative routines

Fluid volume deficit Risk factors: Loss of fluid through abnormal routes, hypermetabolic state, decreased intake secondary to *Pain* and *Impaired swallowing*

Grieving, anticipatory/dysfunctional Related factors: Actual loss of function, change in appearance, threat of dying

Infection, risk for Risk factors: Tissue destruction and increased environmental exposure, loss of normal filtration systems in the mouth and nose secondary to use of artificial airway, immunosuppression secondary to chemotherapy and malignancies

Injury (falls), risk for Risk factors: Sensory dysfunction, integrative dysfunction, vascular insufficiency, altered mobility

Mobility: physical, impaired Related factors: Limited shoulder and head movement secondary to removal of muscles and nerves, flap graft reconstruction

Nutrition: less than body requirements, altered Related factors: *Pain*, *Impaired swallowing*, loss of appetite, *Nausea*/vomiting, loss of sense of smell, cachexia secondary to malignancy, accelerated metabolic rate (eg, from thyroidectomy)

Oral mucous membrane, altered Related factors: Inadequate oral hygiene, tubes, surgery in oral cavity, infection, radiation therapy to head and neck

Pain Related factor: Surgical procedure, edema, tracheostomy tube irritation

Role performance, altered Related factors: Surgery, treatment side effects, *Impaired physical mobility*

Self-esteem disturbance See *Body image disturbance*

Skin integrity, impaired Related factors: Mechanical factors, radiation, altered nutritional state

Social isolation Related factors: Difficulty communicating, embarrassment and concern over others' response to disfigurement, avoidance by others

Swallowing, impaired Related factors: Irritated oropharyngeal cavity, mechanical obstruction, edema, cranial nerve damage

Tissue integrity, impaired Related factors: Nutritional deficit, irritants, mechanical factors (eg, tracheostomy tube), radiation

Ventilatory weaning response, dysfunctional (DVWR) Related factors: *Ineffective airway clearance*, lack of motivation secondary to malaise, moderate/severe *Anxiety, Fear*, uncontrolled episodic energy demands or problems

Rectal Surgery

Includes but is not limited to fissurectomy, hemorrhoidectomy, pilonidal cystectomy, and polypectomy.

Potential Complications (Collaborative Problems)

PC of rectal surgery: Hemorrhage, infection, stricture formation

Nursing Diagnoses

Constipation Related factors: Dietary changes, decreased motility secondary to medication and inactivity, *Fear* of painful defecation
Incontinence, bowel Related factor: Loss of sphincter integrity
Infection, risk for Risk factors: Loss of primary line of defense secondary to surgery, fecal contamination
Pain Related factors: Surgical procedure, passage of stool

Skin Graft

Includes but is not limited to excision of lesion with flap, excision of lesion with full-thickness graft, excision of lesion with split-thickness graft, and excision of lesion with synthetic graft.

Potential Complications (Collaborative Problems)

PC of skin graft: Edema, flap necrosis, hematoma, infection

Nursing Diagnoses

Body image disturbance Related factor: Results of reconstructive surgery not as anticipated by patient
Constipation Related factor: Decreased activity secondary to prescribed positioning
Diversional activity deficit Related factors: Prolonged bed rest, prescribed positioning
Fear Related factors: Real or imagined threat to own well-being, fear of flap failure, fear of others' reactions to appearance
Mobility: physical, impaired Related factors: *Pain*/discomfort, prescribed position
Pain Related factors: Surgical procedure, paresthesia
Peripheral neurovascular dysfunction, risk for Risk factors: Immobilization, burns, edema
Tissue perfusion, altered (specify) Related factors: Restricted blood flow secondary to edema, blood clot, or tension on the flap

Spinal Surgery

Includes but is not limited to Harrington rod implant, laminectomy, Luque rod implant, and spinal fusion.

Potential Complications (Collaborative Problems)

PC of laminectomy/spinal fusion: Displacement of bone graft

PC of spinal surgery: Bladder and bowel dysfunction, cerebrospinal fistula, hematoma, hemorrhage, infection, nerve root injury, paralytic ileus, sensorineural impairments, spinal cord edema or injury

Nursing Diagnoses

Activity intolerance Related factors: *Fear* of damaging surgical site, *Pain*, weakness/*Fatigue*, sedentary lifestyle, enforced inactivity

Caregiver role strain Related factors: Premature birth/congenital defect, developmental delay or retardation of the care receiver/caregiver, duration of caregiving required

Constipation Related factors: Decreased activity, medications (eg, opiates), inability to assume normal position for defecation, change in daily routine, temporary loss of parasympathetic function innervating the bowels

Injury (falls), risk for Risk factors: Sensory dysfunction, loss of balance, muscle weakness secondary to recent inactivity, vertigo secondary to postural hypotension

Mobility: physical, impaired Related factors: *Pain*, neuromuscular impairment, stiffness in fused area, prescribed activity and position limitations

Nutrition: more than body requirements, altered Related factors: increased appetite when pain subsides, sedentary lifestyle, decreased activity

Pain, acute/chronic Related factors: Bed rest, muscle cramps, paresthesia, surgical procedure (eg, graft site), inflammation, localized edema, muscle spasms

Peripheral neurovascular dysfunction Risk factors: Fractures, mechanical compression, trauma, immobilization

Self-care deficit: (specify) Related factors: Prescribed postoperative immobility, *Pain*

Skin integrity, impaired Related factors: Prescribed activity restrictions, diminished/interrupted blood flow secondary to edema, hematoma, or hypovolemia

Urinary retention Related factors: Swelling in operative area, inability to assume usual position for voiding

<u>Urologic Surgery</u>

Includes but is not limited to cystocele repair, rectocele repair, removal of bladder tumor, cystoscopy, nephrectomy, penile implant, percutaneous nephrostomy, retroperitoneal lymphadenotomy, prostatectomy, transurethral resection of the prostate, ureterolithotomy, urostomy, and vasectomy.

Potential Complications (Collaborative Problems)

PC of prostate resection/prostatectomy: Retrograde ejaculation

PC of urologic surgery: Bladder neck constriction, bladder perforation (intraoperative), epididymitis, hemorrhage, paralytic ileus, urethral stricture, urinary tract infection

PC of urostomy/nephrostomy: Stomal necrosis, stenosis, obstruction

Nursing Diagnoses

Anxiety Related factors: Threat to self-concept, change in health status, change in body appearance or function, threat to or change in role functioning, threat to or change in interaction pattern

Body image disturbance Related factors: Surgery, depression, treatment side effects (eg, impotence), appearance of ostomy (eg, urostomy)

Grieving, anticipatory/dysfunctional Related factor: Potential loss of body parts or function

Incontinence, urinary, stress. Related factors: Incompetent bladder outlet, overdistention between voidings, weak pelvic muscles and structural supports

Incontinence, urinary, urge Related factors: Decreased bladder capacity, surgery, irritation of bladder stretch receptors causing spasms, overdistention of bladder

Infection, risk for Risk factors: Stasis of body fluids, change in pH of secretions, suppressed inflammatory response, tissue destruction and increased environmental exposure, invasive procedures and lines (eg, catheters, irrigation, suprapubic drains)

Mobility: physical, impaired Related factor: *Pain*

Pain Related factors: Muscle cramps, surgical procedure, coughing and deep breathing (eg, renal surgeries), bladder spasms, back and leg pain, clot in drainage devices (eg, from transurethral resection)

Sexual dysfunction Related factors: Side effects of surgery, *Pain*, altered body function or structure, *Body image disturbance*, reaction of partner to ostomy, erectile dysfunction (male), inadequate vaginal lubrication (female)

Social isolation Related factors: Concern about others' reaction to ostomy, worry about odor and leaking from appliance

Urinary retention Related factors: Inhibition of reflex arc, blockage secondary to edema or inflammation

Vascular Surgery

Includes but is not limited to aortic aneurysm resection, aortoiliac bypass graft, embolectomy, femoroiliac bypass graft, portacaval shunt, sympathectomy, and vein ligation.

Potential Complications (Collaborative Problems)

PC of aortic aneurysm resection: Renal failure, myocardial infarction, hemorrhage, emboli, spinal cord ischemia, congestive heart failure, rupture of suture line

PC of vascular surgery: Cardiac dysrhythmia, compartmental syndrome, failure of anastomosis, infection, lymphocele, occlusion of graft

Nursing Diagnoses

Activity intolerance Related factors: *Anxiety*, *Pain*, weakness secondary to inactivity, imbalance between oxygen supply and demand

Caregiver role strain Related factors: Illness severity of care receiver, unpredictable illness course or instability in the care receiver's health, complexity/amount of caregiving tasks

Fear Related factor: Real or imagined threat to own well-being (eg, surgery, failure of graft, loss of limb, death)

Fluid volume deficit Related factors: Loss of fluid through abnormal routes, medications, third spacing, hematoma, diuresis secondary to contrast media given for angiography

Fluid volume excess Related factor: Decreased urine output secondary to heart failure

Grieving, anticipatory/dysfunctional Related factor: Potential loss of body part or function

Injury, risk for Risk factors: Tissue hypoxia, abnormal blood profile, *Impaired mobility*

Mobility: physical, impaired Related factors: *Pain*, nerve injury secondary to ischemia

Pain, acute/chronic Related factors: Surgical procedure, increased tissue perfusion to previously ischemic tissue, peripheral nerve ischemia, paresthesias

Peripheral neurovascular dysfunction, risk for Related factors: Immobilization, vascular obstruction

Sexual dysfunction Related factors: Impotence and retrograde ejaculation secondary to aortic aneurysm resection

Tissue integrity, impaired Related factors: Chronically compromised peripheral tissue perfusion, decreased activity postoperatively, multiple surgical procedures

Tissue perfusion, altered: (specify) Related factors: Interruption of venous blood flow, exchange problems, graft occlusion, edema, compartmental syndrome, inadequate anticoagulation, progressive arterial disease

Psychiatric Conditions

Assaultive patient

Borderline personality

Eating disorders

Mania

Paranoia

Phobias

Psychosis

Severe depression

Substance abuse

Suicide

Withdrawn patient

Assaultive Patient

Associated psychiatric diagnoses include but are not limited to bipolar disorder, manic; disorganized schizophrenia; substance use disorders; organic mental disorders; drug-induced psychoses; personality disorders; panic disorder; and post-traumatic stress disorder.

Nursing Diagnoses

Coping: defensive Related factors: Psychologic impairment (specify), situational crisis (specify), neurologic alteration, other physical factors (specify)

Post-trauma syndrome Related factors: Abuse, incest, rape, participation in combat

Self-esteem, chronic low Related factors: Psychologic impairment (specify), repeatedly unmet expectations

Self-esteem, situational low Related factor: Situational crisis (specify)

Sensory/perceptual alterations: (specify) Related factors: Alcohol/substance abuse (specify); altered sensory reception, transmission, and/or integration; sensory deficit (specify); sensory overload (specify)

Social interaction, impaired Related factors: Developmental disability, communication barriers, psychologic impairment (specify)

Thought processes, altered Related factors: Mental disorder (specify), organic mental disorder (specify), personality disorder (specify), substance abuse

Violence: self-directed or directed at others, risk for Risk factors: Manic excitement, panic states, rage reaction, history of violence, drug/alcohol intoxication/withdrawal, temporal lobe epilepsy, paranoid ideation, organic brain syndrome, arrest/conviction pattern, toxic reaction to medications, command hallucinations

Borderline Personality

Nursing Diagnoses

Anxiety Related factors: Threat to or change in role functioning, situational crises (specify), maturational crisis (specify), unmet needs, change in environment, threat to or change in interaction patterns, unconscious conflict about values/beliefs, negative self-talk, post-traumatic experience

Coping: family, ineffective, disabling Related factors: Conflicting coping styles, highly ambivalent family relationships, chronically unresolved feelings (specify), role changes, and ongoing family disorganization secondary to patient's illness

Coping: individual, ineffective Related factors: Personal vulnerability in situational or maturational crisis (specify); procrastination, stubbornness, and inefficiency in performing social roles; unrealistic perceptions; unmet expectations; disregard for social norms; inadequate support system; no assertion or recognition of own needs; poor impulse control; mood shifts, use of splitting and projection

Personal identity disturbance Related factors: Situational crises, psychologic impairment (eg, borderline personality disorder), developmental impairment

Powerlessness Related factor: Pattern of helplessness

Role performance, altered Related factors: Situational crises, psychologic impairment (eg, borderline personality disorder)

Self-esteem, chronic low Related factors: Psychologic impairment (eg, borderline personality disorder), repeatedly unmet expectations of others, inability to meet role expectations, learned helplessness

Self-Mutilation, risk for Risk factors: Inability to cope with increased psychologic/physiologic tension in a healthy manner; feelings of depression, rejection, self-hatred, separation anxiety, guilt, and depersonalization; fluctuating emotions; drug/alcohol abuse; history of self-injury; history of physical, emotional, or sexual abuse

Sexuality patterns, altered Related factors: Conflict with sexual orientation, sexual abuse, impaired relationship with significant person

Social interaction, impaired Related factors: Psychologic impairment (eg, borderline personality disorder), low self-esteem, misinterpretation of internal/external stimuli, hypervigilance in social situations, dysfunctional interactions, withdrawal, inability to maintain attachments, fear of abandonment

Violence: self-directed or directed at others, risk for Risk factors: Rage reaction, suicidal ideation, history of self-mutilation, substance abuse (specify)

Eating Disorders

Associated psychiatric diagnoses are limited to anorexia nervosa and bulimia.

Potential Complications (Collaborative Problems)

PC of eating disorders: Amenorrhea, anemia, dysrhythmias

Nursing Diagnoses

Activity intolerance Related factor: Weakness/*Fatigue* secondary to malnutrition

Anxiety Related factors: Threat to self-concept, worry about being overweight, change in environment, situational/maturational crises, unmet needs

Body image disturbance Related factors: Eating disorder (see *Anxiety*), dysfunctional family system

Constipation Related factors: Less than adequate amounts of fiber and bulk-forming foods in diet, chronic use of medication and enemas, inadequate fluid intake

Coping: family, ineffective, disabling Related factors: Arbitrary disregard for patient's needs, chronically unresolved feelings (specify guilt, anxiety, hostility, despair, and so on), conflicting coping styles, highly ambivalent family relationships, effect of marital discord on family members

Coping: individual, ineffective Related factors: Personal vulnerability in a maturational or situational crisis (specify), feelings of loss of control, inaccurate perception of weight status, anxiety about maturing body

Fluid volume deficit Related factors: Extreme weight loss, self-induced vomiting, abuse of laxatives/diuretics

Management of therapeutic regimen: individual, ineffective Related factors: *Decisional conflict*, family conflict, mistrust of regimen and/or health care personnel, denial of illness, perceived lack of benefits of treatment, *Powerlessness*

Noncompliance Related factors: Denial of illness, negative perception of treatment regimen, perceived benefits of continued illness

Nutrition: less than body requirements, altered Related factors: Psychologic impairment (eg, bulimia, anorexia), refusal to eat, self-induced vomiting, laxative abuse, need for more calories because of physical exertion (eg, excessive exercising)

Self-esteem, chronic low Related factors: Psychologic impairment (specify), repeatedly unmet expectations, perception of self as fat

Sexuality patterns, altered Related factors: Ineffective or absent role models, *Body image disturbance*, impaired relationship with significant other, *Self-esteem disturbance*

Social interaction, impaired Related factor: Psychologic impairment (eg, anorexia, bulimia), fear and mistrust of relationships

Mania

Associated psychiatric diagnoses include but are not limited to bipolar disorders (manic, mixed), schizophrenia (undifferentiated type, catatonic type), schizoaffective disorder, and substance use disorders.

Potential Complications (Collaborative Problems)

PC of lithium therapy: Lithium toxicity

Nursing Diagnoses

Anxiety Related factors: Change in role functioning, change in environment, change in interaction patterns, unmet needs, threats to self-concept

Communication, impaired verbal Related factors: Hyperactivity, pressured speech

Coping, defensive Related factors: Ideas of grandiosity/self-importance/ abilities secondary to feelings of inferiority

Coping: individual, ineffective Related factor: Personal vulnerability in a situational crisis (specify)

Family processes, altered Related factors: Illness/disability of family member, exhaustion of family members, situational crises (eg, financial difficulty, role changes), patient's euphoria and grandiose ideas, manipulative behavior, limit testing, patient's refusal to take responsibility for own actions

Fluid volume deficit Related factors: Inadequate fluid intake secondary to manic behaviors, medication-induced *Diarrhea* and vomiting, polyuria

Health maintenance, altered Related factors: Significant alteration in communication skills, lack of ability to make deliberate and thoughtful judgments

Injury, risk for Risk factors: Orientation; drugs (eg, alcohol, caffeine, nicotine); cognitive, affective, and psychomotor factors

Nutrition: less than body requirements, altered Related factor: Inadequate intake to balance excessive (ie, manic) activity

Personal identity disturbance Related factor: Psychologic impairment (specify)

Role performance, altered Related factor: Psychologic impairment (specify), see *Altered family processes*

Sensory/perceptual alterations (specify) Related factors: *Sleep deprivation*, endogenous chemical alteration, stress

Sleep pattern disturbance Related factors: Psychologic impairment (specify), inability to recognize *Fatigue* and need for sleep, hyperactivity, denial of need to sleep

Social interaction, impaired Related factors: Psychologic impairment (specify), others' unwillingness to tolerate patient's behaviors

Thought processes, altered Related factor: Mental disorder (specify), delusions, hallucinations, euphoria, flight of ideas

Violence: self-directed or directed at others, risk for Risk factors: Manic excitement, rage reaction, history of violence, irritability, impulsive behavior, delusional thinking, command hallucinations, impaired reality testing

Paranoia

Associated psychiatric diagnoses include but are not limited to schizophrenia (undifferentiated type, paranoid type), mood disorders (major depression [eg, single episode, recurrent]), bipolar disorders (eg, mixed, manic, depressed), schizoaffective disorder, paranoid disorders, substance abuse disorders, organic mental disorders, and personality disorders.

Nursing Diagnoses

Anxiety (severe) Related factors: Failure to master developmental task of trust versus mistrust, delusions

Coping, defensive Related factor: Psychologic impairment (specify)

Coping: individual, ineffective Related factors: Personal vulnerability in situational crisis, use of projection to control fears and anxieties

Family processes, altered Related factors: Illness/disability of family member, temporary or long-term family disorganization, exhausted family patient's behaviors

Fear Related factor: Imagined threat to own well-being

Health maintenance, altered Related factors: Significant alteration in communication skills, lack of ability to make deliberate and thoughtful judgments

Noncompliance Related factors: Denial of illness, negative perception of treatment regimen, mistrust of caregivers

Powerlessness Related factors: Health care environment, treatment regimen, feelings of inadequacy, maladaptive interpersonal relationships (eg, use of force, abusive relationships), *Self-esteem disturbance*, feelings that he/she has no control over situations

Self-esteem disturbance Related factor: Psychologic impairment (specify), failure of relationships, feelings of *Powerlessness*

Sexuality patterns, altered Related factors: Impaired relationship with significant other secondary to manipulative, violent, or other unacceptable behaviors; conflicts with sexual orientation

Sleep pattern disturbance Related factor: Psychologic impairment, *Fear* of danger, hypervigilance

Social interaction, impaired Related factors: Psychologic impairment (specify), delusions, suspiciousness, *Fear* and mistrust of others

Thought processes, altered Related factors: Mental disorder (specify), organic mental disorder (specify), personality disorder (specify), poor reality testing secondary to mistrust of others, delusions, hallucinations

Violence: self-directed or directed at others, risk for Risk factors: Panic states, drug/alcohol intoxication/withdrawal, delusions, feelings of *Anxiety*, perceived danger

Phobias

Associated psychiatric diagnoses include but are not limited to agoraphobia, simple phobia, and social phobia.

Nursing Diagnoses

Anxiety Related factors: Threat to or change in role functioning, change in environment, threat to self-concept, threat to or change in interaction pattern, unmet needs

Coping: individual, ineffective Related factor: Personal vulnerability in situational or maturational crisis (specify)

Diversional activity deficit Related factors: Impaired perception of reality, fear of loss of control if dreaded object/situation is encountered

Fear Related factors: Real or imagined threat to own well-being, learned irrational response to objects or situations

Role performance, altered Related factors: Psychologic impairment (eg, phobic disorder), inability to perform role behaviors secondary to irrational fears

Social interaction, impaired Related factors: Psychologic impairment (eg, phobic disorder), *Fear* of encountering dreaded object/situation, *Fear* of loss of control

Social isolation Related factors: Psychologic impairment (eg, phobic disorder), others' reactions to irrational behaviors

Psychosis

Associated psychiatric diagnoses include but are not limited to schizophrenia (disorganized, catatonic, paranoid, and undifferentiated types) schizophreniform disorder; bipolar disorders (mixed, manic, and depressed) organic mental disorders; substance abuse disorders; and medical conditions.

Nursing Diagnoses

Anxiety (severe, panic) Related factors: Continuation of maladaptive coping learned early in life, unconscious conflicts, unmet needs, threats to self-concept

Communication, impaired verbal Related factors: Psychologic impairment (specify), incoherent/illogical speech, medication side effects

Coping: family, ineffective, disabling Related factors: Long-term pattern of multiple stressors, significant others exhausted by prolonged illness

Health maintenance, altered Related factors: Lack of ability to make deliberate and thoughtful judgments

Home maintenance management, impaired Related factors: Psychologic impairment (specify), *Altered thought processes*, impaired judgment/decision making

Noncompliance Related factors: Denial of illness, negative perception of treatment regimen, *Altered thought processes*, responding to delusions and hallucinations

Personal identity disturbance Related factors: Psychologic impairment (specify), psychologic conflicts, childhood abuse, underdeveloped ego, threats to self-concept, threats to physical integrity

Self-care deficit: (specify) Related factors: Psychologic impairment (specify), severe *Anxiety*, *Altered thought processes*, inability to make decisions, feelings of worthlessness, lack of energy

Self-mutilation, risk for Risk factors: Fluctuating emotions, command hallucinations, patients in psychotic state—frequently males in young adulthood

Sensory/perceptual alterations (auditory, visual) Related factors: Escalating *Anxiety*, withdrawal

Social interaction, impaired Related factor: Psychologic impairment (specify)

Thought processes, altered Related factors: Mental disorder (specify), organic mental disorder (specify), dementia, delirium

Violence: self-directed or directed at others, risk for Risk factors: Paranoid ideation, suicidal ideation, history of violence, substance abuse (specify), responding to delusions and hallucinations

Severe Depression

Associated psychiatric diagnoses include but are not limited to bipolar disorder (depressed) and major depression.

Nursing Diagnoses

Activity intolerance Related factors: Weakness/*Fatigue*, depression, inadequate nutrition

Anxiety Related factors: Psychologic conflicts, unmet needs, unconscious values/goals conflicts, change in role functioning, change in interaction patterns, threat to self-concept

Constipation Related factors: Decreased activity, lack of exercise, inadequate intake of fiber and fluids, medications (specify)

Coping: family, ineffective, disabling Related factors: Role conflicts, marital discord secondary to long-term depression (see *Family processes, altered*)

Coping: individual, ineffective Related factors: Personal vulnerability in situational or maturational crisis, guilt, low self-esteem, feelings of rejection, unconscious conflicts

Family processes, altered Related factor: Illness/disability of family member, changes in roles/responsibilities, family disorganization, *Impaired verbal communication*, difficulty accepting or receiving help

Grieving, dysfunctional Related factors: Actual loss (specify), anticipated loss (specify), perceived loss (specify), unresolved grief secondary to prolonged *Ineffective denial*, repressed feelings

Health maintenance, altered Related factors: Lack of ability to make deliberate and thoughtful judgments, significant alteration in communication skills, lack of energy, feelings of worthlessness

Home maintenance management, impaired Related factors: Psychologic impairment (specify), inability to concentrate, impaired decision making, lack of energy

Hopelessness Related factors: Long-term stress, lack of social supports, abandonment by others

Injury, risk for Risk factors: Orientation; drugs (eg, alcohol, caffeine, nicotine); cognitive, affective, and psychomotor factors; electroconvulsive therapy and anesthesia effects on cardiovascular and respiratory systems; medication side effects such as sedation/blurred vision

Nutrition: less than body requirements, altered Related factors: Psychologic impairment (specify), loss of appetite, feelings of worthlessness, emotional stress/*Anxiety*

Powerlessness Related factors: Psychologic impairment (specify), negative beliefs about own abilities, past failures, lack of energy, feelings of worthlessness

Role performance, altered Related factors: Psychologic impairment (specify), lack of energy, *Powerlessness*, helplessness

Self-care deficit: (specify) Related factors: Depression, lack of energy

Self-esteem, chronic low Related factors: Psychologic impairment (specify), repeatedly unmet expectations, past failures, feelings of worthlessness

Sexuality patterns, altered Related factors: *Self-esteem disturbance*, lack of energy, loss of interest, decreased sex drive

Sleep pattern disturbance Related factors: *Anxiety*, psychologic impairment (eg, depression), decreased serotonin, daytime inactivity, naps, difficulty falling asleep at night, hypersomnia, early awakening

Social interaction, impaired Related factors: Psychologic impairment (depression), failure to initiate interactions secondary to decreased energy/inertia, poor self-concept, lack of social skills, feelings of worthlessness

Social isolation Related factors: Others' responses to depressed mood, *Altered thought processes*, lack of social skills, feelings of unworthiness

Thought processes, altered Related factors: Mental disorder (specify), overgeneralizing, negative thinking, dichotomous thinking

Violence: self-directed, risk for Risk factors: Suicidal ideation/intent secondary to feelings of worthlessness and *Hopelessness, Loneliness*

Substance Abuse

Associated psychiatric diagnoses include alcohol/drug intoxication withdrawal and dependence.

Potential Complications (Collaborative Problems)

PC of alcoholism: Delirium tremens

PC of substance abuse: Hallucinations, hypertension, sepsis, toxic overdose

PC of substance abuse or withdrawal: Seizures

Nursing Diagnoses

Anxiety Related factors: Change in health status, change in role functioning, situational crisis, unmet needs, *Impaired memory*, loss of control, fear of withdrawal, legal implications

Coping: family, ineffective, compromised/disabling Related factors: Temporary family disorganization and role changes, unrealistic expectations/demands, lack of mutual decision-making skills, inadequate information/understanding by family member, arbitrary disregard for patient's needs, chronically unresolved feelings (specify guilt, anxiety, hostility, despair, and so on), conflicting coping styles, inconsistent limit setting, highly ambivalent family relationships, violence

Coping: individual, ineffective Related factors: Personal vulnerability in situational or maturational crisis (specify), anger, denial, dependence, inability to manage stressors

Decisional conflict (specify) Related factor: Chemical dependence

Denial, ineffective Related factors: Feelings of vulnerability, ambivalence about withdrawal, inability to cope without alcohol/drugs, *Anxiety*, *Fear*

Diarrhea Related factors: Excessive alcohol/drug intake, withdrawal

Family processes: alcoholism, altered Related factor: Alcohol abuse by a family member

Fluid volume deficit Related factors: Excessive, continuous consumption of alcohol, vomiting, *Diarrhea*

Home maintenance management, impaired Related factors: Insufficient family organization or planning, psychologic impairment (eg, substance abuse), decreased motivation, *Altered thought processes*, depression, severe *Anxiety*

Injury, risk for Risk factors: Orientation; affective factors; impaired judgment; *Confusion, acute/chronic*; delirium; substance intoxication

Memory, impaired Related factor: Organic brain damage

Noncompliance Related factors: Denial of illness, negative perception of treatment regimen, inability to ask for or accept help, lack of social support, inability to cope with stressors without alcohol/drugs

Nutrition: less than body requirements, altered Related factors: Chemical dependence (specify), anorexia, hypermetabolism secondary to stimulants, no money for food

Nutrition: more than body requirements, altered Related factor: Increased appetite secondary to drug taking (eg, marijuana)

Parenting, altered Related factors: Dysfunctional relationship between parents, change in marital status, psychologic impairment (substance abuse) (see *Family coping* and *Family processes*)

Post-trauma syndrome Related factors: Abuse, accidents, assault, disaster, epidemic, incest, kidnapping, torture, terrorism, participation in combat

Powerlessness Related factors: Pattern of helplessness, failed attempts to abstain, changes in personal/social life

Role performance, altered Related factor: Psychologic impairment (eg, substance abuse)

Self-esteem, chronic low Related factors: Repeatedly unmet expectations, guilt, failed withdrawal, ambivalence

Sensory/perceptual alterations (auditory, kinesthetic, tactile, visual) Related factors: Alcohol intoxication, substance intoxication (specify)

Sexual dysfunction/Sexuality patterns, altered Related factors: *Self-esteem disturbance*, impotence, loss of libido secondary to substance abuse, neurologic damage, debilitation from drug use, embarrassment about changes in appearance (eg, testicular atrophy, spider angiomas)

Sleep pattern disturbance Related factors: Chemical dependence (specify, eg, stimulants), nightmares, difficulty sleeping at night secondary to sleeping during the day

Social interaction, impaired Related factors: Chemical dependence (specify), inability to focus on others, emotional immaturity, aggressiveness, *Anxiety*

Social isolation Related factors: Others' responses to impulsive behaviors, avoidance behaviors and anger, job loss, perceived difference from others

Violence: self-directed or directed at others, risk for Risk factors: Substance intoxication (specify), substance withdrawal (specify), disorientation, impaired judgment, altered perceptions, poor impulse control

Suicide

Suicide actually represents a nursing diagnosis that can be associated with any of the psychiatric diagnoses (eg, schizophrenia, substance abuse). The following nursing diagnoses may also occur for patients who are suicidal.

Nursing Diagnoses

Anxiety Related factors: Threat to self-concept, threat to/change in role functioning, situational/maturational crises, unmet needs, changes in social supports

Coping: individual, ineffective Related factors: Personal vulnerability in situational or maturational crisis (specify)

Decisional conflict Related factors: Perceived threat to value system, lack of support system

Hopelessness Related factors: Abandonment, lack of social supports, lost spiritual belief

Personal identity disturbance Related factor: Situational crisis (specify)

Post-trauma syndrome Related factors: Abuse, accidents, assault, disaster, epidemic, incest, kidnapping, terrorism, torture, catastrophic illness or accident, participation in combat

Rape-trauma syndrome Related factor: Patient's biopsychosocial response to event

Self-esteem, chronic low Related factors: Psychologic impairment (specify), repeatedly unmet expectations

Self-mutilation, risk for Risk factors: Inability to cope with increased psychologic/physiologic tension in a healthy manner; feelings of depression, rejection, self-hatred, separation anxiety, guilt, and depersonalization; fluctuating emotions; drug/alcohol abuse

Sensory/perceptual alterations: (specify) Related factor: Alcohol/substance abuse (specify)

Spiritual distress Related factor: Challenged beliefs and values systems

Thought processes, altered Related factors: Mental disorders (specify), organic mental disorders (specify), personality disorders (specify), substance abuse

Violence: self-directed, risk for Risk factors: History of suicide attempt, command hallucinations, battered women, panic states, history of abuse by others, suicidal ideation, substance abuse

Withdrawn Patient

Associated psychiatric diagnoses include but are not limited to major depression; schizophrenia: disorganized, catatonic, paranoid, and undifferentiated types; schizophreniform disorder; phobic disorders; schizoid personality disorder; avoidant personality disorder; substance use disorders; and organic mental disorders.

Nursing Diagnoses

Anxiety Related factors: Threat to or change in role functioning, real or perceived threat to physical self or to self-concept, unconscious conflicts (eg, values, beliefs), negative self-talk, feelings of apprehension and uneasiness, altered perceptions

Communication, impaired verbal Related factors: Psychologic impairment (specify), refusal to speak or make eye contact

Coping: individual, ineffective Related factor: Personal vulnerability in situational or maturational crisis (specify)

Diversional activity deficit Related factors: Lack of motivation, deficit in social skills, impaired perception of reality

Family processes, altered Related factors: Illness/disability of family member, inability to communicate secondary to withdrawal

Fear Related factors: *Powerlessness*, real or imagined threat to own well-being

Grieving, dysfunctional Related factors: Actual loss (specify), anticipated loss (specify), perceived loss (specify)

Health maintenance, altered Related factors: Lack of ability to make thoughtful and deliberate judgments, significant alteration in communication skills, lack of awareness of environment and own needs

Parenting, altered Related factors: Psychologic impairment (specify), situational crisis (specify), see *Altered family processes*

Personal identity disturbance Related factor: Psychologic impairment (specify)

Role performance, altered Related factor: Psychologic impairment (specify)

Self-esteem disturbance Related factor: Psychologic impairment (specify)

Self-mutilation, risk for Risk factors: Inability to cope with increased psychologic/physiologic tension in a healthy manner; feelings of depression, rejection, self-hatred, separation anxiety, guilt, and depersonalization; need for sensory stimuli

Social interaction, impaired Related factors: Psychologic impairment (specify), *Fear* of social situations, *Anxiety*, depression

Social isolation Related factors: Psychologic impairment (specify), others' difficulty communicating with patient

Thought processes, altered Related factors: Mental disorders (specify), organic mental disorders (specify), personality disorders (specify)

Antepartum and Postpartum Conditions

Abortion, spontaneous or induced

Change in birthing plans

Gestational diabetes

Hyperemesis gravidarum

Maternal infection

Painful breast

Perinatal loss

Postpartum care, uncomplicated

Pregnancy-induced hypertension

Suppression of preterm labor

Uterine bleeding

Abortion, Spontaneous or Induced

Potential Complications (Collaborative Problems)

PC of abortion: Hemorrhage, infection

Nursing Diagnoses

Anxiety Related factors: Threat to health status, ambivalence, *Knowledge deficit* regarding procedures and postprocedural care, unfamiliar sights and sounds, *Fear* of implications for future pregnancies

Coping: individual, ineffective Related factors: Unresolved feelings (eg, guilt) about elective abortion; societal, moral, religious, and family conflicting values; unresolved feelings over loss of baby

Decisional conflict Related factors: Values conflicts, inadequate support system

Family processes, altered Related factors: Effects of elective procedure or spontaneous loss on relationships, inability of family members to agree on decisions, adolescent identity conflicts, preexisting personal or marital conflicts

Grieving, anticipatory/dysfunctional Related factors: Perinatal loss, perceived or actual loss of cultural and/or religious approval

Health maintenance, altered Related factor: *Knowledge deficit* (eg, of contraception, "safer sex")

Infection, risk for Risk factors: Invasive procedures, traumatized tissue, incomplete expulsion of uterine contents

Pain Related factor: Strong uterine contractions

Powerlessness Related factors: Treatment regimen, inability to change the course of events or prevent the loss, perception that there are limited/no options

Self-esteem disturbance Related factors: Unmet expectations for pregnancy, unmet expectations for child, preexisting low self-esteem

Sexual dysfunction/Sexuality patterns, altered Related factors: *Self-esteem disturbance*, fear of pregnancy, unstable relationship with significant others, *Body image disturbance*

Spiritual distress Related factors: Test of spiritual beliefs, unresolved feelings about elective abortion, inability to find meaning in spontaneous abortion

Change in Birthing Plans

May include any deviation from a couple's original birthing plans. Such a change may include but is not limited to use of analgesia, anesthesia, or forceps; limitation of visitors; episiotomy, and cesarean birth.

Nursing Diagnoses

Family processes, altered Related factors: Unmet expectations for childbirth, situational crisis (eg, fetal distress), separation of family members (eg, emergency hysterectomy secondary to uterine rupture)

Fear Related factors: Real or imagined threat to child or to own well-being, unfamiliar equipment, urgency of emergency procedures

Pain Related factors: Surgery, episiotomy, uterine contractions, invasive procedures

Parent/infant/child attachment, risk for altered Risk factors: Unmet expectations for childbirth, separation of family members

Powerlessness Related factors: Complication threatening pregnancy, perceived inability to effect outcome of situation, inability to cope with overwhelming uterine contractions

Self-esteem disturbance Related factors: Unmet expectations for childbirth (eg, inability to "tolerate" uterine contractions, inability to deliver vaginally)

Gestational Diabetes

Potential Complications (Collaborative Problems)

PC of gestational diabetes: Anemia, dystocia, fetal morbidity/mortality, hydramnios, ketoacidosis, pregnancy-induced hypertension, pyelonephritis

Nursing Diagnoses

Family processes, altered Related factors: Hospitalization/change in environment, illness/disability of family member, inadequate finances

Fear Related factors: Environmental stressors/hospitalization, *Powerlessness*, real or imagined threat to own well-being, real or imagined threat to child, implications for future pregnancies

Infection (urinary tract infection, vaginitis), risk for Risk factors: Favorable environment for bacterial growth secondary to glycosuria

Injury, risk for (maternal or fetal) Risk factors: Hypoglycemia, hyperglycemia

Nutrition: less than body requirements, altered Related factors: Inadequate intake to support increased calorie needs of pregnancy, secondary to limited exposure to basic nutritional knowledge; *Nausea*

Nutrition: more than body requirements, altered Related factors: Limited exposure to new basic nutritional knowledge, imbalance between intake and available insulin

Sensory/perceptual alterations (visual) Related factor: Increase in diabetic retinopathy

Hyperemesis Gravidarum

Potential Complications (Collaborative Problems)

PC of hyperemesis: Bleeding secondary to hypothrombinemia, fetal death, fluid/electrolyte imbalance, hypotension, negative nitrogen balance, peripheral neuropathy

Nursing Diagnoses

Activity intolerance Related factors: Inadequate nutrition, dehydration, decreased activity

Coping: individual, ineffective Related factors: Personal vulnerability during health crisis, projected role changes, worry about safety of fetus

Family processes, altered Related factors: Hospitalization/change in environment, illness/disability of family member, threats to job security (of patient or spouse), need for child care for siblings

Fatigue See *Activity intolerance*

Fear Related factor: Real or imagined threat to child

Fluid volume deficit Related factors: Inadequate fluid intake secondary to *Nausea*, abnormal fluid loss secondary to vomiting

Nutrition: less than body requirements, altered Related factors: Limited intake of nutrients secondary to *Nausea*, loss of nutrients secondary to vomiting

Parenting, risk for altered See *Role performance, altered*

Powerlessness Related factors: Complications threatening pregnancy, perceived/actual inability to change the course of events

Role performance, altered Related factors: Unmet expectations for pregnancy, *Nausea*, hospitalization

Self-esteem disturbance Related factors: Unmet expectations for pregnancy, inability to meet role demands (eg, work, mother, spouse)

Maternal Infection

Includes but is not limited to active genital herpes, amnionitis, acquired immune deficiency syndrome (AIDS), and hepatitis B.

Potential Complications (Collaborative Problems)

PC of infection: Fetal morbidity/mortality, sepsis

Nursing Diagnoses

Activity intolerance Related factors: Disease process, malaise

Body image disturbance Related factors: Pregnancy, odors and lesions secondary to infection, precautions regarding hand washing and spread of infection

Breastfeeding, interrupted Related factors: Maternal illness, maternal medications that are contraindicated for the infant

Diversional activity deficit See *Loneliness*

Family processes, altered Related factors: Change in family roles, hospitalization/change in environment, unresolved feelings about how the infection was acquired

Fear Related factor: Real or imagined threat to child

Infection, risk for Risk factor: Presence of lesions (eg, herpes) predispose patient to secondary infections

Infection (transmission), risk for Risk factor: Contagious nature of disease (eg, herpes, hepatitis B)

Loneliness Related factor: Therapeutic isolation

Pain Related factors: Cesarean birth, infection, lesions

Parenting, altered Risk factor: Delayed parent/infant attachment secondary to need for infection precautions

Self-esteem disturbance Related factors: Cesarean birth, inability to assume new role, inability to fulfill usual role requirements (eg, wife, mother, worker)

Social interaction, impaired Related factor: Therapeutic isolation

Painful Breast

Includes but is not limited to sore, cracked nipples, engorgement, and mastitis.

Potential Complications (Collaborative Problems)

PC of cracked nipples, engorgement: Mastitis
PC of mastitis: Abscess

Nursing Diagnoses

Breastfeeding, ineffective. See *Interrupted breastfeeding*

Breastfeeding, interrupted Related factors: *Pain*, engorgement; sore, cracked nipples; mastitis; maternal medications that are contraindicated for the infant

Health maintenance, altered Related factors: Limited exposure to information about breast hygiene, care of nipples, treatments, and/or signs and symptoms of infection

Pain Related factors: Sore nipples, breast engorgement, edema and inflammation of breast tissues

Parent/infant/child attachment, risk for altered Risk factors: *Pain*, unmet expectations

Role performance, altered Related factors: Assumption of new role, unmet expectations for childbirth, *Pain*/discomfort, *Interrupted breastfeeding*

Skin integrity (nipples), impaired Risk factors: Inadequate breast care, improper positioning of baby at breast, incorrect sucking by infant

Perinatal Loss

Includes but is not limited to less-than-perfect baby, miscarriage, stillbirth, adoption, and elective abortion.

Nursing Diagnoses

Coping: family, ineffective, compromised/disabling Related factor: Chronically unresolved feelings about loss

Coping: individual, ineffective Related factor: Personal vulnerability in a situational crisis

Family processes, altered Related factors: Illness/disability of baby, fetal demise, stillbirth, lack of adequate support system, *Dysfunctional grieving*, conflicting styles of grieving among family members, guilt, blaming

Fear Related factors: Real or imagined threat to child, environmental stressors/hospitalization, *Powerlessness*, implications for future pregnancies

Grieving, anticipatory Related factors: Imminent loss of child, anticipated loss of perfect child

Grieving, dysfunctional Related factors: Inability to resolve feelings about actual or anticipated loss of child or of perfect child, marital discord, lack of support system

Parenting, altered Related factors: Interruption in bonding process, unrealistic expectations of self or partner (see *Altered family processes*)

Powerlessness Related factors: Complication threatening pregnancy, inability to change course of events

Role performance, altered Related factors: *Dysfunctional grieving* secondary to loss of child, birth of less-than-perfect baby, guilt, blame

Self-esteem disturbance Related factors: Unmet expectations for child, feelings of failure (eg, to produce a perfect child)

Sexual dysfunction Related factors: Medically imposed restrictions, *Fear* of harming fetus, *Self-esteem disturbance*, *Fear* of another pregnancy

Spiritual distress Related factors: Test of spiritual beliefs, intense suffering

Postpartum Care, Uncomplicated

Potential Complications (Collaborative Problems)

PC of Childbirth: Hematoma; hemorrhage secondary to uterine atony, retained placental fragments, lacerations; infection/sepsis

Nursing Diagnoses

Anxiety Related factors: Changes in role functioning, inexperience

Body image disturbance Related factors: Lack of or inaccurate information about body's adjustment after delivery, change in body appearance (eg, striae)

Breastfeeding, effective Related factors: Basic breastfeeding knowledge, normal breast structure, normal infant oral structure, gestational age of more than 34 weeks, supportive resources, maternal confidence

Breastfeeding, ineffective Related factors: *Interrupted breastfeeding*, inexperience, cultural influences, breast engorgement, infant factors (eg, inability to latch on or suck)

Constipation Related factors: *Fear* of painful defecation, decreased peristalsis after delivery, decreased activity, decreased fluid intake, effects of analgesics, decreased tone of abdominal muscles

Family processes, altered Related factors: Transition in family roles, change in family structure, lack of adequate support systems

Health maintenance, altered Related factors: *Knowledge deficit* (eg, hygiene, contraception, nutrition, infant care, symptoms of complications), lack of support from partner

Home maintenance management, impaired Related factors: Inadequate support system, lack of organizational skills, *Ineffective individual coping*

Incontinence, urinary, stress Related factor: Tissue trauma during delivery

Nutrition: less than body requirements, altered Related factor: Lack of basic nutritional knowledge concerning lactation

Pain Related factors: Episiotomy, sore nipples, breast engorgement, hemorrhoids, sore muscles, uterine contractions (afterpains)

Parent/infant/child attachment, risk for altered See *Altered parenting*

Parenting, altered Related factors: Lack of knowledge/skill regarding effective parenting; unrealistic expectations of self, infant, and partner; unwanted child; no role models; inexperience

Role performance, altered Related factor: Assumption of new role

Sexuality patterns, altered Related factors: *Pain*, *Fear* of pain, *Body image disturbance*, demands of infant, lack of sleep

Sleep pattern disturbance Related factors: Excessive social demands, role demands (eg, frequent breastfeeding), *Pain*, *Anxiety*, exhilaration/excitement

Urinary retention Related factors: Local tissue edema, effects of medication/anesthesia, *Pain*, inability to assume normal voiding position secondary to effects of epidural anesthesia/analgesia

Pregnancy-Induced Hypertension (PIH)

PIH is sometimes referred to as toxemia of pregnancy, preeclampsia, and eclampsia.

Potential Complications (Collaborative Problems)

PC of magnesium sulfate therapy: Magnesium toxicity

PC of PIH: Cerebral edema, coma, fetal morbidity/mortality, HELLP syndrome (<u>h</u>emolysis, <u>e</u>levated <u>l</u>iver enzymes, <u>l</u>ow <u>p</u>latelet count), hypertension (malignant), pulmonary edema, renal insufficiency/damage, seizures

PC of malignant hypertension: Uncontrolled hypertension: cerebral hemorrhage

PC of seizures: Precipitous birth, fetal bradycardia, placental separation

Nursing Diagnoses

Activity intolerance Related factors: Imbalance between oxygen supply and demand; lethargy, weakness, and *Fatigue* secondary to prescribed bed rest and magnesium sulfate side effects; preeclampsia

Body image disturbance Related factors: Changes in appearance related to pregnancy and edema

Breathing pattern, ineffective Related factor: Side effects of magnesium sulfate

Constipation Related factors: Side effects of magnesium sulfate, decreased activity, decreased intake of fiber

Diversional activity deficit Related factor: Prolonged bed rest

Family processes, altered Related factors: Hospitalization/change in environment, illness/disability of family member, enforced bed rest, role changes

Fear Related factors: Changes in birthing plans, real or imagined threat to child (eg, premature labor), environmental stressors/hospitalization, threat to own well-being

Fluid volume deficit (intravascular) Related factors: Intercompartmental fluid shifts secondary to loss of plasma proteins and decreased plasma colloid osmotic pressure

Fluid volume excess (extracellular tissues) Related factors: Sodium and water retention, fluid shift into extracellular spaces secondary to decreased plasma colloid osmotic pressure

Home maintenance management, impaired Related factors: Inadequate support system, *Knowledge deficit*, inability to perform usual roles

Injury, risk for (maternal and fetal) Risk factors: Seizure activity, inadequate placental perfusion, falls secondary to vertigo or postural hypotension, visual disturbances, fetal distress secondary to inadequate placental perfusion

Nausea Related factor: Side effect of magnesium sulfate

Noncompliance Related factors: Unable to comply with bed rest secondary to perceived demands of role (eg, care of siblings), perceived negative effects of medical regimen (eg, unpalatable diet), perception that condition is not serious secondary to having no subjectively unpleasant symptoms, *Knowledge deficit* (eg, related to disease, treatments, symptom relief, dietary restrictions)

Nutrition: less than body requirements, altered Related factors: Lack of basic nutritional knowledge, loss of appetite, *Nausea*/vomiting, drowsiness secondary to medications

Pain Related factors: Epigastric (precursor to eclampsia), headache secondary to magnesium sulfate administration

Sensory/perceptual alterations (visual) Related factor: Alterations precede eclampsia

Tissue perfusion, altered: cerebral, renal, placental. Related factors: Vasospasm (spiral arteries), edema, decreased intravascular volume

Suppression of Preterm Labor

Potential Complications (Collaborative Problems)

PC of preterm labor: Preterm delivery of infant, pulmonary edema (secondary to tocolytic medications)

PC of magnesium sulfate therapy: Magnesium toxicity

Nursing Diagnoses

Anxiety Related factors: Outcome of pregnancy, side effects of tocolytics, insufficient time to prepare for labor or infant care

Diversional activity deficit Related factor: Prolonged bed rest

Family processes, altered Related factors: Illness/disability of family member, change in family roles, lack of adequate support systems, enforced bed rest

Fear Related factor: Possibility of early labor and delivery

Home maintenance management, impaired Related factors: Inadequate support system, enforced bed rest

Management of therapeutic regimen management: individual, ineffective Related factors: *Knowledge deficit*s, excessive demands made on individual/family, social support deficits

Nausea Related factor: Side effects of tocolytic medications

Pain (headache) Related factor: Side effects of magnesium sulfate

Powerlessness Related factors: Complications threatening pregnancy, lack of improvement despite complying with bed rest and medication regimen

Self-esteem disturbance Related factors: Unmet expectations for childbirth, inability to fulfill usual roles

Sexual dysfunction Related factors: Medically imposed restrictions, *Fear* of harming fetus, *Fear* of causing uterine contractions

Sleep pattern disturbance Related factors: Frequency of medication and monitoring

Uterine Bleeding

Includes but is not limited to the following conditions. (1) Antepartal bleeding may result from first trimester spotting, placenta previa, abruptio placentae, uterine rupture, or hydatidiform mole; (2) postpartal bleeding may be a consequence of postpartum hemorrhage/shock or uterine atony.

Potential Complications (Collaborative Problems)

PC of uterine bleeding: Anemia, disseminated intravascular coagulation, fetal death, renal failure, sepsis, shock

Nursing Diagnoses

Breastfeeding, interrupted Related factors: Maternal illness, *Fatigue*, *Activity intolerance*, activities of caregivers

Cardiac output, decreased Related factor: Hypovolemia

Diversional activity deficit Related factors: Prolonged bed rest and/or activity limitations

Family processes, altered Related factors: Change in family roles, patient's inability to assume usual role, hospitalization/change in environment

Fear Related factors: Threat to the pregnancy and/or baby, threat to own well-being, *Powerlessness*, environmental stressors/hospitalization, implications for future pregnancies

Grieving, anticipatory Related factors: Possible loss of pregnancy and expected child, possible effect on future childbearing abilities secondary to intractable postpartum hemorrhage

Home maintenance management, impaired Related factors: Inadequate support system, prescribed bed rest, *Activity intolerance* secondary to blood loss and anemia

Infection, risk for Risk factors: Traumatized tissue, invasive procedures, blood loss, partial separation of placenta

Mobility: physical, impaired Related factors: Increased bleeding in response to activity, presence of lines (eg, intravenous, urinary catheter, fetal monitor)

Pain Related factors: Surgical procedure, uterine contractions, collection of blood between placenta and uterine wall

Powerlessness Related factors: Complications threatening pregnancy or future pregnancies

Self-care deficit: (specify) Related factors: Medically imposed restrictions, *Activity intolerance* secondary to blood loss

Self-esteem disturbance Related factors: Unmet expectations for childbirth, inability to perform usual role functions

Sexual dysfunction Related factors: Medically imposed restrictions, *Fear* of harming fetus, *Fear* of starting labor or increasing bleeding

Tissue perfusion, altered [placental] Related factors: Imbalance between oxygen supply/demand to the fetus secondary to hypovolemia, hypotension, placental separation

Newborn Conditions

Congenital anomalies

Drug withdrawal

Feeding problems

High-risk infant

Hyperbilirubinemia

Hypoglycemia

Hypothermia

Low birth weight/small for gestational age

Normal newborn

Respiratory distress

Congenital Anomalies

Includes but is not limited to infants with serious congenital anomalies (eg, congenital heart disease, meningomyelocele, choanal atresia, tracheoesophageal fistula).

Potential Complications (Collaborative Problems)

PC of congenital heart disease: Congestive heart failure, dysrhythmias

PC of meningomyelocele: Hydrocephalus, neurovascular deficits below lesion

PC of tracheoesophageal fistula: Aspiration pneumonia, choking

Nursing Diagnoses

Activity intolerance Related factor: Imbalance between oxygen supply and demand

Aspiration, risk for Risk factor: Secondary to tracheoesophageal fistula

Breastfeeding, ineffective Related factors: Infant *Fatigue*, inadequate sucking reflex, interrupted or infrequent feeding, difficulty breathing, secondary to cardiac anomaly

Breastfeeding, interrupted Related factor: Infant illness

Breathing pattern, ineffective Related factors: Decreased energy/*Fatigue* secondary to cardiac anomaly, aspiration pneumonia

Cardiac output, decreased Related factors: Increased ventricular workload, hypovolemia, cardiac anomaly (specify)

Caregiver role strain Related factors: Illness severity of the infant; premature birth/congenital defect; unpredictable illness course; situational stressors within the family; complexity and duration of caregiving; caregiver's health; lack of developmental readiness, knowledge, skills, or experience; competing role commitments; ineffective coping styles; isolation; limited opportunity for respite and recreation

Development, risk for altered See *Growth, risk for altered*

Family processes, altered Related factors: Unmet expectations for child, separation of family members, illness/disability of infant, immaturity of parents, lack of resources, lack of social supports, lack of knowledge

Fatigue Related factor: Disease process (eg, cardiac anomaly, aspiration pneumonia)

Fear Related factor: Real threat to child

Gas exchange, impaired Related factors: Decreased pulmonary blood supply secondary to pulmonary hypertension, congestive heart failure, respiratory distress syndrome, decreased functional lung tissue secondary to respiratory distress syndrome, atelectasis

Grieving, anticipatory Related factor: Anticipatory loss of child

Growth, risk for altered Risk factors: Congenital anomaly, fetal distress, prematurity, unhealthy maternal lifestyle during pregnancy, serious illness, delayed bonding secondary to infant's condition or parent's unmet expectations

Infant feeding pattern, ineffective Related factors: Prematurity, neurologic impairment/delay, prolonged NPO status, anatomical abnormalities (eg, of esophagus and stomach), *Fatigue* and difficulty breathing secondary to heart anomaly

Injury, risk for Related factors: Meningomyelocele, omphalocele, other defects creating vulnerability

Nutrition: less than body requirements, altered Related factors: Difficulty in swallowing, inadequate sucking reflex in infant, vomiting, food intolerance

Mobility: physical, impaired Related factors: *Fatigue* secondary to inadequate oxygenation, spinal cord lesions

Skin integrity, impaired Related factors: Impaired circulation, immobility (eg, inability to move lower extremities), altered nutritional status

Sleep pattern disturbance Related factor: Sleep deprivation secondary to frequent therapeutic interventions

Spontaneous ventilation, inability to sustain Related factors: Metabolic factors, respiratory muscle fatigue, pulmonary immaturity

Tissue perfusion, altered (peripheral) Related factors: Imbalance between oxygen supply/demand secondary to high metabolic rate, *Decreased cardiac output, Impaired gas exchange*

Urinary retention Related factor: Congenital anomaly affecting spinal cord (specify)

Ventilatory weaning response, dysfunctional (DVWR) Related factors: Pulmonary immaturity, *Impaired gas exchange*, *Ineffective airway clearance*, ventilator dependence > one week

Drug Withdrawal

Potential Complications (Collaborative Problems)

PC of drug withdrawal: Dehydration, drug/alcohol withdrawal, electrolyte imbalances, respiratory distress syndrome, seizures, sepsis, tachypnea

Nursing Diagnoses

Aspiration, risk for Related factor: Oral feeding of infant with central nervous system irritability

Breastfeeding, ineffective Related factors: Infant fatigue, poor nursing secondary to alcohol/drug exposure in utero and growth-deficient status at birth

Breathing pattern, ineffective Related factors: Depression of respiratory center secondary to _____ (specify drug), meconium aspiration pneumonia

Coping: family, ineffective, disabling Related factors: Arbitrary disregard for patient's needs, overwhelming needs of infant in the presence of poor coping skills and continued drug use by parent(s)

Family processes: alcoholism, altered Related factors: Alcohol use by parent(s), lack of support from others, lack of coping skills

Development, altered (eg, failure to thrive), risk for See *Growth, risk for altered*

Diarrhea Related factor: Hyperperistalsis secondary to narcotic withdrawal

Disorganized infant behavior Related factors: Abnormal structural development and central nervous system dysfunction secondary to alcohol/drug exposure in utero, prematurity secondary to maternal drug use, fetal withdrawal in utero

Fluid volume deficit Related factors: Inadequate fluid intake secondary to inadequate sucking reflex, vomiting secondary to fetal alcohol syndrome or narcotic withdrawal

Growth, risk for altered (eg, small for gestational age) Risk factors: Unhealthy maternal lifestyle during pregnancy, intrauterine exposure to alcohol/drugs

Home maintenance management, impaired Related factors: Physical/psychologic impairment of family member other than infant, inadequate support system, insufficient family organization or planning, continued substance abuse by parent(s)

Infant feeding pattern, ineffective Related factors: Neurologic impairment/delay (see *Breastfeeding, ineffective*), lethargy, failure to thrive secondary to fetal alcohol syndrome

Injury, risk for Risk factors: Psychomotor hyperactivity, seizure activity

Nutrition: less than body requirements, altered Related factors: Chemical dependence/withdrawal, inadequate sucking reflex in infant, vomiting, food intolerance, failure to thrive secondary to fetal alcohol syndrome

Parent/infant/child attachment, risk for altered See *Parenting, altered*

Parenting, altered Related factors: Psychologic/developmental impairment of infant, substance abuse by parent(s), presence of stressors (eg, legal, financial), interrupted bonding process, difficulty interacting with a child with inability to express feelings of pleasure, anger, and so forth

Sensory/perceptual alterations (specify) Related factors: Hypersensitivity to environmental stimuli, inability to maintain alertness and attentiveness to environment, difficulty with attending to and engaging in auditory and visual stimuli

Skin integrity, impaired Related factors: Excoriated buttocks, knees, elbows; facial scratches; pressure point abrasions—all secondary to intrauterine/newborn withdrawal or abstinence syndrome; diaphoresis; *Diarrhea*

Sleep pattern disturbance Related factors: Sleep deprivation secondary to _____ (specify), effect of depressants or stimulants on central nervous system in utero, newborn withdrawal

Feeding Problems

Include but are not limited to food allergies or intolerances, malabsorption, or motor problems that affect the infant's ability to consume food.

Nursing Diagnoses

Breastfeeding, ineffective Related factors: Inadequate sucking reflex in infant, infant fatigue secondary to illnesses such as respiratory distress syndrome or heart anomalies, inability of infant to "latch on," central nervous system anomalies, prematurity

Diarrhea Related factor: Food intolerance

Disorganized infant behavior Related factors: Abnormal structural development and central nervous system dysfunction, prematurity

Family processes, altered Related factors: Illness/disability of family member, separation of family members

Fluid volume deficit Related factors: Inadequate fluid intake, psychomotor immaturity (eg, poor suck-swallow response), inadequate milk production, *Diarrhea*

Infant feeding pattern, ineffective Related factors: Prematurity, neurologic impairment/delay, oral hypersensitivity, prolonged NPO status, anatomical abnormalities

Nutrition: less than body requirements, altered Related factors: Difficulty in swallowing, inadequate sucking reflex in the infant, vomiting, food intolerance, failure to thrive, insufficient maternal milk production

Swallowing, impaired Related factor: Motor problem (specify)

High-Risk Infant

Includes but is not limited to birth asphyxia, meconium aspiration, prematurity, postmaturity, large for gestational age (LGA), small for gestational age (SGA), premature rupture of membranes, maternal infection, infant of diabetic mother, intrauterine growth retardation, infant of adolescent mother, infant of chemically dependent mother, and lack of prenatal care.

Potential Complications (Collaborative Problems)

PC of *in utero* infections: Anemia, cataracts, congenital heart disease, deafness, hepatosplenomegaly, hydrocephalus, hyperbilirubinemia, mental retardation, microcephaly, seizures, septicemia, thrombocytopenic purpura

PC of prematurity: Acidosis, apnea, bradycardia, cold stress, hyperbilirubinemia, hypocalcemia, hypoglycemia, pneumonia, respiratory distress syndrome, seizures, sepsis

PC of postmaturity: Birth asphyxia, birth trauma secondary to LGA status, central nervous system depression, cerebral edema, hypoglycemia, intestinal absorption problems, meconium aspiration, polycythemia (due to SGA status), renal tubular necrosis

Nursing Diagnoses

Activity intolerance Related factors: Inadequate oxygenation secondary to respiratory insufficiency, *Ineffective airway clearance*, respiratory distress syndrome

Airway clearance, ineffective Related factors: Meconium aspiration, tracheobronchial secretions

Aspiration, risk for Risk factors: Immobility, increased secretions, presence of enteral or tracheal tubes

Body temperature, risk for altered See *Thermoregulation, ineffective*

Breastfeeding, ineffective Related factors: Infant *Fatigue*, inadequate sucking reflex, interrupted or infrequent feeding

Breastfeeding, interrupted Related factors: Infant illness, prematurity, maternal obligations outside the home, abrupt weaning of infant

Breathing pattern, ineffective Related factors: Decreased energy/*Fatigue* secondary to illness (eg, sepsis, respiratory distress syndrome), medication side effects, immature respiratory center, metabolic imbalances

Cardiac output, decreased Related factors: Increased ventricular workload, hypovolemia, cardiac anomaly (specify)

Caregiver role strain Related factors: Illness severity of the infant; premature birth/congenital defect; unpredictable illness course; situational stressors within the family; chronicity of caregiving; caregiver's health; lack of developmental readiness, knowledge, skills, or experience; competing role commitments; ineffective coping styles; isolation; limited opportunity for respite and recreation

Constipation Related factors: Decreased activity and decreased motility secondary to prematurity

Diarrhea Related factor: Increased intestinal motility secondary to inflammation

Disorganized infant behavior Related factors: Immature central nervous system and excess environmental stimulation

Development, risk for altered. See *Growth, risk for altered.*

Family processes, altered Related factors: Illness/disability of family member, separation of family members

Fear (parental) Related factor: Threat to child

Fluid volume deficit Related factors: Abnormal blood loss, abnormal fluid loss (specify, eg, diarrhea, diaphoresis), inadequate fluid intake secondary to _____ (specify, eg, poor sucking reflex)

Fluid volume excess Related factor: Decreased urinary output secondary to heart failure

Gas exchange, impaired Related factors: Decreased functional lung tissue secondary to pneumonia, chronic lung disease, atelectasis, alveolar capillary membrane changes secondary to inadequate surfactant, cold stress, immature central nervous system

Grieving, anticipatory (parental) Related factor: Imminent loss of child

Growth, risk for altered Risk factors: Congenital anomaly, fetal distress, prematurity, unhealthy maternal lifestyle during pregnancy, serious illness

Home maintenance management, impaired Related factors: Inadequate support system, insufficient family organization or planning, complex needs of infant

Infant feeding pattern, ineffective Related factors: Prematurity, neurologic impairment/delay, prolonged NPO status, anatomical abnormalities, lethargy

Infection, risk for Risk factors: Inadequate immune system; lack of normal flora; insufficient family knowledge, organization, or planning; invasive treatments/lines; open wounds (eg, circumcision, umbilical cord), *in utero* infection

Infection (transmission), risk for Risk factor: Contagious nature of organism acquired *in utero*

Nutrition: less than body requirements, altered Related factors: Inadequate sucking reflex in the infant, vomiting, food intolerance, high metabolic rate

Skin integrity, impaired Related factors: Fragility of skin, immobility, susceptibility to infections, and lack of normal skin flora secondary to prematurity; absence of vernix and prolonged exposure to amniotic fluid secondary to postmaturity and LGA status

Spontaneous ventilation, inability to sustain Related factors: Metabolic factors, respiratory muscle fatigue, pulmonary immaturity

Thermoregulation, ineffective Related factors: Prematurity (immature central nervous system, decreased body-mass to body-surface ratio, minimal subcutaneous fat, limited brown fat, inability to shiver or sweat), transition to extrauterine environment, exposure to environment secondary to need for frequent treatments/interventions

Ventilatory weaning response, dysfunctional (DVWR) Related factors: Pulmonary immaturity, *Impaired gas exchange, Ineffective airway clearance*, ventilator dependence > one week

Hyperbilirubinemia

Potential Complications (Collaborative Problems)

PC of hyperbilirubinemia: Anemia, hepatosplenomegaly, hydrops fetalis (including hepatosplenomegaly, anasarca, hydrothorax, ascites, thrombocytopenia, hypoglycemia secondary to adrenal and pancreatic hyperplasia), kernicterus, renal failure

PC of kernicterus: Athetosis, hearing loss, intellectual deficits

PC of phototherapy: Dehydration, diarrhea, hyperthermia, hypothermia, weight loss, retinal damage, corneal abrasions)

Nursing Diagnoses

Breastfeeding, ineffective Related factor: Poor sucking reflex secondary to kernicterus

Breastfeeding, interrupted Related factor: Infant illness

Diarrhea Related factors: Dietary changes, phototherapy

Family processes, altered Related factor: Separation of family members

Fluid volume deficit Related factors: Abnormal fluid loss (specify, eg, *Diarrhea* and insensible loss secondary to phototherapy), inadequate fluid intake secondary to _____ (specify)

Injury, risk for Related factor: Reabsorption of bilirubin secondary to decreased defecation

Nutrition: less than body requirements, altered Related factors: Lethargy, inadequate sucking reflex in infant

Parent/infant/child attachment, risk for altered Related factors: Lack of visual stimulation and contact secondary to phototherapy, *Fear* of hurting infant or displacing tubes/lines

Parenting, altered Related factor: Interruption in bonding process

Sensory/perceptual alterations: (visual, tactile) Related factor: Sensory deficit secondary to use of eye patches for protection of eyes during phototherapy, lack of tactile stimulation

Skin integrity, impaired Related/risk factors: *Diarrhea*, drying of skin secondary to phototherapy, pruritus, excretion of bilirubin in urine and feces, exposure to phototherapy

Sleep pattern disturbance Related factors: Sleep deprivation secondary to frequent assessment and treatments, discomfort, environmental stimuli

Tissue integrity, impaired (corneal) Related factors: Phototherapy, continuous wearing of eye pads

Hypoglycemia

Potential Complications (Collaborative Problems)

PC of hypoglycemia: Apnea, central nervous system damage, respiratory distress, seizures, tremors, jerkiness

Nursing Diagnoses

Cardiac output, decreased Related factor: Poor cardiac contractility

Family processes, altered Related factors: Illness of infant, separation of family members, ineffective coping, *Knowledge deficit*s

Injury, risk for Risk factor: Seizure activity

Nutrition: less than body requirements, altered Related factors: Inadequate sucking reflex in infant, high metabolic rate/physiologic stress, vomiting, loss of swallowing reflex

Hypothermia

Potential Complications (Collaborative Problems)

PC of hypothermia: Atelectasis, hyperbilirubinemia, hypoglycemia, hypoxemia, metabolic acidosis

Nursing Diagnoses

Breathing pattern, ineffective Related factor: Decreased energy/*fatigue*, atelectasis

Cardiac output, decreased Related factor: Bradycardia

Family processes, altered Related factor: Separation of family members, *Anxiety, Ineffective coping*

Nutrition: less than body requirements, altered Related factor: Loss of/decreased appetite

Tissue perfusion, altered (peripheral) Related factors: Imbalance between oxygen supply/demand, hypoxemia secondary to atelectasis and pulmonary vasoconstriction

Low Birth Weight/Small for Gestational Age

Potential Complications (Collaborative Problems)

PC of SGA: Aspiration syndrome; hypocalcemia; hypoglycemia, causing central nervous system abnormalities, and mental retardation; hypothermia; perinatal asphyxia; polycythemia

Nursing Diagnoses

Activity intolerance Related factor: Weakness/*Fatigue*

Airway clearance, ineffective Related factors: Decreased energy/*Fatigue*, meconium aspiration

Body temperature, risk for altered Risk factors: Diminished subcutaneous fat, large body surface compared to body mass, decreased brown fat stores

Breastfeeding, ineffective Related factors: Infant *Fatigue*, inadequate sucking reflex, interrupted or infrequent feeding

Breastfeeding, interrupted Related factor: Illness of infant

Breathing pattern, ineffective Related factor: Decreased energy/*Fatigue*

Family processes, altered Related factors: Illness/disability of family member, separation of family members, feelings of guilt, blame

Fatigue Related factors: Decreased energy, high metabolic rate, poor oxygenation

Fluid volume deficit Related factor: Inadequate fluid intake

Gas exchange, impaired Related factors: Decreased pulmonary blood supply secondary to respiratory distress syndrome; decreased functional lung tissue secondary to atelectasis, respiratory distress syndrome, and meconium aspiration

Grieving, dysfunctional Related factor: Anticipated or perceived loss of the perfect child

Home maintenance management, impaired Related factors: Inadequate support system, insufficient family organization or planning, lack of resources, lack of support

Infant feeding pattern, ineffective See *Altered nutrition: less than body requirements*

Nutrition: less than body requirements, altered Related factors: Inadequate sucking reflex in infant, food intolerance, high metabolic rate, decreased glycogen stores

Parent/infant/child attachment, risk for altered Risk factors: Infant's illness, need for technologic support, long hospitalization

Parenting, altered Related factor: Prolonged separation of newborn and parents

Skin integrity, impaired Related factors: Fragile, dry, desquamating skin; lack of subcutaneous fat

Sleep pattern disturbance Related factor: Sleep deprivation secondary to frequent therapeutic interventions

Tissue perfusion, altered (peripheral) Related factors: Imbalance between oxygen supply/demand, increased blood viscosity

Normal Newborn

Potential Complications (Collaborative Problems)

PC of adjustment to extrauterine life: Bleeding secondary to circumcision, cold stress, hemorrhagic disease of newborn, hyperbilirubinemia, hypoglycemia, meconium aspiration pneumonia

Nursing Diagnoses

Airway clearance, ineffective Related factors: Oropharynx secretions, obligatory nose breather, apnea

Body temperature, risk for altered Risk factors: Large body surface-to-mass ratio, inability to shiver, extrauterine transition

Fluid volume deficit Related factors: Inadequate oral intake, increased metabolic rate secondary to excessive handling of newborn

Infection, risk for Risk factors: Lack of acquired immunity, inadequate primary defenses (eg, open wound such as circumcision) and secondary defenses (eg, altered phagocytosis), lack of normal flora, exposure to pathogens (eg, *Neisseria gonorrhoeae*) during passage through birth canal

Nutrition: less than body requirements, altered Related factors: *Ineffective breastfeeding*, inadequate breast milk production, inadequate glucose stores, parental *Knowledge deficit*

Pain Related factors: Circumcision, gastroesophageal reflux, colic

Parent/infant attachment, risk for altered Risk factors: *Anxiety* about parenting, unmet expectations of parents for labor, delivery, and infant; lack of early parent-infant contact; marital discord; lack of privacy during immediate postpartum period

Parenting, altered Related factors: *Knowledge deficit* (eg, related to infant care, follow-up visits), *Anxiety* over new roles, lack of support, financial problems, marital problems

Skin integrity, impaired Related/risk factors: Lack of normal skin flora, inadequate primary or secondary defenses, relative fragility of skin

Thermoregulation, ineffective See *Body temperature, risk for altered*

Urinary retention Related factor: Urethral obstruction secondary to postcircumcision edema

Respiratory Distress

Includes but is not limited to bronchopulmonary dysplasia, respiratory distress syndrome/hyaline membrane disease, meconium aspiration, pneumonia, pneumothorax, and transient tachypnea.

Potential Complications (Collaborative Problems)

PC of respiratory distress: Acidosis, atelectasis, cardiopulmonary shunting, hypoxemia, respiratory failure

Nursing Diagnoses

Activity intolerance Related factor: Weakness/*Fatigue* secondary to inadequate oxygenation and respiratory difficulty

Airway clearance, ineffective Related factors: Decreased energy/*Fatigue*, tracheobronchial secretions

Aspiration, risk for Risk factors: Presence of enteral or tracheal tubes, increased oropharyngeal secretions

Breastfeeding, interrupted Related factors: Prematurity, infant illness

Breathing pattern, ineffective Related factors: Decreased energy/*Fatigue*, dependence on ventilator

Cardiac output, decreased Related factors: Increased ventricular workload, cardiac anomaly (specify), hypotension

Caregiver role strain Related/risk factors: Life-threatening illness, premature birth/congenital defect; unpredictable illness course; situational stressors within the family; chronicity of caregiving; caregiver's health; lack of developmental readiness, knowledge, skills, or experience; competing role commitments; ineffective coping styles; isolation; limited opportunity for respite and recreation; financial difficulties

Constipation Related factor: Decreased fluid intake

Coping: family, ineffective, compromised/disabling Related factors: Life-threatening illness, ineffective communication among family members, lack of support, lack of resources (see *Caregiver role strain*)

Family processes, altered Related factors: Illness/disability of family member, separation of family members (see *Caregiver role strain* and *Coping: family, ineffective, compromised/disabling*)

Fatigue Related factor: Disease process

Fear (parental) Related factor: Real threat to child

Fluid volume deficit Related factors: Inadequate fluid intake secondary to *Fatigue* with oral feedings, prescribed fluid restrictions (eg, to treat cerebral edema), abnormal fluid loss (insensible water loss secondary to rapid respiratory rate)

Gas exchange, impaired Related factors: Decreased pulmonary blood supply secondary to pulmonary hypertension/persistent fetal circulation, respiratory distress syndrome, decreased functional lung tissue secondary to pneumonia, atelectasis, respiratory distress syndrome, diaphragmatic hernia

Grieving, anticipatory (parental) Related factor: Anticipated or perceived loss of child

Home maintenance management, impaired Related factors: Inadequate support system, insufficient family planning or organization, overwhelming demands of caregiving and maintaining usual roles

Infant feeding pattern, ineffective Related factors: Prematurity, anatomical abnormalities

Infection, risk for Risk factors: Inadequate immune system, invasive procedures, break in primary defenses (eg, circumcision, umbilical cord)

Nutrition: less than body requirements, altered Related factors: Inadequate sucking reflex in infant, food intolerance, high metabolic rate of stressed infant, lethargy

Skin integrity, impaired Related/risk factors: Decreased peripheral perfusion, fragility of skin, lack of normal skin flora

Sleep pattern disturbance Related factor: Sleep deprivation secondary to frequent therapeutic interventions

Spontaneous ventilation, inability to sustain Related factors: Metabolic factors, respiratory muscle fatigue, pulmonary immaturity

Thermoregulation, ineffective Related factors: Increased respiratory effort secondary to respiratory distress syndrome

Tissue perfusion, altered peripheral Related factors: Imbalance between oxygen supply/demand, compensatory responses

Ventilatory weaning response, dysfunctional (DVWR) Related factors: Pulmonary immaturity, *Impaired gas exchange*, *Ineffective airway clearance*, ventilator dependence > one week

Pediatric Conditions

Developmental problems/needs related to illness for
all conditions

Burns

Cancer (see Medical Conditions: Cancer, pp. 533–535)

Casts and traction

Child abuse

Cleft lip/cleft palate: surgical repair

Coagulation disorders

Congenital malformations of the central nervous system:
surgical repair

Diabetes mellitus (see Medical Conditions: Diabetes
Mellitus/Hypoglycemia, p. 541)

Failure to thrive

Gastroenteritis

Gastrointestinal obstruction: Surgical repair

Infection of central nervous system

Ingestion/accidental poisoning

Juvenile rheumatoid arthritis (see Medical Conditions:
Arthritis, pp. 528–529)

Obese child

Osteomyelitis

Pregnancy in adolescence

Renal failure, Acute (see Medical Conditions: Renal failure,
Acute, pp. 549–550)

Renal failure, Chronic (see Medical Conditions: Renal failure,
Chronic, pp. 550–552)

Respiratory disorder, chronic

Respiratory infection, acute

Rheumatic fever (see Medical Conditions:
Pericarditis/endocarditis, p. 538)

Seizure disorders

Sepsis

Sickle cell crisis

Suicidal adolescent (see Psychiatric Conditions: Suicidal
patient, p. 576)

Tonsillectomy

Developmental Problems/Needs Related to Illness

The following nursing diagnoses (as well as *Knowledge deficit*) should be considered for all pediatric medical/surgical conditions. For nursing diagnoses specific to a medical condition (eg, burns, gastroenteritis), add the nursing diagnoses in that section to the following general illness/development-related diagnoses that apply.

Nursing Diagnoses

Activity intolerance Related factors: Decreased strength and endurance, Weakness/*Fatigue*, imbalance between oxygen supply and demand, *Pain* (acute or chronic), *Altered nutrition: less than body requirements*, limited mobility, frail/debilitated state, chronic illness, decreased hemoglobin

Adjustment, impaired Related factors: Incomplete grieving, *Dysfunctional grieving*, necessity for major lifestyle/behavior change, pattern of dependence, inadequate support systems, failure to accomplish developmental tasks

Anxiety Related factors: Threat to or change in role functioning and interaction patterns, unmet needs, separation anxiety

Caregiver role strain Related factors: Illness severity of the child, premature birth/congenital defect, developmental delay or retardation of the child or caregiver, marginal caregiver coping patterns, duration of caregiving required, caregiver's competing role commitments, complexity/amount of caregiving tasks, lack of respite and recreation for caregiver

Coping: family, ineffective, compromised/disabling Related factors: Arbitrary disregard for child's needs, conflicting coping styles, highly ambivalent relationships (see *Altered family processes* and *Caregiver role strain*)

Decisional conflict: Related factors: Necessity to make choices about treatments/interventions, weighing needs of ill child against those of healthy siblings

Development, risk for altered See *Growth, altered*

Diversional activity deficit Related factors: Separation from school, friends, and family secondary to hospitalization or disability, *Pain*, illness

Family processes, altered Related factors: Change in family roles, illness/disability of family member, unmet expectations for child, inadequate support systems, overwhelming stressors, emotional and physical exhaustion, financial problems, separation of family members, prolonged illness

Fear Related factors: *Powerlessness*, threat to well-being of self/child

Grieving, anticipatory/dysfunctional Related factors: Loss (actual or anticipated) secondary to the particular condition, chronic illness

Growth, risk for altered Related factors: Inability to achieve developmental tasks secondary to serious illness, prescribed dependence/limitations

Home maintenance management, impaired Related factors: Home environment obstacles, inadequate support system, insufficient family organization or planning, insufficient finances, lack of familiarity with community resources, developmental disability of caregivers, physical/psychologic impairment of family member other than patient, *Knowledge deficits*

Hopelessness Related factor: Failing or deteriorating physical condition of child

Management of therapeutic regimen: individual, ineffective Related factors: *Knowledge deficit*s (eg, illness/surgical procedure, signs and symptoms of complications, medications, home care/treatments, dietary modifications), complex treatments/medication regimens

Noncompliance Related factors: Denial of illness, negative consequence of treatment regimen, perceived benefits of continued illness, lack of parental supervision/support

Parental role conflict Related factors: Separation of family members secondary to hospitalization(s) of child, inability to maintain usual role demands (eg, work, spouse), intimidation with invasive/technical procedures

Parenting, altered Related factors: Interruption in bonding process; treatment-imposed separation; abuse, rejection, or overprotection secondary to inadequate coping skills; lack of knowledge/skill necessary to address the child's special needs; inadequate supports/resources

Powerlessness Related factor: Chronic illness

Role performance, altered Related factors: Chronic illness, *Chronic pain*

Self-care deficit: (specify) Related factors: Specific to illness (eg, depression, *Pain*/discomfort, *Activity intolerance*, decreased strength and endurance)

Self-esteem disturbance Related factors: Chronic illness, *Chronic pain*

Social interaction, impaired Related factors: Self-concept disturbance, limited physical mobility

Social isolation Related factors: Actual or perceived reactions of others to child's disability, intensity of caregiving demands (eg, lack of time, energy)

Spiritual distress Related factor: Test of spiritual beliefs

Burns
Nursing Diagnoses

See "Medical Conditions: Burns," pp. 532–533, and "Pediatric Conditions: Developmental Problems/Needs Related to Illness," pp. 597–598.

Body image disturbance Related factors: Burns, scarring

Body temperature, risk for altered Risk factors: Dehydration secondary to impairment in skin integrity, infection

Constipation Related factors: Decreased gastrointestinal motility, dehydration

Coping: individual, ineffective Related factors: Multiple stressors (eg, severe injury, *Pain*, repeated painful procedures, *Fear* of disfigurement), prolonged treatment period

Fear Related factors: Painful therapeutic procedures, environmental stressors secondary to hospitalization, separation from family

Fluid volume deficit Related factor: Abnormal fluid loss secondary to loss of skin integrity

Infection, risk for Risk factors: Malnutrition, loss of primary defense (ie, *Impaired skin integrity*)

Nutrition: less than body requirements, altered Related factors: High metabolic needs, loss of appetite secondary to *Fear* and *Pain*

Pain Related factors: Injury, *Fear*

Skin integrity, impaired Related factors: Burns, immobility
Social interaction, impaired Related factor: *Fear* of rejection
Social isolation Related factor: Reactions of others to disfigurement

Casts and Traction

Includes but is not limited to orthopedic trauma and congenital hip dysplasia. See "Surgical Conditions: Musculoskeletal Surgery," pp. 561–562, and "Pediatric Conditions: Developmental Problems/Needs Related to Illness," pp. 597–598.

Body image disturbance Related factors: Surgery, appliances, congenital defects
Infection: risk for Risk factors: *Impaired tissue integrity* secondary to trauma or surgery, broken skin (eg, secondary to pins)
Mobility: physical, impaired Related factors: *Pain*/discomfort, medically imposed restrictions, musculoskeletal impairment, casts, traction
Pain Related factors: *Pain* secondary to injury, pain secondary to surgery, muscle cramps secondary to immobilization, muscle soreness (eg, from walking with crutches)
Peripheral neurovascular dysfunction Related factors: Immobilization, tissue trauma
Skin integrity, impaired Related factors: Altered circulation, prescribed immobility, *Impaired mobility* secondary to pain, broken skin (eg, secondary to external pins)
Tissue perfusion, altered (peripheral) Related factors: Interruption of venous flow to _____ (specify) secondary to constriction pressure, interruption of arterial flow to _____ (specify) secondary to compartmental syndrome, tissue trauma
Urinary Incontinence, Functional Related factor: Mobility deficits

Child Abuse

Nursing Diagnoses

See "Pediatric Conditions: Developmental Problems/Needs Related to Illness," pp. 597–598.

Coping: family, ineffective, compromised/disabling Related factors: Chronically unresolved feelings (specify), lack of extended family, financial problems, highly ambivalent family relationships, unwanted child, unwanted characteristics of child (eg, appearance, mental retardation, hyperactivity), substance-abusing family member, emotionally disturbed family member, use of violence to manage conflict, child sexual/physical abuse
Coping, individual (abuser), ineffective Related factors: History of abuse by own family, lack of love from own family, *Social isolation*, lack of support system, *Situational low self-esteem*, mental illness, emotional immaturity, unrealistic expectations of child
Coping, individual (child), ineffective Related factor: Personal vulnerability in situational crisis
Fear (child) Related factors: Real threat to own well-being, *Powerlessness*, possibility of placement in a foster home
Fear (parent) Related factors: Possibility that abuse will be discovered, anticipated reactions of others, loss of child, criminal prosecution

Hopelessness Related factors: Long-term stress/abuse, inability to escape

Injury, risk for Risk factors: Physical/psychologic abuse, parental neglect

Nutrition: less than body requirements, altered Related factor: Parental neglect

Pain Related factor: Trauma

Parenting, altered Related factors: Absent or ineffective role model; interruption in bonding process; lack of knowledge/skill; lack of or inappropriate response of child to parent; lack of support for nurturing figure(s); psychologic impairment; physical illness; unrealistic expectations of self, child, or partner; dysfunctional relationship between parents/nurturing figures; situational crisis (specific to family)

Post-trauma response Related factors: Abuse, assault, torture, accidents, and incest

Self-esteem disturbance. Related factors: Abuse, negative feedback from family members, feelings of abandonment

Sleep pattern disturbance Related factors: *Anxiety*, emotional state

Social interaction, impaired Related factors: *Self-esteem disturbance*, isolation enforced by parents

Social isolation See *Social interaction, impaired*

Trauma (specify; eg, poisoning, physical injury), risk for Risk factors: Vulnerability secondary to congenital problems or chronic illness; lack of support system for caregivers; dysfunctional family interactions

Violence: directed at others, risk for Risk factor: History of physical/mental abuse by others

Cleft Lip/Cleft Palate: Surgical Repair

See "Pediatric Conditions: Developmental Problems/Needs Related to Illness," pp. 597–598.

Potential Complications (Collaborative Problems)

PC of cleft lip/palate: Failure to thrive, otitis media, excessive scar formation, poor cosmetic effect secondary to sloughing of sutures

PC of cleft lip/palate, surgical repair: Hypostatic pneumonia

Nursing Diagnoses

Airway clearance, ineffective Related factor: Edema secondary to surgery

Aspiration, risk for Risk factors: Aspiration of feedings through congenital defect in palate, postoperative aspiration of mucus and blood

Body image disturbance Related factor: Obvious congenital anomaly

Communication, impaired verbal Related factors: Incomplete palate repair, delayed muscle development, dental problems, hearing loss

Fear Related factors: Environmental stressors/hospitalization, separation from parent, parental *Fear* that child will aspirate or suture line will be harmed

Fluid volume deficit Related factor: Deviation affecting access to or intake of fluids secondary to difficult handling of oral fluids

Infant feeding pattern, ineffective Related factors: Anatomical abnormalities, oral hypersensitivity

Infection, risk for Risk factors: Trauma secondary to surgery, aspiration of feedings, difficulty cleaning sutures

Injury, risk for (disruption of surgical site) Risk factors: Limitations of maturational age; tension on suture line secondary to crying, feeding, or cleansing the area, sucking or blowing

Nutrition: less than body requirements, altered Related factors: Difficulty in chewing, difficulty in swallowing secondary to *Acute pain*, postoperative *Nausea* and vomiting, prescribed diet modifications (eg, liquids)

Oral mucous membrane, altered Related factor: Surgery in oral cavity

Pain Related factors: Surgical repair of cleft lip/palate, restraints

Mobility: physical, impaired Related factors: Use of restraints to protect surgical repair

Self-care deficit: feeding Related factors: Age of child and need for adapted feeding

Swallowing, impaired Related factors: *Pain*, unfamiliar method of feeding

Coagulation Disorders

Include but are not limited to hemophilia, von Willebrand's disease, and idiopathic thrombocytopenic purpura. See "Pediatric Conditions: Developmental Problems/Needs Related to Illness," pp. 597–598, and "Medical Conditions: Blood Disorders," pp. 531–532.

Potential Complications (Collaborative Problems)

PC of coagulation disorders: Hemorrhage

Nursing Diagnoses

Coping: individual, ineffective Related factors: Chronic illness and limitations

Fear Related factors: Risks associated with diagnosis (eg, uncontrollable bleeding, potential joint degeneration, transfusion-acquired diseases)

Mobility: physical, impaired Related factors: Joint hemorrhage, swelling, or degenerative changes; muscle atrophy

Pain Related factors: Joint hemorrhage, swelling

Protection, altered Related factors: Abnormal blood profile, medication therapy (eg, corticosteroids)

Congenital Malformations of the Central Nervous System: Surgical Repair

Include but are not limited to spina bifida, meningocele, myelomeningocele, and hydrocephalus. See "Pediatric Conditions: Developmental Problems/Needs Related to Illness," pp. 597–598.

Potential Complications (Collaborative Problems)

PC of hydrocephalus: Increased intracranial pressure

PC of myelomeningocele: Hydrocephalus

PC of congenital malformation or surgery of the CNS: Neurovascular insufficiency, sepsis, urinary tract infections

Nursing Diagnoses

Incontinence, bowel Related factors: Effects of spinal cord anomaly on anal sphincter

Incontinence, urinary, total Related factors: Effects of spinal cord anomaly on bladder

Infection, risk for Risk factor: Loss of intact skin secondary to congenital anomaly or surgery

Injury, risk for Risk factors: Increased intracranial pressure/seizures secondary to shunt malfunction in hydrocephalus, inability to support large head

Mobility: physical, impaired Related factor: Neuromuscular impairment secondary to spinal cord involvement

Nutrition: less than body requirements, altered Related factor: Vomiting secondary to increased intracranial pressure

Pain Related factor: Surgery

Sensory/perceptual alterations (kinesthetic, tactile) Related factors: Sensory deficits secondary to spinal cord involvement

Skin integrity, risk for impaired Risk factors: Immobility (eg, related to limbs, head and neck), incontinence of stool/urine

Failure To Thrive

See "Pediatric Conditions: Developmental Problems/Needs Related to Illness," pp. 597–598.

Potential Complications (Collaborative Problems)

PC of failure to thrive: Dehydration, metabolic disorders

Nursing Diagnoses

Activity intolerance Related factor: Weakness/*Fatigue* secondary to malnutrition

Fluid volume deficit Related factors: Inadequate fluid intake secondary to disinterest in eating/drinking, parental neglect, abnormal fluid loss (loose stools)

Infection, risk for Risk factors: Weakened defenses secondary to malnutrition, parental neglect (eg, hygiene)

Nutrition: less than body requirements, altered Related factors: Food intolerance, malabsorption, loss of appetite, parental neglect, lack of emotional and sensory stimulation, parental *Knowledge deficit*, metabolic disorders, organ dysfunction

Sensory/perceptual alterations (specify) Related factor: Lack of sensory stimulation from caregiver/parents

Skin integrity, impaired Related factors: Altered nutritional status, parental neglect (eg, hygiene)

Sleep pattern disturbance Related factors: *Anxiety*, parental emotional deprivation

Social interaction, impaired Related factors: Developmental disability, limited physical mobility, low self-esteem

Gastroenteritis

See "Pediatric Conditions: Developmental Problems/Needs Related to Illness," pp. 597–598.

Potential Complications (Collaborative Problems)

PC of gastroenteritis: Fluid and electrolyte imbalance

Nursing Diagnoses

Diarrhea Related factors: Food intolerance, infection/inflammation, stress, dietary changes, increased intestinal motility

Fluid volume deficit Related factors: Abnormal fluid loss (*Diarrhea*, vomiting) secondary to infection, food intolerance, malabsorption

Nutrition: less than body requirements, altered Related factors: Loss of appetite, *Nausea*/vomiting

Oral mucous membrane, altered Related factor: Dehydration, vomiting

Pain Related factor: *Diarrhea*, abdominal cramps secondary to inflammation, distention, and hyperperistalsis

Sensory/perceptual alterations: (specify) Related factor: Electrolyte imbalance

Skin integrity, impaired Related/risk factor: Incontinence of stool secondary to *Diarrhea*

Gastrointestinal Obstruction: Surgical Repair

Includes but is not limited to gastroschisis, omphalocele, intestinal atresia, meconium ileus, imperforate anus, Hirschsprung's disease, pyloric stenosis, intussusception, inguinal hernia, and hydrocele. See "Surgical Conditions, Abdominal Surgery," pp. 555–556 and "Pediatric Conditions: Developmental Problems/Needs Related to Illness," pp. 597–598.

Potential Complications (Collaborative Problems)

PC of GI obstruction/surgery: Hemorrhage, ileus, sepsis

Nursing Diagnoses

Body image disturbance Related factors: Effects of condition or surgery on body

Breathing pattern, ineffective Related factor: Acute *Pain*

Fluid volume deficit Related factors: Abnormal blood loss, abnormal fluid loss, NPO status

Nausea Related factors: *Pain*, abdominal distention, obstruction

Nutrition: less than body requirements, altered Related factors: Loss of appetite, *Nausea*/vomiting, dietary changes

Pain Related factor: Surgery

Skin integrity, impaired Related/risk factors: Altered nutritional status, surgical wound

Infection of Central Nervous System (CNS)

Includes but is not limited to meningitis, encephalitis, rabies, Reye's syndrome, and Guillain-Barré syndrome. See "Pediatric Conditions: Developmental Problems/Needs Related to Illness," pp. 597–598 and "Medical Conditions: Neurologic Disorders," pp. 545–548.

Potential Complications (Collaborative Problems)

PC of CNS infection: Atelectasis, Coma, fluid and electrolyte imbalance, hepatic failure, increased intracranial pressure, pneumonia, renal failure, respiratory distress, seizures, sepsis

PC of Reye's syndrome: Diabetes insipidus

Nursing Diagnoses

Airway clearance, ineffective Related factors: Impaired gag reflex, *Impaired swallowing, Fatigue*, weakness/paralysis of respiratory muscles, tracheobronchial obstruction, aspiration pneumonia

Breathing patterns, ineffective See *Airway clearance, ineffective*

Communication, impaired verbal Related factors: Inability to speak secondary to coma, dysarthrias secondary to weakness of speech muscles

Confusion, acute See *Memory, impaired*

Disuse syndrome, risk for Risk factors: Paralysis, coma

Fluid volume deficit Related factors: Inadequate fluid intake secondary to *Nausea*, abnormal fluid loss secondary to vomiting, failure of regulatory mechanisms (eg, diabetes insipidus)

Hyperthermia Related factors: Illness, dehydration, increased metabolic rate secondary to infectious process

Infection, risk for (transmission) Risk factor: Contagious pathogen

Injury, risk for Risk factors: Seizure activity, generalized weakness, reduced coordination, cognitive deficits, sensory deficits, unsteady gait

Memory, impaired Related factors: Decreased cerebral tissue perfusion secondary to edema, hypovolemia, or increased intracranial pressure

Mobility: physical, impaired Related factors: Neuromuscular impairment, coma, *Pain*, partial or complete paralysis, loss of muscle strength and control, muscle rigidity/tremors

Nutrition: less than body requirements, altered Related factors: *Impaired swallowing*, dysphagia/chewing difficulties secondary to cranial nerve involvement

Pain Related factors: *Nausea*/vomiting, headache secondary to meningeal irritation/inflammation, muscle spasms (neck, shoulders), paresthesia

Sensory/perceptual alterations: (specify) Related factors: Sensory deficits secondary to coma; sleep deprivation; altered sensory reception, transmission, and integration; electrolyte imbalance; hypoxia; emotional stress

Skin integrity, impaired Related factor: *Impaired physical mobility*

Suffocation, risk for Risk factors: Decreased level of consciousness, seizures, muscle weakness/paralysis

Swallowing, impaired Related factor: Cerebellar lesions

Tissue perfusion, altered (cerebral) Related factors: Cerebral edema, increased intracranial pressure, hypovolemia, acidosis

Ingestion/Accidental Poisoning

See "Pediatric Conditions: Developmental Problems/Needs Related to Illness," pp. 597–598.

Potential Complications (Collaborative Problems)

PC of lead poisoning: Anemia, aspiration, blindness, burns (eg, acid, alkaline), hemorrhage, metabolic acidosis, respiratory alkalosis
(Carpenito 1997b, p. 536)

Nursing Diagnoses

Anxiety Related factors: Emergency nature of situation, concern about parents' reactions, guilt feelings

Breathing pattern, ineffective Related factor: Depression of respiratory center secondary to _____ (specify drug)

Fluid volume excess Related factors: Decreased urine output secondary to renal dysfunction, vomiting, _Diarrhea_, decreased intake

Injury (eg, falls), risk for Risk factors: Seizures secondary to lead poisoning, aspirin toxicity, seizures, loss of coordination, decreased level of consciousness

Nutrition: less than body requirements, altered Related factors: Chemically induced changes in gastrointestinal tract, anorexia, abdominal _Pain_, anemia secondary to lead poisoning

Pain, chronic Related factor: Deposits of lead in soft tissues and bone

Sensory/perceptual alterations (specify) Related factors: Decreased consciousness, encephalopathy

Thought processes, altered Related factor: Deposit of lead in brain tissue and central nervous system

Obese Child

See "Pediatric Conditions: Developmental Problems/Needs Related to Illness," pp. 597–598.

Nursing Diagnoses

Activity intolerance Related factors: Sedentary lifestyle, difficulty exercising because of extra weight, exertional discomfort

Body image disturbance Related factors: Eating disorder (ie, obesity), view of self in contrast to cultural values

Coping: individual, ineffective Related factor: Use of food to cope with stressors

Family processes, altered Related factors: Effects of therapy (eg, food restriction) on parent-child relationship

Health maintenance, altered Related factors: Cultural beliefs, lack of social supports, inability to make deliberate and thoughtful judgments secondary to maturational age, lack of exercise

Mobility: physical, impaired Related factor: Strain on muscles and joints because of weight

Nutrition: more than body requirements, altered Related factors: Psychologic impairment; sedentary lifestyle; lack of basic nutritional knowledge; ethnic/cultural norms; eating as a way of coping; control, sex, or love issues

Self-esteem disturbance Related factors: Obesity, appearance not culturally valued, response of others to obesity

Social interaction, impaired Related factor: Inability to initiate relationships because of self-concept disturbance, embarrassment, and fear of others' negative responses

Social isolation Related factors: Obesity, reactions of others

Osteomyelitis

See "Pediatric Conditions: Developmental Problems/Needs Related to Illness," pp. 597–598.

Potential Complications (Collaborative Problems)

PC of osteomyelitis: Infective emboli, pathologic fractures

PC of antibiotic therapy: Hematologic, hepatic, and renal problems; anaphylactic shock

Nursing Diagnoses

Constipation Related factors: Immobility, narcotic medications

Hyperthermia Related factors: Infectious process, increased metabolic rate

Injury, risk for Risk factor: Pathologic fractures related to disease process

Mobility: physical, impaired Related factors: *Pain*/discomfort, musculoskeletal impairment, prescribed immobility

Nutrition: less than body requirements, altered Related factors: High metabolic rate, anorexia secondary to infectious process and *Pain*

Pain Related factors: Inflammation, swelling, hyperthermia, tissue necrosis, fractures

Skin integrity, impaired Related factors: Immobility, irritation from cast or splint

Tissue perfusion, altered Related factors: Inflammatory reaction with thrombosis of vessels, edema, abscess formation, tissue destruction

Pregnancy in Adolescence

Includes pregnancy, antepartum and postpartum periods, and parenting. See "Pediatric Conditions: Developmental Problems/Needs Related to Illness," pp. 597–598. See also "Antepartum and Postpartum Conditions," pp. 578–585.

Nursing Diagnoses

Body image disturbance Related factors: Pregnancy and developmental stage

Coping: individual, ineffective Related factors: Adolescent pregnancy, adolescent parenthood

Health maintenance, altered Related factors: Lack of social supports, lack of material resources, cultural beliefs, lack of ability to make deliberate and thoughtful judgments secondary to maturational age

Knowledge deficit (specify) Related factors: Limited exposure to information (eg, about birth control, parenting), limited practice of skills, information misinterpretation

Nutrition: less than body requirements, altered Related factors: High metabolic needs secondary to both adolescence and pregnancy, lack of basic nutritional knowledge, limited access to food, *Nausea*/vomiting

Nutrition: more than body requirements, altered Related factors: Ethnic/cultural norms, lack of basic nutritional knowledge, "fast" food, "junk" food

Parent/infant/child attachment, risk for altered See *Parenting, altered*

Parenting, altered Related factors: Lack of knowledge/skill; lack of support for nurturing figure from own parents; alienation from own parents; unrealistic expectations of self, infant, and partner; situational crisis

Social interaction, impaired Related factors: Sociocultural conflict, self-concept disturbance, embarrassment, withdrawal from school

Social isolation Related factors: Alteration in physical appearance, lifestyle changes

Violence: directed at others (child), risk for Risk factors: Rage reaction, history of physical/mental abuse by others, ineffective coping skills, substance abuse

Respiratory Disorder, Chronic

Includes but is not limited to asthma, bronchopulmonary dysplasia, and cystic fibrosis. See "Pediatric Conditions: Developmental Problems/Needs Related to Illness," pp. 597–598. See also "Medical Conditions: Acute respiratory disorders (eg, pneumonia, pulmonary edema, pulmonary embolism)," and "Chronic respiratory disorders," pp. 552–554.

Potential Complications (Collaborative Problems)

PC of chronic respiratory disorder: Hypoxemia, respiratory acidosis

PC of corticosteroid therapy: Hypertension, hypokalemia, hypoglycemia, immunosuppression, osteoporosis, ulcers

Nursing Diagnoses

Activity intolerance Related factors: Inadequate oxygenation secondary to bronchospasm and/or increased pulmonary secretions

Airway clearance, ineffective Related factors: Tracheobronchial secretions, spasms of the bronchi and bronchioles, ineffective cough secondary to *Fatigue*/weakness

Anxiety Related factors: Air hunger, difficulty breathing, *Fear* of suffocation/dying

Breathing pattern, ineffective Related factors: *Anxiety*, pulmonary infection, decreased energy/*Fatigue*

Fear Related factors: Dyspnea, fear of recurrences

Fluid volume deficit, risk for Risk factors: Inadequate fluid intake secondary to difficulty in breathing, abnormal fluid loss secondary to increased insensible water loss from rapid respirations

Gas exchange, impaired Related factor: Decreased functional lung tissue secondary to fibrotic, nonventilated areas of lung parenchyma in bronchopulmonary dysplasia

Infection, risk for Risk factors: Malnutrition, stasis of respiratory secretions

Nutrition: less than body requirements, altered Related factors: Loss of appetite with chronic illness, high metabolic needs secondary to pulmonary infection, malabsorption of nutrients secondary to cystic fibrosis

Respiratory Infection, Acute

Includes but is not limited to tonsillitis, pharyngitis, croup, laryngotracheobronchitis, epiglottitis, bronchitis, and pneumonia. See "Pediatric Conditions: Developmental Problems/Needs Related to Illness," pp. 597–598. See also "Medical Conditions: Acute respiratory disorders (eg, pneumonia, pulmonary edema, pulmonary embolism) and Chronic respiratory disorders," pp. 552–554.

Potential Complications (Collaborative Problems)

PC of acute respiratory infection: Hypoxemia, respiratory acidosis, respiratory insufficiency, sepsis

PC of corticosteroid therapy: Hypertension, hypokalemia, hypoglycemia, immunosuppression, osteoporosis, ulcers

Nursing Diagnoses

Airway clearance, ineffective Related factors: Edema, increased and/or viscous tracheobronchial/pulmonary secretions, bronchospasm, tracheobronchial inflammation, pleuritic pain, ineffective cough secondary to *Fatigue*

Anxiety Related factors: *Fear* of dying, dyspnea, inadequate oxygenation

Fear Related factors: Real threat to well-being, environmental stressors/ hospitalization, separation from parent, dyspnea, *Fear* of recurring attacks

Fluid volume deficit Related factors: Inadequate fluid intake secondary to difficulty in breathing, abnormal fluid loss secondary to increased insensible water loss from rapid respirations and/or fever

Gas exchange, impaired Related factors: Decreased functional lung tissue secondary to pneumonia, air trapping, impaired exchange of oxygen in alveoli secondary to collected secretions, hypoventilation (see *Airway clearance, ineffective*)

Nutrition: less than body requirements, altered Related factors: Loss of appetite secondary to dyspnea and malaise, high metabolic needs

Pain Related factors: Sore throat, *Pain* with inspiration, pleural *Pain*

Sensory/perceptual alterations: (specify) Related factor: Sensory deficit secondary to time spent in croupette

Skin integrity, risk for impaired Risk factors: Altered nutritional status, hyperthermia, damp therapeutic environment, decreased mobility, diaphoresis

Seizure Disorders

See "Pediatric Conditions: Developmental Problems/Needs Related to Illness," pp. 597–598. See also "Medical Conditions: Neurologic Disorders," pp. 545–548.

Potential Complications (Collaborative Problems)
PC of seizure disorder: Status epilepticus

Nursing Diagnoses
Airway clearance, ineffective Related factors: Loss of tongue and gag reflexes during seizure activity

Injury, risk for Risk factor: Uncontrolled muscle movements during seizure activity

Self-esteem disturbance Related factors: Chronic illness, feelings of being out of control, stigma associated with seizures, perceived "weakness"

Social interaction, impaired Related factors: Embarrassment, fear of having a seizure in public

Suffocation, risk for Risk factors: Weakness, altered level of consciousness, cognitive limitations

Sepsis

See "Pediatric Conditions: Developmental Problems/Needs Related to Illness," pp. 597–598.

Potential Complications (Collaborative Problems)
PC of sepsis: Anemia, edema, hemorrhage, hypotension, hypothermia/hyperthermia, meningitis, respiratory distress, seizures

Nursing Diagnoses

Cardiac output, decreased Related factors: Decreased circulating volume and venous return, increased systemic vascular resistance, effects of hypoxia

Constipation Related factor: Decreased fluid intake

Diarrhea Related factors: Increased intestinal motility, intestinal irritation secondary to infectious process

Fluid volume deficit Related factors: Decreased fluid intake, fever, widespread vasodilation and intercompartmental fluid shifts

Injury, risk for Risk factor: Seizure activity secondary to high fever

Nutrition: less than body requirements, altered Related factors: Inadequate sucking reflex in infant, vomiting, food intolerance, increased metabolic rate, lethargy

Skin integrity, impaired Related factors: Decreased peripheral perfusion, hyperthermia, edema, immobility

Sleep pattern disturbance Related factors: Frequent therapeutic interventions, discomfort secondary to fever, difficulty breathing, diaphoresis

Tissue perfusion, altered (specify) Related factors: Selective vasoconstriction, presence of microemboli, hypovolemia

Sickle Cell Crisis

See "Pediatric Conditions: Developmental Problems/Needs Related to Illness," pp. 597–598.

Potential Complications (Collaborative Problems)

PC of sickle cell crisis: Vaso-occlusive crisis, causing infarctions of vital organs (eg, liver, kidneys, central nervous system); infections (eg, pneumonia, osteomyelitis); aplastic crisis (rapidly developing severe anemia); splenic sequestration, causing circulatory collapse

PC of repeated transfusions: Hemosiderosis

Nursing Diagnoses

Body image disturbance Related factors: Delayed onset of puberty, swelling of the hands and feet, prominence of the bones of the face and skull, *Pain*, need to avoid strenuous activities

Fluid volume deficit Related factor: Increased need for fluid volume in blood to prevent sickling and thrombosis. (**NOTE:** This is a relative deficit. Enough fluid must be ingested to create hemodilution.)

Gas exchange, impaired Related factors: Susceptibility to pneumonia and pulmonary infarctions, decreased oxygen-carrying capacity of the blood

Infection, risk for Risk factors: Chronic illness, defects in immunologic system

Pain Related factors: Sickle cell crisis, causing tissue hypoxia and impaired peripheral circulation

Tissue perfusion, altered (peripheral) Related factors: Imbalance between oxygen supply/demand secondary to anemia, thrombosis secondary to clumping of red blood cells in sickle cell crisis, increased blood viscosity, arteriovenous shunts in peripheral and pulmonary circulation

Tonsillectomy

See "Pediatric Conditions: Developmental Problems/Needs Related to Illness," pp. 597–598

Potential Complications (Collaborative Problems)

PC of tonsillectomy: Airway obstruction, aspiration, hemorrhage

Nursing Diagnoses

Airway clearance, ineffective Related factors: Trauma, edema, *Pain*, tracheobronchial secretions, collection of blood in oropharynx, vomiting, sedation

Fluid volume deficit Related factors: Blood loss secondary to surgery of highly vascular site, decreased intake secondary to painful swallowing

Nutrition: less than body requirements, altered Related factors: Loss of appetite secondary to sore throat and blood swallowing

Pain Related factors: Surgery, packing, edema

Bibliography

Aaronson, L. S., Teel, C. S., Cassmeyer, V., Neuberger, G. B., Pallikkathayil, L., Pierce, J., Press, A. N., Williams, P. D., & Wingate, A. (1999). Defining and measuring fatigue. *Image: Journal of Nursing Scholarship, 31*(1), 45–50.

Abraham, I., & Reel, S. (1993). Cognitive nursing interventions with long-term care residents: Effects on neurocognitive dimensions. *Archives of Psychiatric Nursing, 6*(6), 356–365.

Ackerman, L. L. (1992). Interventions related to neurological care. In G. M. Bulechek & J. C. McCloskey (Eds.), *Symposium on Nursing Interventions. Nursing Clinics of North America, 27*(2), 325–346.

Acute Pain Management Guideline Panel. (1992, Feb.). *Acute pain management: Operative or medical procedures and trauma. Clinical practice guideline.* (AHCPR Publication No. 92-0032). Rockville, MD: Agency for Health Care Policy and Research, Public Health Service, U.S. Department of Health and Human Services.

Agency for Health Care Policy and Research (1996). *Smoking cessation. Clinical practice guideline.* Washington, DC: U.S. Government Printing Office.

Agostinelli, B., Demers, K., Garrigan, D., & Waszynski, C. (1994). Targeted interventions: Use of the mini-mental state exam. *Journal of Gerontological Nursing, 20*(8), 15–23.

Ahrens, T. (1993). Changing perspectives in the assessment of oxygenation. *Critical Care Nurse, 13*(4), 78–83.

Ahrens, T. S. (1993). Respiratory disorders. In M. R. Kinney, D. R. Packa, & S. B. Dunbar (Eds.), *AACN's clinical reference for critical-care nursing* (pp. 701–704). St. Louis: Mosby.

American Academy of Pediatrics & American College of Obstetricians and Gynecologists (1992). Postpartum and follow-up care. In *Guidelines for perinatal care* (3rd ed.) (pp. 91–116). Evanston, IL: Authors.

American Association of Critical-Care Nurses. (1990). *Outcome standards for nursing care of the critically ill.* Laguna Niguel, CA: Author.

American Association of Post-Anesthesia Nurses. (1992). *Standards of post-anesthesia nursing.* Resource 18. Richmond, VA: Author.

American College of Allergy & Immunology (1992). *Interim recommendations to health professionls and organizations regarding latex allergy precautions.* Milwaukee, WI: Author.

American Psychiatric Association Practice Guidelines (1993). *American Journal of Psychiatry, 150*(2), 207–228.

American Public Health Association and the American Academy of Pediatrics. (1992). *Caring for our children: National health and performance standards: Guidelines for out-of-home child care programs.* Washington, DC: Author.

Arnold, E., & Boggs, K. (1995). *Interpersonal relationships: Professional communications skills for nurses* (2nd ed.). Philadelphia: Saunders.

Aronson, M. K. (Ed.). (1994). *Reshaping dementia care.* Thousand Oaks, CA: Sage Publications.

Association of Operating Room Nurses. (1993). *Standards and recommended practices.* Denver: Author.

Association of Women's Health, Obstetric, and Neonatal Nurses (1993). *Fetal heart monitoring principles & practices.* Washington: DC: Author.

Badger, J. M. (1994). Calming the anxious patient. *American Journal of Nursing, 94*(5), 46–50.

Baer, C. L. (1993a). Acid-base balance. In M. R. Kinney, D. R. Packa, & S. B. Dunbar (Eds.), *AACN's clinical reference for critical care nursing* (pp. 209–216). St. Louis: Mosby.

Baer, C. L. (1993b). Fluid & electrolyte balance. In M. R. Kinney, D. R. Packa, & S. B. Dunbar (Eds.), *AACN's clinical reference for critical-care nursing* (pp. 173–208). St. Louis: Mosby.

Baginski, Y. (1994). Roadblocks to home care. *Caring, 13*(12), 18–20, 22, 24.

Bakcr, D. M. (1993). Assessment and management of impairments in swallowing. *Nursing Clinics of North America, 28*(4), 793–806.

Bakker, R. H., Kastermans, M. C., & Dassen, T. W. N. (1995). An analysis of the nursing diagnosis "ineffective management of therapeutic regimen" compared to "noncompliance" and Orem's self-care deficit theory of nursing. *Nursing Diagnosis, 6*(4), 161–166.

Bank, L. J. (1992). Counseling. In G. M. Bulechek & J. C. McCloskey (Eds.), *Nursing interventions: Essential nursing treatments* (pp. 279–291). Philadelphia: Saunders.

Barry, K. (1993). Patient self-medication: An innovative approach to medication teaching. *Journal of Nursing Care Quality, 8*(1), 75–82.

Bates, B. (1991). *A guide to the physical examination and history taking* (5th ed.). Philadelphia: Lippincott.

Bear, K., & Tigges, B. B. (1993). Management strategies for promoting successful breastfeeding. *Nurse Practitioner: American Journal of Primary Health Care, 18,* 50, 53–54, 56–58, 60.

Beck, C. F. (1994). Malignant hyperthermia: Are you prepared? *AORN Journal, 59*(2), 367–390.

Beck, A. T., Steer, R. A., & Brown, G. (1993). Dysfunctional attitudes and suicidal ideation in psychiatric outpatients. *Suicide and Life-Threatening Behavior, 23*(1), 11–20.

Bendorf, K., & Lyman, B. (1993). Transition from the hospital to the home for the infant requiring total parenteral nutrition. *Journal of Perinatal and Neonatal Nursing, 6*(4), 80–90.

Bines, A. S., & Landron, S. L. (1993). Cardiovascular emergencies in the post anesthesia care unit. In K. L. Saleh & V. Brinsko (Eds.), *Nursing Clinics of North America, 28*(3), 493–506.

Blackburn, S. (1993). Assessment and management of neurologic dysfunction. In C. Kenner, A. Brueggemeyer, & L. Gunderson (Eds.), *Comprehensive neonatal nursing.* Philadelphia: Saunders.

Blackburn, S., & Vandenberg, K. (1993). Assessment and management of neonatal neurobehavioral development. In C. Kenner, A. Brueggemeyer, & L. Gunderson (Eds.), *Comprehensive neonatal nursing.* Philadelphia: Saunders.

Bliss-Holtz, J. (1992). Temperature relationships in cold-stressed infants. *Neonatal Network, 11*(2), 72.

Boggs, R. L., & Woolridge-Kim, M. (1993). *AACH procedural manual for critical care* (3rd ed). Philadelphia: Saunders.

Bolton, P. J., & Kline, K. A. (1994). Understanding modes of mechanical ventilation. *American Journal of Nursing, 94*(6), 36–43.

Bossert, E., Holaday, B., Harkins, A., & Turner-Henson, A. (1990). Strategies of normalization used by parents of chronically ill school age children. *Journal of Child and Adolescent Psychiatric and Mental Health Nursing, 3*(2), 57–61.

Bowers, B. (1987). Intergenerational caregiving: Adult caregivers and their aging parents. *Advances in Nursing Science, 9*(2), 20–31.

Boyes, R. J., & Kruse, J. A. (1992), Nasogastric and nasoenteric intubation. *Critical Care Clinics, 8*(4), 865–878.

Bozzette, M. (1993). Observations of pain behavior in the NICU: An exploratory study. *Journal of Perinatal and Neonatal Nursing, 7*(1), 76–87.

Breslin, E. H. (1992). Dyspnea-limited response in chronic obstructive pulmonary disease: Reduced unsupported arm activities. *Rehabilitation Nursing, 17*, 12–20.

Bricker, D. (Ed.). (1993). *AEPS measurement for birth–three years* (Vol. 1). Baltimore: Paul H. Brookes Publishing.

Brooks-Brunn, J. A. (1995). Postoperative atelectasis and pneumonia: Risk factors. *American Journal of Critical Care, 4*, 340.

Brown, D. R., Morgan, W. P., & Raglin, J. S. (1993). Effects of exercise and rest on the state of anxiety and blood pressure of physically challenged college students. *Journal of Sports Medicine and Physical Fitness, 33*(3), 300–305.

Brukwitzki, G., Holmgren, C., & Maibusch, R. M. (1996). Validation of the defining characteristics of the nursing diagnosis "ineffective airway clearance." *Nursing Diagnosis, 7*(2), 63–69.

Brundage, D. J., & Linton, A. D. (1997). Age related changes in the genitourinary system. In M. A. Matteson, E. S. McConnell, & A. D. Linton (Eds.), *Gerontological nursing: Concepts in practice* (2nd ed.). Philadelphia: Saunders.

Bull, M. J. (1994). Patients' and professionals' perceptions of quality in discharge planning. *Journal of Nursing Care Quality, 8*(2), 47–61.

Burnside, I., & Haight, B. (1994). Reminiscence and life review: Therapeutic interventions for older people. *Nurse Practitioner, 19*(4), 55–60.

Burrow, S. (1994). Nursing management of self-mutilation. *British Journal of Nursing, 3*, 8, 382–386.

Caldwell, S. M. (1993). Measuring family well-being: Conceptual model, reliability, validity and use. In C. F. Waltz & O. L. Strickland (Eds.), *Measuring client outcomes.* New York: Springer.

Campbell, J., McKenna, L. S., Torres, S., Sheridan, D., & Landenburger, K. (1993). Nursing care of abused women. In J. Campbell & J. Humphreys (Eds.), *Nursing care of survivors of family violence.* St. Louis: Mosby.

Campus, R. G. (1994). Rocking and pacifiers: Two comforting interventions for heelstick pain. *Research in Nursing & Health, 17*, 321–331.

Carlson-Catalano, J. (1998). Nursing diagnosis and interventions for post-acute-phase battered women. *Nursing Diagnosis: The Journal of Nursing Language and Classification, 9*(3), 101–110.

Carlson-Catalano, J., Lunney, M., Paradiso, C., Bruno, J., Luise, B. K., Martin, T., Massoni, M., & Pachter, S. (1998). Clinical validation of ineffective breathing pattern, ineffective airway clearance, and impaired gas exchange. *Image: Journal of Nursing Scholarship, 30*(3), 243–248.

Carpenito, L. J. (1997a). *Handbook of nursing diagnosis* (7th ed.). Philadelphia: Lippincott.

Carpenito, L. J. (1997b). *Nursing diagnosis: Application to clinical practice* (7th ed.). Philadelphia: Lippincott.

Casaburi, R., & Petty, T. (1993). *Principles and practice of pulmonary rehabilitation.* Philadelphia: Saunders.

Chang, B. L., Uman, G. C., & Hirsch, M. (1998). Predictive power of clinical indicators of self-care deficit. *Nursing Diagnosis: The Journal of Nursing Language and Classification, 9*(2), 71–82.

Chilman, C., Nunnally, E., & Cox, F. (1988). *Chronic illness and disability.* Beverly Hills, CA: Sage Publications, 30–31.

Clark, C. C. (1998). Wellness self-care by healthy older adults. *Image: Journal of Nursing Scholarship, 31*(4), 351–355.

Cohen, R. K., Diegelmann, R. F., & Lindblad, W. L. (1992). *Wound healing: Biochemical and clinical aspects.* Philadelphia: Saunders.

Cole, S. L. (1992). Dress for success: A nurse's knowledge of simple clothing adaptations and dressing aids may make the difference between rehabilitation success and failure. *Geriatric Nursing, 13*(4), 217–221.

Collins, C. E., Given, B. A., & Given, C. W. (1994). Interventions with family caregivers of persons with Alzheimer's disease. *Nursing Clinics of North America, 29*(1), 127–131.

Conn, V., Talor, S., & Casey, B. (1992). Cardiac rehabilitation program participation and outcomes after myocardial infarction. *Rehabilitation Nursing, 17*(2), 58–62.

Cooley, M. E. (1992). Bereavement care: A role for nurses. *Cancer Nursing, 15*(2), 125–129.

Courtens, A. M., & Abu-Saad, H. H. (1998). Nursing diagnoses in patients with leukemia. *Nursing Diagnosis: The Journal of Nursing Language and Classification, 9*(2), 49–61.

Craft, M. J., & Willadsen, J. A. (1992). Interventions related to family. In G. M. Bulechek & J. C. McCloskey (Eds.), *Symposium on Nursing Interventions. Nursing Clinics of North America, 27*(2), 517–540.

Cullen, L. M. (1992). Interventions related to circulatory care. In G. M. Bulechek & J. C. McCLoskey (Eds.), *Symposium on Nursing Interventions. Nursing Clinics of North America, 27*(2), 445–476.

Dean, G. E., & Ferrell, B. R. (1995). Impact of fatigue on quality of life in cancer survivors. *Quality of Life—A Nursing Challenge, 4*(1), 25–28.

Dean-Barr, S. L. (1994). Standards and guidelines: How do they assure quality? In J. McCloskey & H. K. Grace (Eds.), *Current issues in nursing* (4th ed.). St. Louis: Mosby.

Denehy, J. A. (1990). Anticipatory guidance. In M. J. Craft & J. A. Denehy (Eds.), *Nursing interventions for infants and children* (pp. 53–68). Philadelphia: Saunders.

Denehy, J. A. (1992). Interventions related to parent-infant attachment. In G. M. Bulechek & J. C. McCloskey (Eds.), *Symposium on Nursing Interventions. Nursing Clinics of North America, 27*(2), 425–444.

Donnelly, A. J. (1994). Malignant hyperthermia: Epidemiology, pathophysiology, treatment. *AORN Journal, 59*(2), 393–405.

Dougherty, C. M. (1992). Surveillance. In G. M. Bulechek & J. C. McCloskey (Eds.). *Nursing interventions: Essential nursing treatments* (2nd ed.) (pp. 500–511). Philadelphia: Saunders.

Dougherty, C. (1997). Reconceptualization of the nursing diagnosis "decreased cardiac output." *Nursing Diagnosis: The Journal of Nursing Language and Classification, 8*(1), 29–36.

Doughty, D. (Ed.). (1991). *Urinary and fecal incontinence: Nursing management.* St. Louis: Mosby-Year Book.

Dyckoff, D., Goldstein, L., & Levine-Schacht, L. (1996). The investigation of behavioral contracting in patients with borderline personality disorder. *Journal of the American Psychiatric Nurses Association, 2*(3), 71–76.

Eakes, G. G., Burke, M. L., & Hainsworth, M. A. (1998). Middle-range theory of chronic sorrow. *Image: Journal of Nursing Scholarship, 30*(2), 179–184.

El Camino Hospital Clinical Practice Council. (1992). *Management of the adult patient being weaned.* Mountain View, CA: El Camino Hospital.

Elek, S. M., Hudson, D. B., & Fleck, M. L. (1997). Expectant parents' experience with fatigue and sleep during pregnancy. *Birth, 24,* 49–54.

Elsen, J., & Blegen, M. (1991). Social isolation. In M. Maas, K. Buckwalter, & M. Hardy (Eds.), *Nursing diagnoses and interventions in the elderly* (pp. 519–529). Redwood City, CA: Addison-Wesley.

Fearing, M. O., & Hart, L. K. (1992). Dialysis therapy. In G. M. Bulechek & J. C. McCloskey (Eds.), *Nursing interventions: Essential nursing treatments* (2nd ed.) (pp. 587–601). Philadelphia: Saunders.

Ferrell, B. R., Dow, K. H., Leigh, S., Ly, J., & Gulaskekaram, P. (1995). Quality of life in long-term cancer survivors. Part 1. *Oncology Nursing Forum, 22*(6), 915–922.

Fischman, S. (1993). Self-care: Practical periodontal care in today's practice. *International Dental Journal, 43,* 179–183.

Flanagan, M. (1994). Assessment criteria. *Nursing Times, 90*(35), 76–88.

Folden, S. L. (1993). Definitions of health and health goals of participants in a community-based pulmonary rehabilitation program. *Public Health Nursing, 10*(1), 31–35.

Fontaine, K. L., & Fletcher, J. S. (1998). *Mental health nursing* (4th ed). Menlo Park, CA: Addison-Wesley Nursing.

Fowler, S. B. (1997). Impaired verbal communication during short-term oral intubation. *Nursing Diagnosis: The Journal of Nursing Language and Classification, 8*(3), 93–98.

Frieberg, K. (1992). *Human development: A life span approach* (4th ed.). Boston: Jones and Bartlett.

Friedman, M. M. (1992). *Family nursing: Theory and practice.* Norwalk, CT: Appleton & Lange.

Gardner, D. L., & Campbell, B. (1991). Assessing postpartum fatigue. *Maternal Child Nursing Journal, 16*(5), 264–266.

Geissler, E. (1991). Transcultural nursing and nursing diagnoses. *Nursing and Health Care, 12*(4), 190–192, 203.

Gianino, S., & St. John, R. E. (1993). Nutritional assessment of the patient in the intensive care unit. *Critical Care Nursing Clinics of North America, 5*(1), 1–16.

Giger, J., & Davidhizar, R. (1995). *Transcultural nursing.* St. Louis: Mosby-Year Book.

Gill, L., & Flenstein, A. R. (1994). A critical appraisal of the quality of quality-of-life measurements. *Journal of the American Medical Association, 272,* 619–626.

Gillis, A. J. (1993). Determinants of health promoting lifestyle: An integrative review. *Journal of Advanced Nursing, 18,* 345–353.

Glennon, S. (1993). Mechanical support of ventilation. In M. R. Kinney, D. R. Backa, & S. B. Dunbar (Eds.), *AACN's clinical reference for critical-care nursing* (pp. 828–840). St. Louis: Mosby.

Glick, O. J. (1992). Interventions related to activity and movement. In G. M. Bulechek & J. C. McCloskey (Eds.), *Symposium on Nursing Interventions. Nursing Clinics of North America, 27*(2), 541–568.

Glick, D., Kronenfeld, J., & Jackson, K. (1993). Safety behaviors among parents of preschoolers. *Health Values, 17*(1), 18–27.

Gordon, M. (1987). *Nursing process and application* (2nd ed.). New York: McGraw-Hill.

Gordon, M. (1994). *Nursing process and application* (3rd ed.). New York: McGraw-Hill.

Grancola, P. R., & Zeichner, A. (1993). Aggressive behavior in the elderly: A critical review. *Clinical Gerontologist, 13*(2), 3–22.

Greaves, P., Glik, D. C., Kronenfeld, J. J., & Jackson, K. (1994). Determinants of controllable in-home child safety hazards. *Health Education Research, 9*(3), 307–315.

Green, M. (Ed.). (1994). *Bright futures: Guidelines for health supervision of infants, children and adolescents.* Arlington, VA: National Center for Education in Maternal and Child Health.

Griffin, T., Wishba, C., & Kavanaugh, K. (1998). Nursing interventions to reduce stress in parents of hospitalized preterm infants. *Journal of Pediatric Nursing, 13*(5), 290–295.

Guyton, A. C. (1992). *Human physiology and mechanisms of disease.* Philadelphia: Saunders.

Gyulay, J. (1989). Grief responses. *Issues in Comprehensive Pediatric Nursing, 12*(1), 1–31.

Haber, J., McMahon, A. L., Price-Hoskins, P., & Sideleau, B. F. (1992). *Comprehensive psychiatric nursing* (4th ed.). St. Louis: Mosby.

Halm, M. (1990). The effect of support groups on anxiety of family members during critical illness. *Heart and Lung, 11*(6), 571–576.

Halpern, J. S. (1989). Clinical notebook: Lower extremity peripheral nerve assessment. *Journal of Emergency Nursing, 15*(4), 333–337.

Hartford, M., Karlson, B. W., Sjolin, M., Holmber, S., & Herlitz, J. (1993). Symptoms, thoughts, and environmental factors in suspected acute myocardial infarction. *Heart and Lung, 22*(1), 64–70.

Hawkins-Walsh, E. (1988). Breastfeeding the premature infant. *Pediatric Nursing Forum, 3*(4), 3–13.

Hayden, R. (1992). What keeps oxygenation on track? *American Journal of Nursing, 92*(12), 32–40.

Healthy people 2000: National health promotion and disease prevention objectives. (1990). DHHS Publication (PHS) 91-50213. Washington, DC: U.S. Department of Health and Human Services, Public Health Service.

Hegyvary, S. T. (1993). Patient care outcomes related to management of symptoms. In J. J. Fitzpatrick & J. J. Stevenson (Eds.), *Annual Review of Nursing Research*, 11 (pp. 145–168). New York: Springer.

Henneman, E. A. (1991). The art and science of weaning from mechanical ventilation. *AACN Focus on Critical Care, 18*(6), 490–501.

Herr, K. A., & Mobily, P. R. (1992). Interventions related to pain. In G. M. Bulechek & J. C. McCloskey (Eds.), *Symposium on Nursing Interventions. Nursing Clinics of North America, 27*(2), 347–370.

Hickey, J. V. (1992). *The clinical practice of neurological and neurosurgical nursing.* Philadelphia: Lippincott.

Hoff, L. A. (1993). Battered women—intervention and prevention: A psychosocial cultural perspective. Part 2. *Journal of the American Academy of Nurse Practitioners, 4,* 148–155.

Hogstel, M. O., & Nelson, M. (1992). Anticipation and early detection can reduce bowel elimination complications. *Geriatric Nursing,* January/February, 28–33.

Howells, K., & Hollin, C. R. (1992). *Clinical approaches to violence.* New York: Wiley.

Hurley, M. (Ed.). (1986). *Classification of nursing diagnoses: Proceedings of the Sixth Conference, North American Nursing Diagnosis Association.* St. Louis: Mosby.

Innerarity, S. A., & Stark, J. L. (1994). *Fluids and electrolytes* (2nd ed.). Springhouse, PA: Springhouse.

Iowa Intervention Project Research Team. (1998). *NIC interventions linked to NOC outcomes.* Iowa City, IA: Center for Nursing Classification.

Jacox, A., Ferell, B., Heidrich, G., Hester, N., & Miaskowski, C. (1992). A guideline for the nation: Managing acute pain. *American Journal of Nursing, 92*(5), 49–55.

Janson-Bjerklie, S. (1993). Predicting the outcomes of living with asthma. *Research in Nursing and Health, 16*(4), 241–249.

Jenny, J. (1987). Knowledge deficit: Not a nursing diagnosis. *Image, 19*(4), 184–185.

Jenny, J., & Logan, J. (1991). Analyzing expert nursing practice to develop a new nursing diagnosis: Dysfunctional ventilatory weaning response. In R. M. Carroll-Johnson (Ed.), *Classification of nursing diagnoses: Proceedings of the Ninth Conference* (pp. 133–140). Philadelphia: Lippincott.

Jensen, L., & Allen, M. (1993). Wellness: The dialect of illness. *Image: The Journal of Nursing Scholarship, 25*(3), 220–224.

Jirevec, M. M., Wyman, J. F., & Wells, T. J. (1998). Addressing urinary incontinence with educational continence-care competencies. *Image: Journal of Nursing Scholarship, 30*(4), 375–378.

Johnson, M., & Maas, M. (eds.). (1997). *Nursing Outcomes Classification (NOC)*. St. Louis: Mosby.

Kalbach, L. R. (1991). Unilateral neglect: Mechanisms and nursing care. *Journal of Neuroscience Nursing, 23*(2), 125–129.

Kanak, M. F. (1992). Interventions relted to safety. In G. M. Bulechek & J. C. McCloskey (Eds.), *Symposium on Nursing Interventions. Nursing Clinics of North America, 27*(2), 371–396.

Kelley, M. P., & Henry, P. (1993). Open discussion can lead to acceptance: The psychosocial effects of stoma surgery. *Professional Nurse, 9*(2), 101–110.

King, C. (1998). Enteral feeding for preterm infants: Nutrition and therapy. *Journal of Neonatal Nursing, 4*(5), 6, 8–10.

King, C. (1998). Parenteral nutrition for the preterm infant: Optimal levels of key nutrients. *Journal of Neonatal Nursing, 4*(4), 12–15.

Kluger, M. (1978). Fever versus hyperthermia. *New England Journal of Medicine, 299*(10), 555.

Knebel, A. F. (1991). Weaning from mechanical ventilation: Current controversies. *Heart and Lung, 20*(4), 321–333.

Kozier, B., Erb, G., Blais, K., & Wilkinson, J. (1997). *Fundamentals of nursing* (5th ed.). Menlo Park, CA: Addison-Wesley Nursing.

Krieger, D. (1979). *The therapeutic touch: How to use your hands to help or to heal.* Englewood Cliffs, NJ: Prentice-Hall.

Kulbok, P., & Baldwin, J. (1992). From preventive health behavior to health promotion: Advancing a positive construct of health. *Advances in Nursing Science, 14*(4), 50–64.

Kunz, D., & Krieger, D. (1975–1990). *Annual invitational workshops on therapeutic touch.* Graysville, NY: Pumpkin Hollow Foundation.

Kus, R. J. (1992). Crisis intervention. In G. M. Bulechek & J. C. McCloskey (Eds.), *Nursing interventions: Essential nursing treatments* (2nd ed.) (pp.179–190). Philadelphia: Saunders.

Lane, G. H. (1990). Pulmonary therapeutic management. In L. A. Thelan, J. K. Davie, & L. D. Urden (Eds.). *Textbook of critical care nursing* (pp. 444–471). St. Louis: Mosby.

LeMone, P. (1991). Analysis of a human phenomenon: Self-concept. *Nursing Diagnosis, 2*(3), 129–130.

LeMone, P., & Burke, K. M. (1996). *Medical surgical nursing: Critical thinking in client care.* Menlo Park, CA: Addison-Wesley Nursing.

LeMone, P., & Jones, D. (1997). Nursing assessment of altered sexuality: A review of salient factors and objective measures. *Nursing Diagnosis: The Journal of Nursing Language and Classification, 8*(3), 120–128.

LeMone, P., & Weber, J. (1995). Validating gender-specific defining characteristics of altered sexuality. *Nursing Diagnosis, 6*(2), 64–69.

Lepshy, M. S., & Michael, A. (1993). Chronic diarrhea: Evaluation and treatment. *American Family Physician, 48*(8), 1461–1466.

Lindeman, M., Hokanson, J., & Batek, J. (1994). The alcoholic family. *Nursing Diagnosis, 5*(2), 65–73.

Lindgren, C. L. (1993). The caregiver career. *Image: The Journal of Nursing Scholarship, 25*(3), 214–219.

Loening-Baucke, V. (1994). Management of chronic constipation in infants and toddlers. *American Family Physician, 46*(2), 397–406.

Loeper, J. M. (1992). Positioning. In G. M. Bulechek & J. C. McCloskey (Eds.), *Nursing interventions: Essential nursing treatments* (2nd ed.) (pp. 86–93). Philadelphia: Saunders.

Logan, J., & Jenny, J. (1991). Interventions for the nursing diagnosis "dysfunctional ventilatory weaning response": A qualitative study. In R. M. Carroll-Johnson (Ed.), *Classification of nursing diagnoses: Proceedings of the Ninth Conference* (pp. 141–147). Philadelphia: Lippincott.

Longo, M. B. (1993). Facilitating acceptance of a patient's decision to stop treatment. *Clinical Nurse Specialist, 7*(3), 233–243.

Low, M. B. (1993). Women's body image: The nurse's role in promotion of self-acceptance. *AWHONN's Clinical Issues, 4*(2), 213–219.

Lowe, N. K. (1993). Maternal confidence for labor: Development of the childbirth self-efficacy inventory. *Research in Nursing and Health, 10*, 357–365.

Lowenstein, A. J., & Hoff, P. S. (1994). Discharge planning: A study of nursing staff involvement. *Journal of Nursing Administration, 24*(4), 45–40.

Luiselli, J. K. (1993). Training self-feeding skills in children who are deaf and blind. *Behavior Modification, 17*(4), 457–473.

McCaffrey, M., & Beebe, A. (1989). *Pain: Clinical manual for nursing practice.* St. Louis: Mosby.

McCance, K. L., & Huether, S. E. (1994). *Pathophysiology: The biologic basis for disease in adults and children* (2nd ed.). St. Louis: Mosby.

McCloskey, J. C., & Bulechek, M. C. (Eds.). (1996). *Nursing Interventions Classification (NIC)* (2nd ed.). St. Louis: Mosby.

McFarland, G. K., & McFarlane, E. A. (1993). *Nursing diagnosis and intervention: Planning for patient care* (2nd ed.). St. Louis: Mosby.

McHaffie, H. (1992). The assessment of coping. *Clinical Nursing Research, 1*(1), 67–79.

McHale, J. M., Phipps, M. A., Horvath, K., & Schmelz, J. (1998). Expert nursing knowledge in the care of patients at risk of impaired swallowing. *Image: Journal of Nursing Scholarship, 30*(2), 137–141.

McLane, A. (Ed.). (1987). *Classification of nursing diagnoses: Proceedings of the Seventh Conference, North American Nursing Diagnosis Association.* St. Louis: Mosby.

McLane, A. M., & McShane, R. E. (1992). Bowel management. In G. M. Bulechek & J. C. McCloskey (Eds.), *Nursing interventions: Essential nursing treatments* (2nd ed.), (pp. 73–85). Philadelphia: Saunders.

Maas, M. (1991). Impaired physical mobility. In M. Maas, K. Buckwalter, & M. Hardy (Eds.), *Nursing diagnosis and interventions for the elderly* (pp. 263–284). Redwood City, CA: Addison-Wesley Nursing.

Marshall-Baker, A., Lickliter, R., & Cooper, R. (1998). Prolonged exposure to a visual pattern may promote behavioral organization in preterm infants. *Journal of Perinatal and Neonatal Nursing, 12*(2), 50–62.

Maxfield, M. C., Lewis, R. E., & Connor., S. (1996). Training staff to prevent aggressive behavior of cognitively impaired elderly patients during bathing and grooming. *Journal of Gerontological Nursing, 22*(1), 37–43.

Meehan, T. C. (1991). Therapeutic touch. In G. Bulechek & J. McCloskey (Eds.), *Nursing interventions: Essential nursing treatments.* Philadelphia: Saunders.

Moss, A. B. (1992). Are the elderly safe at home? *Journal of Community Health Nursing, 9*(1), 13–19.

Murphy, T. G., & Bennett, E. J. (1992). Low-tech, high-touch perfusion assessment. *American Journal of Nursing, 92*(5), 36–46.

Murray, M., & Blaylock, B. (1994). Maintaining effective pressure ulcer prevention programs. *Medsurg Nursing, 3*(2), 85–92.

NANDA nursing diagnoses: Definitions and classification 1999–2000. (1999). Philadelphia, PA: NANDA.

Nease, R. (1994). Risk attitudes in gambles involving length of life: Aspirations, variations, and ruminations. *Medical Decision Making, 14*(2), 210–213.

Nelson, D. M. (1992). Interventions related to respiratory care. In G. M. Bulechek & J. C. McCloskey (Eds.), *Symposium on Nursing Interventions. Nursing Clinics of North America, 27*(2), 301–324.

NIC interventions linked to NANDA diagnoses. (1993). Iowa City: IA: Iowa Intervention Project.

Norris, J. (1992). Nursing intervention for self-esteem disturbances. *Nursing Diagnosis, 3*(2), 48–53.

North American Nursing Diagnosis Association. (1986). *Seventh Conference on Classification of Nursing Diagnoses. Syllabus of Conference Proceedings.* St. Louis: Author.

North American Nursing Diagnosis Association. (1988). *Eighth Conference on Classification of Nursing Diagnoses. Syllabus of Conference Proceedings.* St. Louis: Author.

North American Nursing Diagnosis Association. (1999). *NANDA nursing diagnoses: Definitions and classification 1999–2000.* Philadelphia: Author.

Olds, S., London, M., & Ladewig, P. (1996). *Maternal-newborn nursing: A family-centered approach* (5th ed.). Menlo Park, CA: Addison-Wesley Nursing.

Olson, E. V., Johnson, B. J., Thompson, L. F., McCarthy, J. S., Edmonds, R. E., Schroeder, L. M., & Wade, M. (1967). The hazards of immobility. *American Journal of Nursing, 67*(4), 780–797.

Palmer, M. H., McCormick, K. A., Langford, A., Langlais, J., & Alvaran, M. (1992). Continence outcomes: Documentation on medical records in the home environment. *Journal of Nursing Care Quality, 6*(3), 36–43.

Palmer, S. J. (1993). Care of sick children by parents: A meaningful role. *Journal of Advanced Nursing, 18*, 85–191.

Panel for the Prediction and Prevention of Pressure Ulcers in Adults. (1992, May). *Pressure ulcers in adults: Prediction and prevention. Clinical Practice Guideline Number 3.* (AHCPR Publication No. 92-0047.) Rockville,

MD: Agency for Health Care Policy and Research, Public Health Service, U.S. Department of Health and Human Services.

Pawlicki, C. M., & Gaumer, C. (1993). Nursing care of the self-mutilating patient. *Bulletin of the Menninger Clinic, 57*(3), 380–389.

Pehler, S. (1997). Children's spiritual response: Validation of the nursing diagnosis "spiritual distress." *Nursing Diagnosis: The Journal of Nursing Language and Classification, 8*(2), 55–66.

Pender, N. (1996). *Health promotion in nursing practice* (3rd ed.). Stamford, CT: Appleton & Lange.

Peruzzi, W. T., & Smith, B. (1995). Bronchial hygiene therapy. *Critical Care Clinics, 13*, 47.

Pomeroy, V. (1990). Development of an ADL-oriented assessment-of-mobility scale suitable for use for elderly people with dementia. *Physiotherapy, 76*(8), 446–448.

Positioning the surgical patient (1993). In *Standards and Recommended Practices*. Denver: Association of Operating Room Nurses.

Potempa, K. M. (1992). Chronic fatigue. In J. J. Fitzpatrick, R. L. Taunton, & A. K. Jacox (Eds.), *Annual review of nursing research* (Vol. 10, pp. 57–76). New York: Springer.

Pridham, K., Brown, R., Sondel, S., Green, C., Wedel, N., & Lai, H. (1998). Transition time to full nipple feeding for premature infants with a history of lung disease. *Journal of Obstetric, Gynecologic, and Neonatal Nursing, 27*(5), 533–545.

Pugh, L. C., & Milligan, R. (1993). A framework for the study of childbearing fatigue. *Advances in Nursing Science, 15*(4), 60–70.

Puntillo, K., & Weiss, S. J. (1994). Pain: Its mediators and associated morbidity in critically ill cardiovascular surgical patients. *Nursing Research, 43*(1), 31–36.

Rakel, B. A. (1992). Interventions related to patient teaching. In G. M. Bulechek & J. C. McCloskey (Eds.). *Symposium on Nursing Interventions. Nursing Clinics of North America, 27*(2), 397–424.

Rantz, M. J., & McShane, R. E. (1995). Nursing interventions for chronically confused nursing home residents. *Geriatric Nursing, 16*(1), 22–27.

Rasin, J. (1990). Confusion. *Nursing Clinics of North America*, 25, 909–918.

Redman, B. K. (1993). *The process of patient education* (7th ed.). St. Louis: Mosby.

Rhodes, A., & McDaniel, R. (1995). Fatigue and advanced illness. *Quality of Life—A Nursing Challenge, 4*(1), 14–19.

Riordan, J., & Auerbach, K. (1993). *Breastfeeding and human lactation*. Boston: Jones & Bartlett.

Ruzevich, S. (1993). Cardiac assist devices. In J. M. Clochesy, C. Breu, S. Cardin, E. B. Rudy, & A. A. Whittaker (Eds.), *Critical care nursing* (pp. 183–192). Philadelphia: Saunders.

Sachs, B., Hall, L. A., Lutenbacher, M., & Rayens, M. K. (1999). Potential for abusive parenting by rural mothers with low birth weight children. *Image: Journal of Nursing Scholarship, 31*(1), 21–25.

Salazar, M. K., & Primomo, J. (1994). *Taking the lead in environmental health*. American Association of Occupational Health Nurses (AAOHN), *42*(7), 317–324.

Sapala, S. (1994). Pediatric management problems. *Pediatric Nursing, 20*(1), 54–55.

Schainen, J. S. (1991). Environments for nursing care of the older client. In W. C. Chenitz, J. T. Stone, & S. A. Salisbury, *Clinical gerontological nursing*. Philadelphia: Saunders.

Schibler, K. D., & Fay, S. A. (1990). Sleep promotion. In M. J. Craft & J. A. Denehy (Eds.), *Nursing interventions for infants and children* (pp. 285–303). Philadelphia: Saunders.

Schuiling, K. D., & Sampselle, C. M. (1999). Comfort in labor and midwifery art. *Image: Journal of Nursing Scholarship, 31*(1), 77–81.

Schumacher, K. L., Stewart, B. J., & Archbold, P. G. (1998). Conceptualization and measurement of doing family caregiving well. *Image: Journal of Nursing Scholarship, 30*(1), 63–69.

Shaker, C. (1990). Nipple feeding premature infants: A different perspective. *Neonatal Network, 8*(5), 9–17.

Sheppard, M. (1993). Client satisfaction, extended intervention and interpersonal skills in community mental health. *Journal of Advanced Nursing, 18*, 246–259.

Sime, M. (1992). Decisional control. In M. Snyder (Ed.), *Independent nursing interventions* (2nd ed.) (pp. 110–114). Albany: Delmar.

Simon, J. M., Bauman, M. A., & Nolan, L. (1995). Differential diagnosis validation: Acute and chronic pain. *Nursing Diagnosis, 6*(2), 73–79.

Simons, M. R. (1992). Interventions related to compliance. In G. M. Bulechek & J. C. McCloskey (Eds.). *Symposium on Nursing Interventions. Nursing Clinics of North America, 27*(2), 477–494.

Simons-Morton, D. G., Mullen, P. D., Mains, D. A., Tabak, E. R., & Green, L. W. (1992). Characteristics of controlled studies of patient education and counseling for preventive health behaviors. *Patient Education and Counseling, 19*, 174–204.

Smith, J. E., Early, J. A., Green, P. T., Lauck, D. L., Oblaczynski, C., Smochek, M. R., & Wright, G. (1997). Risk for suicide and risk for violence: A case for separating the current violence diagnoses. *Nursing Diagnosis: The Journal of Nursing Language and Classification, 8*(2), 67–77.

Smith, M. (1993). Pediatric sexuality: Promoting normal sexual development in children. *Nurse Practitioner, 18*(8), 37–44.

Snyder, M. (1992). Exercise. In M. Snyder (Ed.), *Independent nursing interventions* (2nd ed.) (pp. 67–77). Albany: Delmar.

Specht, J. P., Maas, M. L., Willett, S., & Myers, N. (1992). Intermittent catheterization. In G. M. Bulechek & J. C. McCloskey (Eds.), *Nursing interventions: Essential nursing treatments* (2nd ed.) (pp. 61–72). Philadelphia: Saunders.

Specht, J., Tunink, P., Maas, M., & Bulecheck, G. (1991). Urinary incontinence. In M. Maas, K. C. Buckwalter, & M. A. Hardy (Eds.). *Nursing diag-*

noses and interventions for the elderly (pp. 181–204). Redwood City, CA: Addison-Wesley.

Sprague-McRae, J. M., Lamb, W., & Homer, D. (1993). Encopresis: A study of treatment alternatives and historical behavioral characteristics. *Nurse Practitioner, 18*(10), 52–63.

Starling, B. P., & Martin, A. C. (1990). Adult survivors of parental alcoholism: Implications for primary care. *Nurse Practitioner, 15*(7), 16–24.

Stephenson, C. (1991). The concept of hope revisited for nursing. *Journal of Advanced Nursing, 16*, 1456–1461.

Stevens, P., & Hall, J. (1993). Environmental health in community health nursing. In J. F. Swanson & M. Albrecht (Eds.). *Community health nursing: Promoting the health of aggregates* (pp. 567–596). Philadelphia: Saunders.

Streitmatter, J. (1993). Gender differences in identity development: An examination of longitudinal data. *Adolescence, 28*(109), 55–66.

Stuart, G. W., & Sundeen, S. J. (1995). *Principles and practice of psychiatric nursing* (5th ed.). St. Louis: Mosby.

Stuifbergen, A. K., & Rogers, S. (1997). The experience of fatigue and strategies of self-care among persons with multiple sclerosis. *Applied Nursing Research, 10*, 2–10.

Sullivan, P., & Markos, P. (1993). *Clinical procedures in therapeutic exercise.* Norwalk, CT: Appleton & Lange.

Szabo, V., & Strang, V. R. (1999). Experiencing control in caregiving. *Image: Journal of Nursing Scholarship, 31*(1), 71–75.

Talashek, M. L., Gerace, L. M., & Starr, K. L. (1994). The substance abuse pandemic: Determinants to guide interventions. *Public Health Nursing, 11*(2), 131–139.

Thelan, L. A., & Urden, L. D. (1993). *Critical care nursing: Diagnosis and management* (2nd ed.). St. Louis: Mosby.

Thompson, E. H., Futterman, A. M., Gallagher-Thompson, D., Rose, J. M., & Lovett, S. B. (1993). Social support and caregiving burden in family caregivers of frail elders. *Journal of Gerontology, 48*, S245-S254.

Tiesinga, L. J., Dassen, T. W. N., & Ruud, J. G. H. (1996). Fatigue: A summary of the definitions, dimensions, and indicators. *Nursing Diagnosis, 7*(2), 51–62.

Titler, M. G. (1992). Interventions related to surveillance. In G. M. Bulechek J. C. McCloskey (Eds.), *Symposium on Nursing Interventions. Nursing Clinics of North America, 27*, 2, 495–516.

Titler, M. G., & Jones, G. (1992). Airway Management. In G. M. Bulechek & J. C. McCloskey (Eds.), *Nursing interventions: Essential nursing treatments* (2nd ed.) (pp. 512–530). Philadelphia: Saunders.

Titler, M. G., & Walsh, S. M. (1992). Visiting critically ill adults: Strategies for practice. *Critical Care Nursing Clinics of North America, 4*(4), 623–633.

Turner, J., & Lovvorn, M. (1992). Communicable diseases and infection control practices in community health nursing. In M. Stanhope and J. Lancaster (Eds.), *Community health nursing* (3rd ed.) (pp. 312–331). St. Louis: Mosby.

U.S. Department of Health and Human Services. (1992). *Pressure ulcers in adults: Prediction and prevention.* Rockville, MD: Public Health Service, Agency for Health Care Policy and Research.

U.S. Department of Health and Human Services. (1994a). *Clinicians handbook of preventive services: Put prevention into practice.* Washington, DC: U.S. Government Printing Office.

U.S. Department of Health and Human Services. (1994b). *Heart failure: Evaluation and care of patients with left-ventricular systolic dysfunction.* (AHCPR Publication No. 94-0612). Rockville, MD: Public Health Service, Agency for Health Care Policy and Research.

U.S. Department of Health and Human Services. (1994c). *Treatment of pressure ulcers.* (AHCPR Publication No. 95-0047). Rockville, MD: Public Health Service, Agency for Health Care Policy and Research.

U.S. Department of Health and Human Services. (1994d). *Unstable angina: Diagnosis and management* (AHCPR Publication No. 94-0602). Rockville, MD: Public Health Service, Agency for Health Care Policy and Research.

Urinary Incontinence Guideline Panel. (1992, March). *Urinary incontinence in adults: Clinical practice guideline. (*AHCPR Publication No. 92-0038). Rockville, MD: Public Health Service, Agency for Health Care Policy and Research.

Van Wynsberghe, D., Noback, C. R., & Carola, R. (1995). *Human anatomy and physiology* (3rd ed.). New York: McGraw-Hill.

Walker, C. (1995). When to wean: Whose advice do mothers find helpful? *Health Visitor, 68,* 109–111.

Wallhagen, M. I., & Kagan, S. H. (1993). Staying within bounds: Perceived control and the experience of elderly caregivers. *Journal of Aging Studies, 7*(2), 197–213.

Wasson, D., & Anderson, M. A. (1995). Chemical dependency and adolescent self-esteem. *Clinical Nursing Research, 4*(3), 274–289.

Watson, D. L., & Tharp, R. G. (1993). *Self-directing behavior: Self-modification for personal adjustment* (2nd ed.). Monterey, CA: Brooks/Cole.

Weitzel, E. A. (1991). Unilateral neglect. In M. Maas, K. Buckwalter, & M. Hardy (Eds.), *Nursing diagnoses and interventions for the elderly* (pp. 387–395). Redwood City, CA: Addison-Wesley.

Whitley, G. G. (1994). Expert validation and differentiation of the nursing diagnoses anxiety and fear. *Nursing Diagnosis, 5*(4), 143–149.

Whitley, G. G., & Tousman, S. A. (1996). A multivariate approach for validation of anxiety and fear. *Nursing Diagnosis, 7*(8), 116–123.

Whitman, G. (1993). Shock. In M. R. Kinney, D. R. Packa, & S. B. Dunbar (Eds.), *AACN's clinical reference for critical-care nursing* (pp. 133–172). St. Louis: Mosby.

Wilkinson, J. (1996). *Nursing process: A critical thinking approach.* Redwood City, CA: Addison-Wesley.

Winslow, E. H., Lane, L. D., & Woods, R. J. (1995). Dangling: A review of relevant physiology, research, and practice. *Heart and Lung, 24,* 263.

Wong, D. L., & Whaley, L. F. (Eds). (1998). *Nursing care of infants and children* (6th ed.). St. Louis: Mosby-Year Book.

Woodtli, A. (1995a). Mixed incontinence: A new nursing diagnosis? *Nursing Diagnosis, 6*(4), 135–142.

Woodtli, A. (1995b). Stress incontinence: Clinical identification and validation of defining characteristics, *Nursing Diagnosis, 6*(3), 115–122.

Wooldridge, J., Herman, J., Garrison, D., Haddock, S., Massey, J., & Tavakoli, A. (1998). A validation study using the case-control method of the nursing diagnosis "Risk for aspiration." *Nursing Diagnosis: The Journal of Nursing Language and Classification, 9*(1), 5–13.

Workman, M. L. (1993). The immune system: Your defensive partner and offensive foe. *AACN Clinical Issues in Critical Care Nursing, 4*(3), 453–570.

Wright, K. B. (1998). Professional, ethical, and legal implications for spiritual care in nursing. *Image: Journal of Nursing Scholarship, 30*(1), 81–83.

Yang, K. L., & Tobin, M. J. (1991). A prospective study of indexes predicting the outcome of trials of weaning from mechanical ventilation. *New England Journal of Medicine, 324*, 1445–1451.

Young, C. K., & While, S. (1992). Preparing patients for tube feedings at home. *American Journal of Nursing, 92*(4), 46–53.

Ziegler, D. B., & Prior, M. M. (1994). Preparation for surgery and adjustment to hospitalization. *Nursing Clinics of North America, 29*(4), 655–669.

Appendix A

1999-2000 NANDA-Approved Nursing Diagnoses

Grouped by Gordon's Functional Health Patterns

*Nutritional/Metabolic**

Autonomic dysreflexia, risk for
Body temperature, risk for altered
Breastfeeding, effective
Breastfeeding, ineffective
Breastfeeding, interrupted
Dentition, altered
Dysreflexia
Failure to thrive, adult
Fluid volume deficit
Fluid volume deficit, risk for
Fluid volume excess
Fluid volume imbalance, risk for
Growth, risk for altered
Hyperthermia
Hypothermia
Infant feeding pattern, ineffective
Nutrition: less than body requirements, altered
Nutrition: more than body requirements, altered
Nutrition: more than body requirements, risk for altered
Oral mucous membrane, altered
Skin integrity, impaired
Skin integrity, risk for impaired
Swallowing, impaired
Thermoregulation, ineffective
Tissue integrity, impaired

*Health-perception/Health Management**

Aspiration, risk for
Denial, ineffective
Health maintenance, altered
Health seeking behaviors (specify)
Infection, risk for
Injury, risk for
Latex allergy response
Latex allergy response, risk for
Management of therapeutic regimen: community, ineffective
Management of therapeutic regimen: families, ineffective
Management of therapeutic regimen: individual, effective
Management of therapeutic regimen: individual, ineffective

Noncompliance (specify)
Poisoning, risk for
Protection, altered
Suffocation, risk for
Surgical recovery, delayed
Trauma, risk for

*Sleep/Rest**

Sleep deprivation
Sleep pattern disturbance

Activity/Exercise

Activity intolerance
Activity intolerance, risk for
Adaptive capacity: intracranial, decreased
Airway clearance, ineffective
Breathing pattern, ineffective
Cardiac output, decreased
Development, risk for altered
Disorganized infant behavior
Disorganized infant behavior, risk for
Disuse syndrome, risk for
Diversional activity deficit
Energy field disturbance
Fatigue
Gas exchange, impaired
Home maintenance management, impaired
Mobility: bed, impaired
Mobility: physical, impaired
Mobility: wheelchair, impaired
Organized infant behavior, potential for enhanced
Perioperative positioning injury, risk for
Peripheral neurovascular dysfunction, risk for
Self-care deficit: bathing/hygiene, dressing/grooming, feeding, toileting, total
Spontaneous ventilation: inability to sustain
Tissue perfusion, altered (specify): cardiopulmonary, cerebral, gastrointestinal, peripheral, renal
Transfer ability, impaired
Ventilatory weaning response, dysfunctional
Walking, impaired

Elimination

Constipation
Constipation, perceived
Constipation, risk for
Diarrhea

Elimination (continued)
Incontinence: bowel
Incontinence: urinary, functional
Incontinence: urinary, reflex
Incontinence: urinary, stress
Incontinence: urinary, total
Incontinence: urinary, urge
Incontinence: urinary, urge, risk for
Urinary elimination, altered
Urinary retention

Value/Belief*

Decisional conflict
Grieving, anticipatory
Grieving, dysfunctional
Sorrow, chronic
Spiritual distress (distress of the human spirit)
Spiritual distress, risk for
Spiritual well-being, potential for enhanced

Sexuality-Reproductivity*

Sexual dysfunction
Sexuality patterns, altered

Self-perception/Self-concept*

Anxiety
Anxiety, death
Body image disturbance
Environmental interpretation syndrome, impaired
Fear
Hopelessness
Personal identity disturbance
Powerlessness
Self esteem, chronic low
Self esteem disturbance
Self esteem, situational low

Cognitive/Perceptual*

Communication, impaired verbal
Confusion, acute
Confusion, chronic
Decisional conflict
Knowledge deficit
Memory, impaired
Nausea
Pain
Pain, chronic

Sensory/perceptual alterations (specify): auditory, gustatory, kinesthetic, olfactory, tactile, visual

Thought processes, altered

Unilateral neglect

*Coping/Stress Tolerance**

Adjustment, impaired

Coping: community, ineffective

Coping: community, potential for enhanced

Coping, defensive

Coping: family, compromised, ineffective

Coping: family, disabling, ineffective

Coping: family, potential for growth

Coping: individual, ineffective

Denial, ineffective

Post-trauma syndrome

Post-trauma syndrome, risk for

Rape-trauma syndrome

Rape-trauma syndrome, compound reaction

Rape-trauma syndrome, silent reaction

Relocation stress syndrome

Self-mutilation, risk for

Violence, risk for: directed at self

*Role-relationship**

Caregiver role strain

Caregiver role strain, risk for

Family processes, altered

Family processes, altered, alcoholism

Loneliness, risk for

Parent/infant/child attachment, risk for altered

Parenting, altered

Parenting, risk for altered

Role conflict, parental

Role performance, altered

Social interaction, impaired

Social isolation

Violence, risk for: directed at others

*The diagnosis, "Altered growth and development can occur in any of the Functional Health Patterns.

Used by permission of NANDA

Adapted from Functional Health Patterns, Gordon, M. (1994). *Nursing diagnosis: Process and application,* 3rd ed. St. Louis: Mosby.

Appendix B

NANDA-Approved Nurses Diagnoses (1999-2000)

This taxonomically organized list represents the NANDA-approved nursing diagnoses for clinical use and testing

* New diagnoses accepted in 1998.

‡ Revised diagnoses submitted and approved in 1998.

\# Diagnoses revised by small work groups at the 1996 Biennial Conference on the Classification of Nursing Diagnoses; changes approved and added in 1998.

Pattern 1. Exchanging

	1.1.2.1	Altered Nutrition: More Than Body Requirements
	1.1.2.2	Altered Nutrition: Less Than Body Requirements
	1.1.2.3	Altered Nutrition: Risk for More Than Body Requirements
	1.2.1.1	Risk for Infection
	1.2.2.1	Risk for Altered Body Temperature
	1.2.2.2	Hypothermia
	1.2.2.3	Hyperthermia
	1.2.2.4	Ineffective Thermoregulation
	1.2.3.1	Dysreflexia
*	1.2.3.2	Risk for Autonomic Dysreflexia
‡	1.3.1.1	Constipation
	1.3.1.1.1	Perceived Constipation
	~~1.3.1.1.2~~	~~Colonic Constipation~~ (Deleted in 1998)
‡	1.3.1.2	Diarrhea
‡	1.3.1.3	Bowel Incontinence
*	1.3.1.4	Risk for Constipation
	1.3.2	Altered Urinary Elimination
	1.3.2.1.1	Stress Incontinence
‡	1.3.2.1.2	Reflex Urinary Incontinence
	1.3.2.1.3	Urge Incontinence
‡	1.3.2.1.4	Functional Urinary Incontinence
	1.3.2.1.5	Total Incontinence
*	1.3.2.1.6	Risk for Urinary Urge Incontinence
	1.3.2.2	Urinary Retention
\#	1.4.1.1	Altered Tissue Perfusion (Specify Type): Renal, Cerebral, Cardiopulmonary, Gastrointestinal, Peripheral
*	1.4.1.2	Risk for Fluid Volume Imbalance
	1.4.1.2.1	Fluid Volume Excess
	1.4.1.2.2.1	Fluid Volume Deficit
	1.4.1.2.2.2	Risk for Fluid Volume Deficit
	1.4.2.1	Decrease Cardiac Output
‡	1.5.1.1	Impaired Gas Exchange
‡	1.5.1.2	Ineffective Airway Clearance

‡ 1.5.1.3   Ineffective Breathing Pattern
   1.5.1.3.1   Inability to Sustain Spontaneous Ventilation
   1.5.1.3.2   Dysfunctional Ventilatory Weaning Response (DVWR)
   1.6.1   Risk for Injury
   1.6.1.1   Risk for Suffocation
   1.6.1.2   Risk for Poisoning
   1.6.1.3   Risk for Trauma
   1.6.1.4   Risk for Aspiration
   1.6.1.5   Risk for Disuse Syndrome
* 1.6.1.6   Latex Allergy Response
* 1.6.1.7   Risk for Latex Allergy Response
   1.6.2   Altered Protection
1.6.2.1   Impaired Tissue Integrity
‡ 1.6.2.1.1   Altered Oral Mucous Membrane
# 1.6.2.1.2.1   Impaired Skin Integrity
# 1.6.2.1.2.2   Risk for Impaired Skin Integrity
* 1.6.2.1.3   Altered Dentition
   1.7.1   Decreased Adaptive Capacity: Intracranial
   1.8   Energy Field Disturbance

Pattern 2. Communicating

2.1.1.1   Impaired Verbal Communication

Pattern 3. Relating

   3.1.1   Impaired Social Interaction
   3.1.2   Social Isolation
   3.1.3   Risk for Loneliness
‡ 3.2.1   Altered Role Performance
‡ 3.2.1.1.1   Altered Parenting
‡ 3.2.1.1.2   Risk for Altered Parenting
   3.2.1.1.2.1   Risk for Altered Parent/Infant/Child Attachment
   3.2.1.2.1   Sexual Dysfunction
‡ 3.2.2   Altered Family Processes
‡ 3.2.2.1   Caregiver Role Strain
   3.2.2.2   Risk for Caregiver Role Strain
   3.2.2.3.1   Altered Family Process: Alcoholism
   3.2.3.1   Parental Role Conflict
   3.3   Altered Sexuality Patterns

Pattern 4. Valuing

   4.1.1   Spiritual Distress (Distress of the Human Spirit)
* 4.1.2   Risk for Spiritual Distress
   4.2   Potential for Enhanced Spiritual Well-Being

Pattern 5. Choosing

‡ 5.1.1.1   Ineffective Individual Coping
‡ 5.1.1.1.1   Impaired Adjustment
   5.1.1.1.2   Defensive Coping

5.1.1.1.3 Ineffective Denial
5.1.2.1.1 Ineffective Family Coping: Disabling
5.1.2.1.2 Ineffective Family Coping: Compromised
5.1.2.2 Family Coping: Potential for Growth
5.1.3.1 Potential for Enhanced Community Coping
‡ 5.1.3.2 Ineffective Community Coping
5.2.1 Ineffective Management of Therapeutic Regimen: Individuals
5.2.1.1 Noncompliance (Specify)
5.2.2 Ineffective Management of Therapeutic Regimen: Families
5.2.3 Ineffective Management of Therapeutic Regimen: Community
5.2.4 Effective Management of Therapeutic Regimen: Individual
5.3.1.1 Decisional Conflict (Specify)
5.4 Health-Seeking Behaviors (Specify)

Pattern 6. Moving

‡ 6.1.1.1 Impaired Physical Mobility
6.1.1.1.1 Risk for Peripheral Neurovascular Dysfunction
6.1.1.1.2 Risk for Perioperative Positioning Injury
* 6.1.1.1.3 Impaired Walking
* 6.1.1.1.4 Impaired Wheelchair Mobility
* 6.1.1.1.5 Impaired Transfer Ability
* 6.1.1.1.6 Impaired Bed Mobility
6.1.1.2 Activity Intolerance
‡ 6.1.1.2.1 Fatigue
6.1.1.3 Risk for Activity Intolerance
‡ 6.2.1 Sleep Pattern Disturbance
* 6.2.1.1 Sleep Deprivation
6.3.1.1 Diversional Activity Deficit
6.4.1.1 Impaired Home Maintenance Management
6.4.2 Altered Health Maintenance
* 6.4.2.1 Delayed Surgical Recovery
* 6.4.2.2 Adult Failure to Thrive
‡ 6.5.1 Feeding Self-Care Deficit
‡ 6.5.1.1 Impaired Swallowing
6.5.1.2 Ineffective Breastfeeding
6.5.1.2.1 Interrupted Breastfeeding
6.5.1.3 Effective Breastfeeding
6.5.1.4 Ineffective Infant Feeding Pattern
‡ 6.5.2 Bathing/Hygiene Self-Care Deficit
‡ 6.5.3 Dressing/Grooming Self-Care Deficit
‡ 6.5.4 Toileting Self-Care Deficit
6.6 Altered Growth and Development
* 6.6.1 Risk for Altered Development
* 6.6.2 Risk for Altered Growth

	6.7	Relocation Stress Syndrome
	6.8.1	Risk for Disorganized Infant Behavior
‡	6.8.2	Disorganized Infant Behavior
	6.8.3	Potential for Enhanced Organized Infant Behavior

Pattern 7. Perceiving

#	7.1.1	Body Image Disturbance
	7.1.2	Self-Esteem Disturbance
	7.1.2.1	Chronic Low Self-Esteem
	7.1.2.2	Situational Low Self-Esteem
	7.1.3	Personal Identity Disturbance
#	7.2	Sensory/Perceptual Alterations (Specify): Visual, Auditory, Kinesthetic, Gustatory, Tactile, Olfactory
	7.2.1.1	Unilateral Neglect
	7.3.1	Hopelessness
	7.3.2	Powerlessness

Pattern 8. Knowing

	8.1.1	Knowledge Deficit (Specify)
	8.2.1	Impaired Environmental Interpretation Syndrome
	8.2.2	Acute Confusion
	8.2.3	Chronic Confusion
	8.3	Altered Thought Processes
	8.3.1	Impaired Memory

Pattern 9. Feeling

	9.1.1	Pain
	9.1.1.1	Chronic Pain
*	9.1.2	Nausea
	9.2.1.1	Dysfunctional Grieving
	9.2.1.2	Anticipatory Grieving
*	9.2.1.3	Chronic Sorrow
	9.2.2	Risk for Violence: Directed at Others
	9.2.2.1	Risk for Self-Mutilation
	9.2.2.3	Risk for Violence: Self-Directed
‡	9.2.3	Post-Trauma Syndrome
‡	9.2.3.1	Rape-Trauma Syndrome
	9.2.3.1.1	Rape-Trauma Syndrome: Compound Reaction
	9.2.3.1.2	Rape-Trauma Syndrome: Silent Reaction
*	9.2.4	Risk for Post-Trauma Syndrome
#	9.3.1	Anxiety
*	9.3.1.1	Death Anxiety
#	9.3.2	Fear

Appendix C

Diagnosis Qualifiers (NANDA)

(Suggested/not limited to the following)

Qualifier	Definition
Acute	Severe but of short duration
Altered	A change from baseline
Chronic	Lasting a long time; recurring; habitual; constant
Decreased	Lessened; lesser in size, amount, or degree
Deficient	Inadequate in amount, quality, or degree; defective; not sufficient; incomplete
Depleted	Emptied wholly or in part; exhausted of
Disturbed	Agitated; interrupted, interfered with
Dysfunctional	Abnormal, incomplete functioning
Excessive	Characterized by an amount or quantity that is greater than necessary, desirable, or useful
Impaired	Made worse, weakened; damaged, reduced; deteriorated
Increased	Greater in size, amount, or degree
Ineffective	Not producing the desired effect
Intermittent	Stopping or starting again at intervals; periodic; cyclic
Potential for	(For use with wellness diagnoses) made
Enhanced	greater, to increase in quality, or more desired

Reference: *NANDA Nursing Diagnoses: Definitions and Classification 1999-2000* by the North American Nursing Diagnosis Association, 1999, Philadelphia: Author.

Appendix D
Multidisciplinary (Collaborative) Problems
Associated with Diseases and Other
Physiologic Disorders

Cancer

*_Potential Complications of cancer:_ Anemia, bowel obstruction, cachexia, clotting disorders, electrolyte imbalance, pathologic fractures, hemorrhage, obstructive uropathy, metastasis to vital organs (eg, brain, lungs), pericardial effusions, tamponade, sepsis→septic shock, spinal cord compression, superior vena cava syndrome, tissue anoxia→necrosis

Potential Complications of antineoplastic medications: Specify for each drug (eg, anemia, bone marrow depression, cardiac toxicity, CNS toxicity, congestive heart failure, electrolyte imbalance, enteritis, leukopenia, necrosis at IV site, pneumonitis, renal failure, thrombocytopenia)

Potential Complications of narcotic medications: Depressed respirations, consciousness, and blood pressure; cardiovascular collapse, biliary spasm

Potential Complications of radiation therapy: Increased intracranial pressure, myelosuppression, inflammation, fluid/electrolyte imbalances

*Also see specific disorders, such as "Gastrointestinal Function Disorders," for effects of cancer on those patterns.

Cardiac Function Disorders

Potential Complications of angina/coronary artery disease: Myocardial infarction

Potential Complications of congestive heart failure: Ascites, severe cardiac decompensation, cardiogenic shock, deep vein thrombosis, gastrointestinal congestion→malabsorption, hepatic failure, acute pulmonary edema, renal failure

Potential Complications of digitalis administration: Toxicity

Potential Complications of dysrhythmias: Decreased cardiac output→decreased myocardial perfusion→heart failure, severe atrioventricular conduction blocks, thromboemboli formation→stroke, ventricular fibrillation

Potential Complications of myocardial infarction: Cardiogenic shock, dysrhythmia, infarct extension or expansion, myocardial rupture, pulmonary edema, pulmonary embolism, pericarditis, thromboembolism, ventricular aneurysm

Potential Complications of pericarditis/endocarditis: Cardiac tamponade, congestive heart failure, emboli (pulmonary, cerebral, renal, splenic, cardiac), valvular stenosis

Potential Complications of rheumatic fever/rheumatic heart disease: Congestive heart failure, decreased ventricular function, endocarditis, pericardial effusion, valvular changes

Endocrine Function Disorders

Potential Complications of adrenal gland disorders:

Potential Complications of Addison's disease: Addisonian crisis (shock, coma), diabetes mellitus, thyroid disease

Potential Complications of Cushing's disease: Congestive heart failure, hyperglycemia, hypertension, pancreatic tumors, potassium and sodium imbalance, psychosis

Potential Complications of parathyroid gland disorders:
Coma, coronary artery disease, hypoglycemia, infections, ketoacidosis, nephropathy, peripheral vascular disease, retinopathy.

Potential Complications of parathyroid gland disorders:

Potential Complications of hyperparathyroidism: Hypercalcemia→cardiac dysrhythmias, hypertension, metabolic acidosis, pathologic fractures, peptic ulcers, psychosis, renal calculi, renal failure

Potential Complications of hypoparathyroidism: Hypocalcemia→Cardiac dysrhythmias, convulsions, malabsorption, psychosis, tetany

Potential Complications of pituitary gland disorders:

Potential Complications of anterior pituitary disorders: Acromegaly, congestive heart failure, seizures

Potential Complications of posterior pituitary disorders: Loss of consciousness, hypernatremia, seizures

Potential Complications of thyroid gland disorders:

Potential Complications of hyperthyroidism: Exophthalmos, heart disease, negative nitrogen balance, thyroid crisis

Potential Complications of hypothyroidism: Adrenal insufficiency, cardiovascular disorders, myxedema coma, psychosis

Gastrointestinal (GI) Function Disorders

Potential Complications of esophageal disorders:

Potential Complications of esophageal diverticula: Obstruction, pulmonary aspiration of regurgitated food

Potential Complications of esophageal surgery: Reflux esophagitis, stricture formation

Potential Complications of hiatal hernia: Incarceration, necrosis→hemorrhage

Potential Complications of gallbladder, liver, and pancreatic disorders

Potential Complications of cirrhosis: Ascites, anemia, diabetes mellitus, disseminated intravascular coagulation (DIC), esophageal varices, GI bleeding/hemorrhage, hepatic encephalopathy, hyperbilirubinemia, hypokalemia, splenomegaly, peritonitis, renal failure

Potential Complications of cholelithiasis and cholecystitis: Fistula, gallbladder perforation, intestinal ileus/obstruction, obstruction of common bile duct→liver damage, pancreatitis, peritonitis

Potential Complications of hepatic abscess: Fluid/electrolyte, imbalance, hyperbilirubinemia

Potential Complications of metronidazole or iodoquinol administration: Bone marrow suppression

Potential Complications of hepatitis: Cirrhosis, hepatic encephalopathy, hepatic necrosis

Potential Complications of pancreatitis: Ascites, cardiac failure, coma, delirium tremens, diabetes mellitus, hemorrhage, hypovolemic shock, hypocalcemia, hyperglycemia/hypoglycemia, pancreatic abscess, pancreatic pseudocyst, pleural effusion/respiratory failure, psychosis, renal failure, tetany

Potential Complications of GI infections

Potential Complications of appendicitis: Abscess, gangrenous appendicitis, perforated appendix, peritonitis, pylephlebitis

Potential Complications of bacterial or viral infections (eg, food poisoning): Bowel perforation, dehydration, hemolytic uremic syndome, hypokalemia, hypovolemic shock, metabolic acidosis, metabolic alkalosis, peritonitis, respiratory muscle paralysis, thrombotic thrombocytopenic purpura

Potential Complications of helminthic infections: Anemia; bowel, biliary, or pancreatic duct obstruction; migration to liver or lungs

Potential Complications of peritonitis: Hypovolemic shock, septicemia, septic shock

Potential Complications of GI inflammatory diseases (eg, diverticulitis, gastritis, peptic ulcer, ulcerative colitis):
Abscess, anal fissure, anemia, colorectal carcinoma, fistula, fluid/electrolyte imbalances, GI bleeding/hemorrhage, intestinal obstruction, intestinal perforation, peritonitis, pyloric obstruction, toxic megacolon

Potential Complications of gastrectomy, pyloroplasty: Dumping syndrome

Potential Complications of structural and obstructive GI disorders:

Potential Complications of hemorrhoids and anorectal lesions: Anemia, infection, thrombosed hemorrhoid, sepsis

Potential Complications of hernias: Bowel infarction, bowel perforation, hernia incarceration and strangulation, peritonitis

Potential Complications of intestinal obstruction: Bowel wall necrosis, gangrene, fluid and electrolyte imbalance, hypovolemic or septic shock, intestinal perforation, peritonitis

Potential Complications of malabsorption syndromes:
Anemia, bleeding, delayed maturity, lack of growth, muscle wasting, rickets (and other nutrient deficiencies), tetany

Hematologic Disorders

Potential Complications of aplastic anemia: Congestive heart failure, hemorrhage, infections

Potential Complications of coagulation disorders:
Hemorrhage (specific effects are determined by site of bleeding, eg, increased intracranial pressure in the brain, adult respiratory distress syndrome in the cardiovascular system), joint deformity/disability

Potential Complications of leukemias: Anemia, bleeding difficulties/internal hemorrhage, bone infarctions, coma, hepatomegaly, infections, renal failure, seizures, splenomegaly, tachycardia

Potential Complications of nutritional anemias: Impaired neurologic function (eg, problems with proprioception), impaired cardiac function

Potential Complications of iron therapy: Hypersensitivity, toxicity (cardiovascular collapse, liver necrosis, metabolic acidosis)

Potential Complications of cyanocobalamin therapy: Hypersensitivity, hypokalemia, peripheral vascular thrombosis, pulmonary edema

Potential Complications of polycythemia: bone marrow fibrosis, gastrointestinal bleeding and ulcers, splenomegaly, thrombosis (various organs)

Potential Complications of sickle cell anemia: Multisystem organ failure (eg, congestive heart failure, hyperuricemia, hepatomegaly, hepatic abscesses/fibrosis, hyperbilirubinemia, gallstones, bone marrow aplasia, osteomyelitis, aseptic bone necrosis, skin ulcers, vitreous hemorrhage, retinal detachment), sickle cell crisis

Potential Complications of sickle cell crisis: Aplastic crisis, cerebrovascular accident, hemosiderosis (from repeated transfusions), infections (eg, pneumonia), seizures, splenic sequestration→circulatory collapse

Immune Function Disorders

Potential Complications of altered immune function: Allergic reactions→anaphylaxis, autoimmune disorders (eg, systemic lupus erythematosus), delayed wound healing, infections (eg, nosocomial, opportunistic), sepsis→septicemia, acute/chronic tissue inflammation (eg, granulomas), transplant/graft rejection

Potential Complications of autoimmune deficiency syndrome (AIDS): HIV wasting syndrome; malignancies (cervical cancer, Kaposi's sarcoma, lymphomas); neurologic (dementia complex, meningitis); opportunistic infections (eg, candidiasis, cytomegalovirus infection, herpes infection, *Mycobacterium avium* infection, *Pneumocystis carinii* pneumonia, toxoplasmosis, tuberculosis)

Immobilized Patient

Potential Complications of immobility: Contractures, decreased cardiac output, decubitus ulcers, embolus, hypostatic pneumonia, joint ankylosis, orthostatic hypotension, osteoporosis, renal calculi, thrombophlebitis

Musculoskeletal Disorders and Trauma

Potential Complications of amputation: Contracture, delayed healing, edema of the stump, infection

Potential Complications of fractures: Compartment syndrome, deep vein thrombosis, delayed union, fat embolism, infection, necrosis, reflex sympathetic dystrophy, shock

Potential Complications of gout: Nephropathy, uric acid stones →renal failure

Potential Complications of osteoarthritis: Contractures, herniated disk

Potential Complications of osteomyelitis: Cutaneous sinus tract formation, necrosis, soft tissue abscesses

Potential Complications of osteoporosis, osteomalacia: Fractures, neuropathies, post-traumatic arthritis

Potential Complications of Paget's disease: Bone tumors, cardiovascular complications (eg, arteriosclerosis, hypertension, congestive heart failure), degenerative osteoarthritis, dementia, fractures, renal calculi

Potential Complications of rheumatoid arthritis: Anemia, bony and/or fibrous ankylosis, carpal tunnel syndrome, contractures, episcleritis or scleritis of the eye, Felty's syndrome, muscle atrophy, neuropathy, pericarditis, pleural disease, vasculitis

Potential Complications of corticosteroid intra-articular injections: Intra-articular infection, joint degeneration

Potential Complications of corticosteroid systemic administration: Atherosclerosis, cataract formation, congestive heart failure, Cushing's syndrome, delayed wound healing, depressed immune response, edema, growth retardation (children), hyperglycemia, hypertension, hypokalemia, muscle wasting, osteoporosis, peptic ulcers, psychotic reactions, renal failure, thrombophlebitis

Potential Complications of nonsteroidal anti-inflammatory medications: Gastric ulcers/bleeding, nephropathy

Neurologic Disorders

Potential Complications of organic brain diseases (eg, Alzheimer's disease): Aspiration pneumonia, dehydration, delusions, depression, falls, malnutrition, paranoid reactions, pneumonia

Potential Complications of brain injury and intracranial hemorrhage: Brain ischemia, herniation, increased intracranial pressure

Potential Complications of brain tumor: Hyperthermia, increased intracranial pressure, paralysis, sensorimotor changes

Potential Complications of cerebrovascular accident (CVA): Behavioral changes, brain stem failure, cardiac dysrhythmias, coma, elimination disorders, increased intracranial pressure, language disorders, motor deficits, respiratory infection, seizures, sensory-perceptual deficits (**NOTE:** The manifestations and complications of a CVA vary according to the area of the brain affected. Also, it is difficult to determine which effects are manifestations/symptoms and which are actually complications. Furthermore, many of the complications of CVA are due to the resulting immobility rather than to the pathophysiology of the CVA itself. Refer to "Immobilized Patient" on page 639.)

Potential Complications of increased intracranial pressure (eg, cerebral edema, hydrocephalus): CNS ischemic response (increased mean arterial pressure, increased pulse pressure, and bradycardia), coma, failure of autoregulation of cerebral blood flow, hyperthermia resulting from impaired hypothalamic function, motor impairment (decorticate or decerebrate posturing)

Potential Complications of intracranial aneurysm: Hydrocephalus, hypothalamic dysfunction, rebleeding, seizures, vasospasm

Potential Complications of meningitis and encephalitis: Arthritis, brain infarction, coma, cranial nerve damage, hydrocephalus, increased intracranial pressure, seizures

Potential Complications of multiple sclerosis: Pneumonia; dementia; sudden progression of neurologic symptoms (convulsions, coma), urinary tract infection

Potential Complications of myasthenia gravis: Aspiration, cholinergic crisis, dehydration, myasthenic crisis, pneumonia

Potential Complications of Parkinson's disease: Depression and social isolation, falls, infections related to immobility (eg, pneumonia), malnutrition related to dysphagia and immobility, oculogyric crisis, paranoia and hallucinations, pressure ulcers

Potential Complications of seizure disorder: Accidental trauma (eg, burns, falls), aspiration, head injury, status epilepticus→ acidosis, hyperthermia, hypoglycemia, hypoxia

Potential Complications of spinal cord injury: Autonomic dysreflexia, cardiac dysrhythmias, complications due to immobility (see "Immobilized Patient"), hypercalcemia, necrosis of spinal cord tissue, paralytic ileus, respiratory infection secondary to decreased cough reflex, spinal shock

Peripheral Vascular and Lymphatic Disorders

Potential Complications of aortic aneurysm: Dissection, hemiplegia and lower extremity paralysis (with dissection), rupture→hypovolemic shock

Potential Complications of femoral and popliteal aneurysms: Embolism, gangrene, rupture, thrombosis

Potential Complications of hypertension: Aortic dissection, cerebrovascular accident, congestive heart failure, hypertensive crisis, malignant hypertension, myocardial ischemia, papilledema, renal insufficiency, retinal damage

Potential Complications of lymphedema: Cellulitis, lymphangitis

Potential Complications of peripheral arterial disease: Arterial thrombosis, cellulitis, cerebrovascular accident, hypertension, ischemic ulcers, tissue necrosis→gangrene

Potential Complications of thrombophlebitis: Chronic leg edema, pulmonary embolism, stasis ulcers

Potential Complications of varicose veins: Cellulitis, hemorrhage, vascular rupture, venous stasis ulcers

Respiratory Function Disorders

Potential Complications of asthma: Atelectasis, cor pulmonale, dehydration, pneumothorax, respiratory infection, status asthmaticus

   Potential Complications corticosteroid therapy: Hypertension, hypokalemia, hypoglycemia, immunosuppression, osteoporosis, ulcers

   Potential Complications of methylxanthine therapy: Toxicity (seizures, circulatory failure, respiratory arrest)

Potential Complications of chronic obstructive pulmonary disease (COPD): Hypoxemia, respiratory acidosis, respiratory failure, respiratory infection, right-sided heart failure, spontaneous pneumothorax

Potential Complications of pneumonia: Bacteremia→endocarditis, meningitis, peritonitis; lung abscess and empyema; lung tissue necrosis; pleuritis

Potential Complications of pulmonary edema: Cerebral hypoxia, multisystem organ failure, right-sided heart failure

Potential Complications of pulmonary embolism: Pulmonary infarction with necrosis, right ventricular heart failure, sudden death

Potential Complications of tuberculosis: Bacteremia→extrapulmonary tuberculosis (eg, genitourinary tuberculosis, meningitis, peritonitis, pericarditis), bronchopleural fistula, empyema

>***Potential Complications of medications for tuberculosis:*** Hepatotoxicity, hypersensitivity, nephrotoxicity, peripheral neuropathy (isoniazid), optic neuritis (ethambutol)

Sexually Transmitted Disease

Potential Complications of chlamydial infections:

Females: Abortion, infertility, pelvic abscesses, pelvic inflammatory disease, postpartum endometritis, spontaneous abortion, stillbirth

Males: Epididymitis, prostatitis, urethritis

Neonates: Ophthalmia neonatorum, pneumonia

Potential Complications of genital herpes:

All: Herpes keratitis

Females: Cervical cancer

Males: Ascending myelitis, lymphatic suppuration, meningitis, neuralgia, urethral strictures

Neonates: Potentially fatal infections; infections of eyes, skin, mucous membranes, and central nervous system.

Potential Complications of genital warts:

All: Urinary obstruction and bleeding

Females: Increased risk of cancer of the cervix, vagina, vulva, and anus; obstruction of the birth canal during labor; transmission to neonate

Neonates: Respiratory papillomatosis

Potential Complications of gonorrhea:

All: Secondary infection of lesions; fistulas; chronic ulcers; sterility

Females: Abdominal adhesions, ectopic pregnancy, pelvic inflammatory disease

Males: Epididymitis, nephritis, prostatitis, urethritis

Neonates: Ophthalmia neonatorum

Potential Complications of syphilis: Blindness, paralysis, heart failure, liver failure, mental illness

Shock

Potential Complications of shock: Cerebral hypoxia→coma, multiple organ system failure, paralytic ileus, pulmonary emboli, renal failure

Skin Integrity Disorders

Potential Complications of burns: Airway obstruction (inhalation injury), Curling's ulcer, hypothermia, hypovolemic shock, hypervolemia, infection secondary to suppression of immune system, negative nitrogen balance, paralytic ileus, renal failure, sepsis, stress ulcers

Potential Complications of skin lesions/dermatitis/acne: Cyst formation, malignancy, infection

Potential Complications of Herpes zoster: Dissemination→ visceral lesions, encephalitis, loss of vision

Potential Complications of pressure ulcer: Necrotic damage to muscle, bone, tendons, joint capsule; infection, sepsis

Urinary Elimination Disorders

Potential Complications of cystitis: Bladder ulceration, bladder wall necrosis, renal infection

Potential Complications of polycystic kidney disease: Renal calculi, urinary tract infection, renal failure

Potential Complications of pyelonephritis: Bacteremia, chronic pyelonephritis, renal insufficiency, renal failure

Potential Complications of acute renal failure: Electrolyte imbalance, fluid overload, metabolic acidosis, pericarditis, platelet dysfunction, secondary infections

Potential Complications of chronic renal failure: Anemia, cardiac tamponade, pericarditis, congestive heart failure, fluid and electrolyte imbalance, gastrointestinal bleeding, hyperparathyroidism, infections, medication toxicity, metabolic acidosis, pleural effusion, pulmonary edema, uremia

Potential Complications of urolithiasis: Hydronephrosis, hydroureter, infection, pyelonephritis, renal insufficiency

Appendix E
Multidisciplinary (Collaborative) Problems
Associated with Tests and Treatments

Test or Treatment	Potential Complications (Collaborative Problems)
Arteriogram	Allergic reaction, embolism, hemorrhage; hematoma, paresthesia, renal failure, thrombosis at site
Bone marrow studies	Bleeding, infection
Bronchoscopy	Airway obstruction/bronchoconstriction, hemorrhage
Cardiac catheterization	Cardiac dysrhythmias, infarction, perforation, embolism, thrombus formation, hypervolemia, hypovolemia, paresthesia, site hemorrhage or hematoma
Casts and traction	Bleeding, edema, impaired circulation, misalignment of bones, neurologic compromise
Chest tubes	Bleeding→hemothorax, blockage or displacement→pneumothorax, septicemia
Foley catheter	Bladder distention (tube not patent), urinary tract infection
Hemodialysis	Air embolism, bleeding, dialysis dementia, electrolyte imbalance, embolism, fluid shifts, hepatitis B, infection/septicemia, shunt clotting; fistulas, transfusion reactions
Intravenous therapy	Fluid overload, infiltration, phlebitis
Medications	Allergic reactions, side effects (specify), toxic effects/overdose (specify)
Nasogastric suction	Electrolyte imbalance, gastric ulceration→hemorrhage
Radiation therapy	Fistulas, tissue necrosis, hemorrhage, radiation burns, radiation pneumonia
Tracheal suctioning	Bleeding, hypoxia
Ventilation, assisted	Acid–base imbalance, airway obstruction (tube plugged or displaced), ineffective O_2–CO_2 exchange, pneumothorax, respirator dependence, tracheal necrosis

Adapted from *Nursing Process: A Critical Thinking Approach* (2nd ed) (p. 99) by J. Wilkinson, 1996, Menlo Park, CA: Addison-Wesley.

Appendix F
Multidisciplinary (Collaborative) Problems Associated with Surgical Treatments

Format for problem statement:

"Potential Complication of [*column 1*]: [*column 2*],"

For example, *Potential Complication of general surgery: Atelectasis, bronchospasm, and so on.*

Column 1 **Type of Surgery "Potential Complication of"**	*Column 2* **Potential Complications (Multidisciplinary Problems)**
General surgery *(Complications that* *can occur regardless* *of type of surgery)*	Atelectasis, bronchospasm or laryngospasm on extubation (with general anesthesia), electrolyte imbalance, excessive bleeding→ shock, fluid imbalance, headache from leakage of cerebrospinal fluid (with regional anesthesia), hypotension (with regional anesthesia), ileus, infection, stasis pneumonia, urinary retention→bladder distention, venous thrombosis→pulmonary embolism, wound dehiscence→evisceration

Instructions: Choose complications from "General surgery" above; then choose those that apply to patient's particular type of surgery. Potential complications of various types of surgery follow; these complications are in addition to those of "General surgery."

Abdominal surgery	Dehiscence, fistula formation, paralytic ileus, peritonitis, renal failure, surgical trauma (eg, to ureter, bladder, or rectum)
Breast surgery	Cellulitis, hematoma, lymphedema, seroma
Chest surgery: Coronary *artery bypass graft*	Cardiovascular insufficiency, renal insufficiency, respiratory insufficiency
Chest surgery: *Thoracotomy*	Adult respiratory distress syndrome, bronchopleural fistula, cardiac dysrhythmias, empyema of the chest cavity, hemothorax, infection at chest tube sites, mediastinal shift, myocardial infarction, pneumothorax, pulmonary edema, subcutaneous emphysema

Craniotomy	Cardiac dysrhythmias, cerebral/cerebellar dysfunction, cerebrospinal fluid leaks, cranial nerve impairment, gastrointestinal bleeding, hematomas, hydrocephalus, hygromas, hyperthermia/hypothermia, hypoxemia, increased intracranial pressure, meningitis/encephalitis, residual neurologic defects, seizures
Eye surgery	Endophthalmus, hyphema, increased intraocular pressure, lens implant dislocation, macular edema, retinal detachment, secondary glaucoma
Musculoskeletal surgeries	Bone necrosis, fat embolus, flexion contractures, hematoma, joint dislocation/displacement of prosthesis, nerve damage, sepsis, synovial herniation
Neck surgeries	Airway obstruction, aspiration, cerebral infarction, cranial nerve damage, fistula formation (eg, between hypopharynx and skin), flap rejection (in radical neck dissection), hypertension/hypotension, hypoparathyroidism (in thyroidectomy/parathyroidectomy), local nerve damage (eg, to the laryngeal nerve), respiratory distress, tetany (in thyroidectomy), thyroid storm, tracheal stenosis, vocal cord paralysis
Rectal surgery	Fistula formation, stricture formation
Skin grafts	Edema, flap necrosis, graft rejection, hematoma
Spinal surgery	Displacement of bone graft (in laminectomy/spinal fusion), bladder or bowel dysfunction, cerebrospinal fistula, hematoma, nerve root injury, paralytic ileus, sensorineural impairments, spinal cord edema or injury
Urologic surgery	Bladder neck constriction, bladder perforation (intraoperative), epididymitis, paralytic ileus, retrograde ejaculation (in prostate resection/prostatectomy), stomal necrosis, stenosis, obstruction (in urostomy/nephrostomy), urethral stricture, urinary tract infection
Vascular surgery: Aortic aneurysm resection	Congestive heart failure, myocardial infarction, renal failure, rupture of the suture line→hemorrhage, spinal cord ischemia
Vascular surgery: Other	Cardiac dysrhythmia, compartment syndrome, failure of anastomosis, lymphocele, occlusion of graft

Index

A
Abdominal pain/irritable bowel syndrome, 543
Abdominal surgery, 555–556
Abuse cessation
    post-trauma syndrome and, 351
    rape-trauma syndrome and, 365
Abuse protection: child
    altered parenting and, 330
    risk for altered parenting and, 334–335
Abuse protection
    altered protection and, 360
    post-trauma syndrome and, 351
    rape-trauma syndrome and, 365
Abuse recovery: emotional
    post-trauma syndrome and, 351, 352
    rape-trauma syndrome and, 365
    risk for altered parenting, 333
Abuse recovery: sexual
    altered sexuality patterns and, 418
    post-trauma syndrome and, 351
    rape-trauma syndrome and, 365
    sexual dysfunction and, 414, 415
Abusive behavior self-control, risk for violence directed at others, 514
Acceptance: health status
    defensive coping and, 92
    impaired adjustment and, 13
    ineffective denial and, 112, 113
Acquired immune deficiency syndrome (AIDS)
    nursing diagnoses of, 527–528
    potential complications (collaborative problems) of, 527
Active listening, 67
Activity intolerance
    nursing diagnoses, **2–5**
    risk for, 6–8
Activity therapy, 4
Acute renal failure, 549–550
Acute respiratory disorders, 552–553
Adaptive capacity, intracranial, decreased, 8–12
Adherence behavior
    effective therapeutic regimen management and, 267, 268
    health seeking behaviors and, 193
    noncompliance and, 290–291
Adjustment, impaired, 12–14
Aggression control
    anxiety and, 23
    risk for self-mutilation and, 403–404

risk for violence directed at others, 514
Airway clearance, ineffective, 15–18
Airway management
    ineffective airway clearance and, 17
    ineffective breathing pattern and, 51
    risk for suffocation and, 459
Airway suctioning, 17
Ambulation: walking
    impaired, 522
    impaired physical mobility and, 280
Ambulation: wheelchair, 283
Analgesic administration
    chronic pain and, 316
    pain and, 312
Anger control assistance
    risk for self-directed violence and, 518
    risk for self-mutilation and, 404
    risk for violence directed at others, 515
Antepartum and postpartum conditions
    abortion, spontaneous or induced, 578–579
    change in birthing plans, 579
    gestational diabetes, 579
    hyperemesis gravidarum, 580
    maternal infection, 580–581
    painful breast, 581
    perinatal loss, 581–582
    postpartum care, uncomplicated, 582–583
    pregnancy-induced hypertension (PIH), 583–584
    suppression of preterm labor, 584
    uterine bleeding, 585
Anticipatory guidance, 268
Anxiety
    death and, **25–27**
    fear vs., 21–22
    nursing diagnoses and, **19–25**
Anxiety control
    anxiety and, 23
    ineffective denial and, 112
    sensory/perceptual alterations and, 410
Anxiety reduction
    fatigue and, 158
    ineffective denial and, 113
Arthritis, 528–529
Artificial airway management, 455
Aspiration precautions

impaired swallowing and, 466
risk for aspiration and, 29
Aspiration, risk for, 27–30
Assaultive patient, 567–568
Attachment promotion
altered parenting and, 330
risk for altered parent-infant attachment and, 319
risk for altered parenting, 335
Autoimmune disorders, 529–531
Autotransfusion, 165

B
Bathing, 383
Behavior management: self-harm, risk for self-mutilation and, 404
Behavior modification, ineffective therapeutic regimen management and, 271
Blood disorders, 531–532
Body image
altered sexuality patterns and, 418
body image disturbance and, 32
sensory/perceptual alterations and, 410
unilateral neglect and, 500
Body image disturbance, 30–34
Body image enhancement, 33
Body mechanics promotion, sensory/perceptual alterations and, 411
Body positioning: self-initiated
risk for perioperative, 338
unilateral neglect and, 500
Body temperature, risk for altered, 34–37
Borderline personality, 568–569
Bottle feeding, 47
Bowel continence, 210
Bowel elimination
altered tissue perfusion and, 479, 481
constipation and, 79
diarrhea and, 121, 122
perceived constipation and, 82
Bowel incontinence care: encopresis, 210
Bowel incontinence care, 210
Bowel management, delayed surgical recovery and, 461
Bowel training, 210
Breastfeeding
establishment
infant, 38, 42, 43, 46
maternal, 38, 42, 46
knowledge of, 42, 46
maintenance of, 38, 42, 46
parent-infant attachment, 46
Breastfeeding, effective, 37–40

Breastfeeding establishment: infant, ineffective feeding pattern and, 237
Breastfeeding, ineffective, 41–44
Breastfeeding, interrupted, 45–48
Breastfeeding maintenance, ineffective feeding pattern and, 237
Breastfeeding weaning, 38, 42
Breast, painful, 581
Breast surgery, 557
Breathing pattern, ineffective, 49–52
Burns
nursing diagnoses of, 532–533
pediatric conditions, 598–599

C
Cancer, 533–535
Cardiac care, 55
Cardiac care, acute
altered tissue perfusion and, 483
decreased cardiac output and, 55
Cardiac disorders, 535–536
Cardiac output, decreased, 52–57
Cardiac pump effectiveness
altered tissue perfusion and, 478
decreased cardiac output and, 54
risk for activity intolerance and, 6
Caregiver adaptation to patient institutionalization, 322
Caregiver emotional health, 59
Caregiver home care readiness, 59, 322
Caregiver lifestyle disruption
altered role performance and, 378
caregiver role strain and, 59
Caregiver-patient relationship, 59
Caregiver performance: direct care, 60
Caregiver performance: indirect care, 60
Caregiver physical health, 60
Caregiver role strain
nursing diagnoses for, **57–63**
risk for, **63–64**
Caregiver stressors
risk for altered parenting, 333
role strain and, 60
Caregiver support, 61
Caregiver well-being, 60
Caregiving endurance potential, 60
Casts and traction, pediatric conditions, 599
Cerebral edema management, 10
Cerebral perfusion promotion
altered tissue perfusion and, 483
decreased intracranial adaptive capacity and, 10
Cerebrovascular accident (stroke), 545–546

Change in birthing plans, 579
Chest surgery, 557–558
Chest trauma, 538
Child abuse, 599–600
Child adaptation to hospitalization, 374
Child development: adolescence (12-17 years)
  altered parenting and, 328
  altered sexuality patterns and, 418
  body image disturbance and, 32
  defensive coping and, 92
  impaired memory and, 274
  impaired social interaction and, 437, 438
  risk for impaired skin integrity and, 424
  self-esteem disturbance and, 402
  sexual dysfunction and, 415
Child development: early (birth to 5 years)
  altered parenting and, 328
  body image disturbance and, 32
  disorganized infant behavior, 228
  impaired memory and, 274
  impaired social interaction and, 437, 438
  potential for enhanced organized infant behavior and, 233, 234
  risk for altered parent/child attachment, 319
  risk for disorganized infant behavior and, 231
  self esteem disturbance and, 402
Child development: middle childhood (6-11 years)
  altered parenting and, 328
  altered sexuality patterns and, 418
  body image disturbance and, 32
  impaired memory and, 274
  impaired social interaction and, 437, 438
  risk for altered parent/child attachment, 319
  self-esteem disturbance and, 402
Chronic renal failure, 550–552
Chronic respiratory disorders, 553–554
Circulation status
  altered tissue perfusion and, 478, 479, 480, 481, 482
  decreased cardiac output and, 54
  peripheral neurovascular dysfunction and, 341
  risk for activity intolerance and, 6
  risk for perioperative positioning injury and, 338, 339
Circulatory care: mechanical assist device, 55

Circulatory care
  altered tissue perfusion and, 483
  peripheral altered tissue perfusion and, 491
  risk for peripheral neurovascular dysfunction and, 342
Cleft lip/cleft palate: surgical repair, 600–601
Coagulation disorders, 601
Cognitive ability
  acute confusion and, 70
  altered thought processes and, 470
  altered tissue perfusion and, 479, 480
  chronic confusion and, 73, 74
  risk for aspiration and, 28
  risk for perioperative positioning injury and, 338
  sensory/perceptual alterations and, 410
Cognitive orientation
  altered thought processes and, 470
  chronic confusion and, 73
  environmental interpretation syndrome and, 139
  impaired memory and, 274
  risk for perioperative positioning injury and, 338
  sensory/perceptual alterations and, 410–411
Comfort level
  chronic pain and, 316
  nausea and, 286
  pain and, 312
  risk for disorganized infant behavior and, 231
  sleep pattern disturbance and, 434
Communication
  expressive ability, 66
  impaired verbal, **65–68**
  receptive ability, 66
Communication ability, 66
Communication enhancement
  hearing deficit, 67, 411
  speech deficit, 67
  visual deficit, 411
Compliance behavior
  effective therapeutic regimen management and, 267
  noncompliance and, 290
Concentration
  altered thought processes and, 470
  chronic confusion and, 73
  fatigue and, 153
Confusion, acute, 69–72
Confusion, chronic, 72–77
Congenital anomalies, 591–592

Congenital malformations of the central nervous system: surgical repair, 601–602
Conscious sedation, 312
Constipation
  nursing diagnoses of, **77–81**
  perceived, **81–83**
  risk of, **83–85**
Coping: community
  ineffective, **86–88**
  potential for enhanced, **88–91**
Coping: family
  ineffective, compromised, **94–98**
  ineffective, disabling, **98–101**
  potential for growth, **102–104**
Coping: individual, ineffective, 105–108
Coping
  anticipatory grieving and, 176
  anxiety and, 23
  defensive coping and, 92
  dysfunctional grieving and, 179
  impaired adjustment and, 13
  ineffective individual coping and, 106
  parent role conflict and, 322–323
  post-trauma syndrome and, 351
  rape-trauma syndrome and, 365–366
  relocation stress syndrome and, 374
  risk for activity intolerance and, 6
  risk for altered parenting and, 333, 334
Coping, defensive, 91–94
Coping enhancement
  fatigue and, 158
  impaired adjustment and, 14
  ineffective individual coping and, 107
  relocation stress syndrome and, and, 375
Counseling
  ineffective denial and, 113
  post-trauma syndrome and, 352
  rape-trauma syndrome: compound reaction and, 369
  rape-trauma syndrome: silent reaction and, 372
  sexual dysfunction and, 415
  See also Teaching
Craniotomy, 558–560
Crisis intervention
  parent role conflict and, 323
  rape-trauma syndrome and, 366
Cushing's disease, 540–541

D
Death
  anticipatory grieving and perinatal, 176

  anxiety and, 25–27
  dysfunctional grieving and, 180
  spiritual distress and dignified, 447
  See also Dying patients
Decisional conflict (specify), 109–111
Decision making
  altered thought processes and, 471
  chronic confusion and, 73
  decisional conflict and, 110
  hopelessness and, 200
  ineffective individual coping and, 106
  situational low self-esteem and, 399
  See also Participation: health care decisions
Decision-making support
  decisional conflict and, 110
  ineffective individual coping and, 107
  personal identity disturbance and, 345
Delirium management, 71
Delusion management
  acute confusion and, 71
  altered thought processes and, 472
Dementia management
  altered thought processes and, 472
  impaired environmental interpretation syndrome and, 139
Denial, ineffective, 111–114
Dentition, altered, 114–117
Development enhancement
  altered growth and development and, 187
  altered parenting and, 330
  potential for family coping growth and, 103
  risk for altered parenting and, 335
Development problems/needs related to illness, 597–598
Development, risk for altered, 117–120
Diabetes mellitus/hypoglycemia, 541
Diarrhea, 120–123
Dignified dying, 447
  See also Death

Discharge planning, relocation stress syndrome and, 375
Distorted thought control
  acute confusion and, 70
  altered thought processes and, 471
  body image disturbance and, 32
  chronic confusion and, 74
  sensory/perceptual alterations and, 410
Disuse syndrome, risk for, 123–127
Diversional activity deficit, 127–130

Dressing self-care deficit, 386
Drug withdrawal (newborn condition), 586–587
DVWR (ventilatory weaning response, dysfunctional), 507–512
Dying patients, 539–540
See also Death
Dysrefelxia, risk for autonomic, 133–135
Dysreflexia, 130–133
Dysreflexia management, 132

E
Ear surgery, 560
Eating disorders
  body image disturbance and, 32
  less than body requirements altered nutrition and, 298–299
  as psychiatric condition, 569–570
Eating disorders management
  less than body requirements altered nutrition and, 295
  more than body requirements altered nutrition and, 301
Education. *See* Health education
Electrolyte and acid-base balance
  altered tissue perfusion and, 382, 479, 481
  decreased intracranial adaptive capacity and, 9
  diarrhea and, 121
  fluid volume deficit and, 161
  fluid volume excess and, 167
  risk for fluid volume deficit, 164
Electrolyte management
  fluid volume deficit and, 162
  risk for fluid volume deficit and, 165
Electronic fetal monitoring: intrapartum
  altered protection and, 360
  risk for injury and, 246
Emotional support
  breastfeeding and, 47
  risk for activity intolerance and, 7
Endocrine disorders, 540–542
Endurance
  activity intolerance and, 3
  fatigue and, 153
  inability to sustain spontaneous ventilation and, 454
Energy conservation
  activity intolerance and, 3
  fatigue and, 153, 154
  risk for activity intolerance and, 6
  sensory/perceptual alterations and, 410
Energy field disturbance, 135–137

Energy management
  activity intolerance and, 4
  delayed surgical recovery and, 461
  risk for activity intolerance and, 7
  risk for disuse syndrome and, 126
Enteral tube feeding, 238
Environmental factors, ineffective airway clearance and, 15
Environmental interpretation syndrome, impaired, 138–140
Environmental management: attachment process, 319
  potential for enhanced organized infant behavior and, 234
Environmental management: violence prevention
  risk for self-directed violence and, 519
  risk for violence directed at others, 515
Environmental management
  deficit in self-care tioleting and, 394
  disorganized infant behavior and, 229
  impaired environmental interpretation syndrome and, 139
  risk for disorganized infant behavior and, 232
  sensory/perceptual alterations and, 411
Environmental management, community
  ineffective therapeutic regimen management and, 262
  potential for enhanced coping and, 90
Environmental management, safety
  risk for poisoning and, 348
  risk for self-mutilation and, 404
  risk for suffocation and, 459
  risk for trauma and, 498
Environmental management, violence prevention, 360
Exercise therapy: balance, 494
Exercise therapy: muscle control, 494
Exercise therapy, ambulation
  impaired physical mobility and, 280
  impaired walking and, 522
Exercise therapy, joint mobility
  impaired physical mobility and, 280
  impaired walking and, 342, 522
  impaired wheelchair mobility and, 284

F
Failure to thrive
  adult, **141–143**
  child, 602

Fall prevention, 246
Family integrity promotion
    altered family processes and, 150
    altered parenting and, 330
    risk for altered parenting and, 335
    risk for loneliness and, 260
Family involvement
    ineffective, compromised family
        coping and, 96
    ineffective family therapeutic regi-
        men management and, 265
Family mobilization
    ineffective, compromised family
        coping and, 96
    ineffective family therapeutic regi-
        men management and, 265
**Family processes: alcoholism,
    altered, 144–148**
Family processes, altered, 148–156
Family process maintenance
    alcoholism and altered, 146
    altered family processes and, 150
    ineffective family therapeutic regi-
        men management and, 265
    parent role conflict and, 323
Family support
    ineffective, compromised family
        coping and, 96
    potential for family coping growth
        and, 103
Fatigue, 152–159
Fear
    anxiety vs., 21–22
    nursing diagnoses of, **156**
Fear control, 157
Feeding problems, 587–588
Feeding self-care deficit, 390
Fever treatment, 204
Fluid balance
    altered tissue perfusion and, 479,
        481, 482
    decreased intracranial adaptive
        capacity and, 9
    diarrhea and, 121
    fluid volume deficit and, 161
    fluid volume excess and, 167,
        167–168
    nausea and, 286
    peripheral altered tissue perfusion
        and, 490
    risk for fluid volume deficit and, 164
Fluid/electrolyte management, 483
Fluid management
    altered tissue perfusion and, 483
    fluid volume deficit and, 162
    nausea and, 287
Fluid monitoring
    fluid volume deficit and, 162

    nausea and, 287
    risk for fluid volume deficit and, 165
Fluid volume deficit
    nursing diagnoses of, **159–163**
    risk for, **164–165**
Fluid volume excess, 165–169
**Fluid volume imbalance, risk for,
    169–170**

G
Gas exchange, impaired, 170–174
Gastroenteritis, 602–603
Gastrointestinal disorders, 542–543
Gastrointestinal intubation, 483
Gastrointestinal obstruction: surgical
    repair, 603
Gestational diabetes, 579
GI bleeding, 542
GI inflammation, 542
Grief resolution
    anticipatory grieving and, 176
    body image disturbance and, 32
    impaired adjustment and, 13
    risk for loneliness and, 259
Grief work facilitation: perinatal death
    anticipatory grieving and, 176
    dysfunctional grieving and, 180
Grief work facilitation
    anticipatory grieving and, 176
    dysfunctional grieving and, 180
Grieving, anticipatory, 174–177
Grieving, dysfunctional, 178–181
**Growth and development, altered,
    184–188**
Growth, risk for altered, 181–184

H
Hair care self-care deficit, 387
Harmonious interconnectedness, 452
Health beliefs: perceived ability to
    perform, 356
Health beliefs: perceived resources
    altered health maintenance and, 190
    powerlessness and, 356
Health beliefs: perceived threat
    ineffective denial and, 112
    perceived constipation and, 82
Health beliefs
    health seeking behaviors and, 193
    perceived constipation and, 82
    powerlessness and, 356
Health education
    health seeking behaviors and, 193
    potential for enhanced coping and,
        90
**Health maintenance, altered,
    189–192**
Health orientation, 193

Health policy monitoring
    ineffective community therapeutic
        regimen management and, 263
    potential for enhanced coping and,
        90
Health promoting behavior, 190, 193
Health-seeking behavior
    altered health maintenance and, 190
    impaired adjustment and, 13
**Health seeking behaviors (specify),
    192–195**
Health system guidance
    altered health maintenance and, 191
    effective therapeutic regimen man-
        agement and, 268
    knowledge deficit and, 252
    noncompliance and, 291
Hemodialysis therapy, 483
Hemodynamic regulation, 55
High-risk infant, 588–589
Home maintenance assistance, 198
**Home maintenance management,
    impaired, 195–198**
Hope
    hopelessness and, 200
    potential for enhanced spiritual
        well-being and, 452
    spiritual distress and, 447
Hope instillation
    hopelessness and, 201
    relocation stress syndrome and, 375
Hopelessness, 199–202
Hydration
    altered tissue perfusion and, 479,
        481, 482
    diarrhea and, 121
    fluid volume deficit and, 161
    fluid volume excess and, 167
    risk for altered body temperature,
        35
    risk for fluid volume deficit and, 164
Hyperbilirubinemia, 590
Hyperemesis gravidarum, 580
Hyperthermia
    nursing diagnoses of, **202–205**
    risk for altered body temperature
        and, 35, 36–37
Hyperthryoidism, 541
Hypoglycemia, 590–591
Hypoglycemia/diabetes mellitus, 541
Hypothermia
    newborn condition, 591
    nursing diagnoses of, **205–208**
    risk for altered body temperature
        and, 35, 36, 37
Hypothermia treatment, 207
Hypothyroidism, 541–542

Hypovolemia management
    fluid volume deficit and, 162
    risk for fluid volume deficit and, 165

I
Identity
    altered thought processes and, 471
    chronic confusion and, 74
    personal identity disturbance and,
        344–345
Immobility consequences: physio-
    logical
    risk for aspiration and, 28
    risk for disuse syndrome and, 125
    risk for impaired skin integrity and,
        424, 425
Immobilized patient, 543–544
Immune status
    altered protection and, 360
    risk for infection and, 241
Immunization/vaccination administra-
    tion, 242
Impulse control
    anxiety and, 23
    ineffective individual coping and,
        106, 107
    post-trauma syndrome and, 351
    risk for self-directed violence and,
        518
    risk for self-mutilation and, 404
    risk for violence directed at others,
        514, 515
Incision site care, impaired skin
    integrity and, 421
Incontinence
    bowel, **208–212**
    urinary, functional, **212–215**
    urinary, reflex, **215–218**
    urinary, stress, **216–220**
    urinary, total, **220–222**
    urinary, urge, **222–224**
    urinary, urge, risk of, **225–226**
Infant behavior
    disorganized, **226–230**
    disorganized, risk for, **231–233**
    organized, potential for enhanced,
        233–236
**Infant feeding pattern, ineffective,
    236–240**
Infection
    of central nervous system (CNS),
        603–604
    risk for, **240–243**
Infection control
    altered protection and, 360
    risk for infection and, 242
Infection protection
    altered protection and, 360

risk for infection and, 242
Information processing
  acute confusion and, 70
  altered thought processes and, 471
  chronic confusion and, 74
  decisional conflict and, 110
  environmental interpretation syndrome and, 139
  ineffective individual coping and, 106, 107
Ingestion/accidental poisoning, 604–605
Injury, risk for, 244–248
Inner strength, 452
Intracranial pressure (ICP) monitoring
  altered tissue perfusion and, 483
  decreased intracranial adaptive capacity and, 10
  peripheral altered tissue perfusion and, 491
Intravenous (IV) therapy
  fluid volume deficit and, 162
  risk for fluid volume deficit and, 165
Irritable bowel syndrome, 543

J
Joint movement: active
  impaired bed mobility and, 277
  impaired physical mobility and, 280
  impaired transfer ability and, 494
  impaired walking and, 522
  impaired wheelchair mobility and, 283

K
Knowledge: treatment regimen
  altered health maintenance and, 190
  effective therapeutic regimen management and, 267
  ineffective therapeutic regimen management and, 271
Knowledge
  breastfeeding, 42
  diet, 251
  health behaviors, 190
  health resources, 190
  infection control, 241
  medication, altered urinary elimination and, 503
  personal safety, risk for suffocation and, 458
  risk for poisoning and, 347
Knowledge deficit (specify), 249–254

L
Labor induction, 246
Lactation counseling
  ineffective breastfeeding and, 43

ineffective infant feeding pattern and, 238
  interrupted breastfeeding and, 47
  See also Breastfeeding
Latex allergy response
  nursing diagnoses for, **254–256**
  risk for, **256–258**
Latex precautions
  risk for injury and, 246
  risk for latex allergy response and, 257
Leisure participation, 128
Liver disease, 544–545
Loneliness, risk for, 258–261
Loss of appetite, 298
Low birth weight/small for gestational age, 592–593

M
Malignant hyperthermia precautions
  hyperthermia and, 204
  risk for injury and, 247
Management of therapeutic regimen: community, ineffective, 261–264
Management of therapeutic regimen: families, ineffective, 264–266
Management of therapeutic regimen: individual, effective, 267–269
Management of therapeutic regimen: individual, ineffective, 269–272
Mania, 570–571
Maternal infection, 580–581
Mechanical ventilation
  DVWR and, 510
  inability to sustain spontaneous ventilation and, 455
Mechanical ventilatory weaning, 510
Medical conditions
  acute renal failure, 550
  acute respiratory disorders, 552–553
  AIDS, 527–528
  arthritis, 528–529
  autoimmune disorders, 529–531
  blood disorders, 531–532
  burns, 532–533
  cancer, 533–535
  cardiac disorders, 536–538
  chest trauma, 538
  chronic renal failure, 550–552
  dying patients, 539–540
  endocrine disorders, 540–542
  gastrointestinal disorders, 542–543
  immobilized patient, 543–544
  liver disease, 544–545
  neurologic disorders, 545–548
  obesity, 548
  pancreatitis, 549

urologic disorders, 554
vascular disease, 554
Memory
acute confusion and, 70
altered thought processes and, 471
chronic confusion and, 74
environmental interpretation syndrome and, 139
impaired, **273–276**
Mobility: bed, impaired, 276–277
Mobility: physical, impaired, 278–282
Mobility: wheelchair, impaired, 282–285
Mobility level
impaired bed mobility and, 277
impaired physical mobility and, 280
impaired transfer ability and, 494
impaired walking and, 522
impaired wheelchair mobility and, 283–284
risk for disuse syndrome and, 125
Mood equilibrium
hopelessness and, 200
social isolation and, 441
Muscle function
disorganized infant behavior and, 228
impaired swallowing and, 466
inability to sustain spontaneous ventilation and, 454
ineffective feeding pattern and, 237
peripheral altered tissue perfusion and, 490
risk for perioperative positioning injury and, 338
Musculoskeletal surgery, 561–562

N
NANDA (North American Nursing Diagnosis Association), 1
Nausea
less than body requirements altered nutrition and, 297
nursing diagnoses for, **285–288**
Neck surgery, 562–564
Neurological status: central motor control, 454
Neurological status: consciousness
acute confusion and, 70
altered thought processes and, 471
chronic confusion and, 74
decreased intracranial adaptive capacity and, 9
impaired environmental interpretation syndrome, 139

impaired memory and, 274
impaired swallowing and, 466
risk for disuse syndrome and, 125
Neurological status: cranial sensory/motor function
impaired swallowing and, 466
peripheral neurovascular dysfunction and, 341
Neurological status: spinal sensory/motor function, 341
Neurological status
altered tissue perfusion and, 479
decreased intracranial adaptive capacity and, 9
disorganized infant behavior, 228
disorganized infant behavior and, 228–229
dysreflexia and, 131
peripheral neurovascular dysfunction and, 341
potential for enhanced organized infant behavior and, 234
risk for aspiration and, 28
risk for disorganized infant behavior and, 231, 232
Neurologic disorders, 545
Neurologic monitoring
altered tissue perfusion and, 483
decreased intracranial adaptive capacity and, 10
peripheral altered tissue perfusion and, 491
Newborn conditions
congenital anomalies, 591–592
drug withdrawal, 586–587
feeding problems, 587–588
high-risk infant, 588–589
hyperbilirubinemia, 590
hypoglycemia, 590–591
hypothermia, 591
low birth weight/small for gestational age, 592–593
normal newborn, 593–594
respiratory distress, 594–595
Newborn monitoring, 232
NIC (Nursing Interventions Classification), 1
NOC (Nursing Outcomes Classification), 1
Noncompliance (specify), 288–292
Nonnutritive sucking, 238
Normalization promotion
altered family processes and, 150
potential for family coping growth and, 103
risk for altered parenting and, 335
Normal newborn, 593–594

Nursing diagnoses
  antepartum and postpartum conditions
    abortion, spontaneous or induced, 578–579
    change in birthing plans, 579
    gestational diabetes, 579
    hyperemesis gravidarum, 580
    maternal infection, 580–581
    painful breast, 581
    perinatal loss, 581–582
    postpartum care, uncomplicated, 582–583
    pregnancy-induced hypertension (PIH), 583–584
    suppression of preterm labor, 584
    uterine bleeding, 585
  medical conditions
    acute renal failure, 550
    acute respiratory disorders, 552–553
    AIDS, 527–528
    arthritis, 528–529
    autoimmune disorders, 529–531
    blood disorders, 531–532
    burns, 532–533
    cancer, 533–535
    cardiac disorders, 536–538
    chest trauma, 538
    chronic renal failure, 550–552
    dying patients, 539–540
    endocrine disorders, 540–542
    gastrointestinal disorders, 542–543
    immobilized patient, 543–544
    liver disease, 544–545
    neurologic disorders, 545–548
    obesity, 548
    pancreatitis, 549
    urologic disorders, 554
    vascular disease, 554
  newborn conditions
    congenital anomalies, 591–592
    drug withdrawal, 586–587
    feeding problems, 587–588
    high-risk infant, 588–589
    hyperbilirubinemia, 590
    hypoglycemia, 590–591
    normal newborn, 593–594
    respiratory distress, 594–595
  pediatric conditions
    burns, 598–599
    casts and traction, 599
    child abuse, 599–600
    cleft lip/cleft palate: surgical repair, 600–601
    coagulation disorders, 601
    congenital malformations of the central nervous system: surgical repair, 601–602
    developmental problems/needs related to illness, 597–598
    failure to thrive, 602
    gastroenteritis, 602–603
    gastrointestinal obstruction: surgical repair, 603
    infection of central nervous system (CNS), 603–604
    ingestion/accidental poisoning, 604–605
    obese child, 605
    osteomyelitis, 605–606
    pregnancy in adolescence, 606
    respiratory disorder, chronic, 607
    respiratory infection, acute, 607–608
    seizure disorders, 608
    sepsis, 609
    sickle cell crisis, 609
    tonsillectomy, 610
  psychiatric conditions
    assaultive patient, 568
    borderline personality, 568–569
    eating disorders, 569–570
    mania, 570–571
    paranoia, 571–572
    phobias, 572
    psychosis, 572–573
    severe depression, 573–574
    substance abuse, 574–576
    suicide, 576
    withdrawn patient, 577
  surgical conditions
    abdominal surgery, 555–556
    breast surgery, 557
    chest surgery, 557–558
    craniotomy, 558–560
    ear surgery, 560
    eye surgery, 560–561
    musculoskeletal surgery, 561–562
    neck surgery, 562–564
    rectal surgery, 564
    skin graft, 564
    spinal surgery, 564–565
    urologic surgery, 565–566
    vascular surgery, 566–567
Nutrition: less than body requirements, altered, 292–299
Nutrition: more than body requirements, altered, 299–303
Nutrition: more than body requirements, risk for altered, 303–305
Nutritional management
  delayed surgical recovery and, 461

risk for more than body requirements altered nutrition and, 305

Nutritional monitoring
  altered growth and development and, 187
  nausea and, 287

Nutritional status: energy, 153

Nutritional status: food and fluid intake
  fluid volume deficit and, 161
  hopelessness and, 200
  ineffective infant feeding pattern and, 237
  less than body requirements altered nutrition and, 295
  more than body requirements altered nutrition and, 301
  nausea and, 286
  risk for fluid volume deficit and, 164
  risk for more than body requirements altered nutrition and, 304

Nutritional status: nutrient value
  less than body requirements altered nutrition and, 295
  more than body requirements altered nutrition and, 301

Nutritional status
  altered tissue perfusion and, 479
  less than body requirements altered nutrition and, 295
  risk for impaired skin integrity and, 424

Nutrition management
  altered tissue perfusion and, 483
  less than body requirements altered nutrition and, 295
  more than body requirements altered nutrition and, 301
  sensory/perceptual alterations and, 411

Nutrition therapy, 187

O
Obese child, 605
Obesity, 548
Obstructed airway, 15
Oral health, 308
Oral health restoration, 308
Oral mucous membrane, altered, 306–309
Osteomyelitis, 605–606

P
Pain: disruptive effects
  chronic pain and, 316
  pain and, 312

Pain
  chronic, **315–317**
  nursing diagnoses for, **309–314**

Pain control behavior
  chronic pain and, 316
  pain and, 312

Painful breast, 581

Pain level
  chronic pain and, 316
  noncompliance and, 290
  pain and, 312
  risk for disorganized infant behavior and, 231, 232
  risk for disuse syndrome and, 125
  sleep pattern disturbance and, 434

Pain management
  chronic pain and, 316
  delayed surgical recovery and, 461
  pain and, 313

Pancreatitis, 549

Paranoia, 571–572

Parental role conflict, 321–324

Parent/child attachment, risk for altered, 317–321

Parent education: childbearing family, 319

Parent-infant attachment
  altered parenting and, 328–329
  interrupted breastfeeding and, 46
  risk for altered and, 318
  risk for altered parenting and, 333, 334
  See also Breastfeeding

Parenting: social safety
  altered parenting and, 328
  impaired home maintenance management and, 197
  risk for injury and, 245

Parenting
  altered, **324–331**
  impaired home maintenance management and, 197
  parent role conflict and, 322, 323
  risk for altered, **331–337**
  risk for altered parent-infant attachment and, 318
  risk for altered parenting, 333

Participation: health care decisions
  altered health maintenance and, 190, 191
  decisional conflict and, 110
  effective therapeutic regimen management and, 267, 268
  impaired adjustment and, 13
  ineffective therapeutic regimen management and, 271
  powerlessness and, 356
  See also Decision making

Participation health care decisions, 357

Pass facilitation, 103

Patient-controlled analgesia (PCA) assistance

chronic pain and, 317

pain and, 313

Patient/family teaching

caregiver role strain and, 61–62

impaired verbal communication and, 67

See also Teaching

Patients

assaultive, 567–568

dying, 539–540

immobilized, 543–544

pass facilitation for, 103

visitation facilitation for, 260

withdrawn, 577

Pediatric conditions

burns, 598–599

casts and traction, 599

child abuse, 599–600

cleft lip/cleft palate: surgical repair, 600–601

coagulation disorders, 601

congenital malformations of the central nervous system: surgical repair, 601–602

development problems/needs related to illness, 597–598

failure to thrive, 602

gastroenteritis, 602–603

gastrointestinal obstruction: surgical repair, 603

infection of central nervous system (CNS), 603–604

ingestion/accidental poisoning, 604–605

obese child, 605

osteomyelitis, 605–606

pregnancy in adolescence, 606

respiratory disorder, chronic, 607

respiratory infection, acute, 607–608

seizure disorders, 608

sepsis, 608–609

sickle cell crisis, 609

tonsillectomy, 610

Pelvic floor exercise, 219

Perinatal loss, 581–582

Perioperative positioning injury, risk for, 337–340

Peripheral neurovascular dysfunction, 340–344

Peripheral sensation management

altered tissue perfusion and, 483

peripheral altered tissue perfusion and, 491

risk for peripheral neurovascular dysfunction and, 342

Peritoneal dialysis therapy, 483

Personal identity disturbance, 344–346

Phobias, 572

Physical aging status

altered growth and development and, 186

sexual dysfunction and, 415

Physical maturation: female, 186

Physical maturation: male, 186

Physiological factors, ineffective airway clearance and, 15

Play participation

diversional activity deficit and, 128

impaired social interaction and, 437, 438

social isolation and, 442

Poisoning, risk for, 346–349

Positioning: intraoperative, 339

Positioning

disorganized infant behavior and, 229

impaired physical mobility and, 281

wheelchair, impaired wheelchair mobility and, 284

Postanesthesia care, 360

Postpartum care, uncomplicated, 582–583

Post-trauma syndrome, 349–352

Post-trauma syndrome, risk for, 353–354

Potential complications (collaborative problems)

antepartum and postpartum conditions

abortion, spontaneous or induced, 578

gestational diabetes, 579

hyperemesis gravidarum, 580

maternal infection, 580

painful breast, 581

postpartum care, uncomplicated, 582

pregnancy-induced hypertension (PIH), 583

suppression of preterm labor, 584

uterine bleeding, 585

medical conditions

acute renal failure, 549–550

acute respiratory disorders, 552–553

AIDS, 527

arthritis, 528–529

autoimmune disorders, 529

blood disorders, 531

burns, 532

cancer, 533
cardiac disorders, 535–536
chest trauma, 538
chronic renal failure, 550
chronic respiratory disorders, 553
endocrine disorders, 540
gastrointestinal disorders, 542
immobilized patients, 543
liver disease, 544
neurologic disorders, 545
obesity, 548
pancreatitis, 549
urologic disorders, 554
vascular disease, 554–555
newborn conditions
congenital anomalies, 591
drug withdrawal, 586
high-risk infant, 588
hyperbilirubinemia, 590
hypoglycemia, 590
hypothermia, 591
low birth weight/small for gestational age, 592
normal newborn, 593
respiratory distress, 594
pediatric conditions
cleft lip/cleft palate: surgical
repair, 600
congenital malformations of the
central nervous system: surgical repair, 601
failure to thrive, 602
gastroenteritis, 602
gastrointestinal obstruction: surgical repair, 603
infection of central nervous system (CNS), 603
ingestion/accidental poisoning,
604
osteomyelitis, 605–606
respiratory disorder, chronic, 607
respiratory infection, acute, 607
seizure disorders, 608
sepsis, 608
sickle cell crisis, 609
tonsillectomy, 610
psychiatric conditions
eating disorders, 569
mania, 570
substance abuse, 574
surgical conditions
abdominal surgery, 555
breast surgery, 557
chest surgery, 557
craniotomy, 558
ear surgery, 560
eye surgery, 560–561
musculoskeletal surgery, 561

neck surgery, 562
rectal surgery, 564
spinal surgery, 564–565
urologic surgery, 565
vascular surgery, 566
Powerlessness, 355–358
Pregnancy in adolescence, 606
Pregnancy-induced hypertension
(PIH), 583–584
Pressure management, 425
Pressure ulcer prevention, 425
Protection, altered, 358–363
Psychiatric conditions
assaultive patient, 568
borderline personality, 568–569
eating disorders, 569–570
mania, 570–571
paranoia, 571–572
phobias, 572
psychosis, 572–573
severe depression, 573–574
substance abuse, 574–576
withdrawn patient, 577
Psychosis, 572–573
Psychosocial adjustment: life change
altered health maintenance and, 190
anticipatory grieving and, 176
body image disturbance and, 32
impaired adjustment and, 13
parent role conflict and, 322
relocation stress syndrome and, 374
sleep pattern disturbance and, 434

Q
Quality of life
hopelessness and, 200
potential for enhanced spiritual
well-being and, 452
relocation stress syndrome and, 374
sleep pattern disturbance and, 434

R
**Rape-trauma syndrome: compound
reaction, 367–370**
**Rape-trauma syndrome: silent reac-
tion, 370–372**
Rape-trauma syndrome, 363–367
Rape-trauma treatment
rape-trauma syndrome: silent reac-
tion and, 372
rape-trauma syndrome and, 366
Reality orientation, 139
Recreation therapy, 128
Rectal surgery, 564
Relocation stress syndrome, 372–376
Renal failure
acute, 549–550
chronic, 550–552

Respiratory disorder, chronic, 607
Respiratory distress, newborn conditions, 594–595
Respiratory infection, acute, 607–608
Respiratory monitoring
    altered tissue perfusion, 483
    inability to sustain spontaneous ventilation and, 455
    ineffective breathing pattern and, 51
    risk for suffocation and, 459
Respiratory status: gas exchange
    DVWR and, 509
    impaired gas exchange and, 172
    ineffective airway clearance and, 16, 17
    risk for activity intolerance and, 6
Respiratory status: ventilation
    DVWR and, 509
    ineffective airway clearance and, 16
    ineffective breathing pattern and, 50
    risk for activity intolerance and, 6
Rest, 434
    See also Sleep
Resuscitation: neonate, 455
Risk control
    caregiver role strain and, 60
    drug use, 347
    effective therapeutic regimen management and, 267, 268
    risk for impaired skin integrity and, 425
    risk for infection and, 241, 242
    risk for injury and, 246
    risk for poisoning and, 347
    risk for trauma and, 497
    sexually transmitted diseases (STDs), 415
    unintended pregnancy, 334
Risk detection
    altered health maintenance and, 190
    risk for infection and, 241
    risk for poisoning and, 347
    risk for self-mutilation and, 404
    risk for suffocation and, 458
Risk for hyperthermia, 35
Risk for hypothermia, 35
Role enhancement
    altered role performance and, 379
    parent role conflict and, 323
Role performance
    altered, **376–380**
    altered parenting and, 328, 329
    altered sexuality patterns and, 418
    caregiver role strain and, 60
    impaired home maintenance management and, 197
    impaired social interaction and, 438
    parent role conflict and, 322, 323

S
Safety behavior: fall prevention
    risk for injury and, 246
    risk for trauma and, 497, 498
Safety behavior: home physical environment
    altered parenting and, 328, 329
    risk for suffocation and, 458
Safety behavior: personal
    acute confusion and, 70
    chronic confusion and, 74
Security enhancement, fatigue and, 158
Seizure disorders, 608
Self-care: activities of daily living (ADLs)
    activity intolerance and, 3
    deficit in bathing/hygiene, 382, 383, 386
    deficit in dressing/grooming, 386, 387
    deficit in feeding, 390
    deficit in toileting, 393
    impaired physical mobility and, 280
    unilateral neglect and, 500
Self-care: eating
    deficit in, 390
    impaired swallowing and, 466
Self-care: instrumental activities of daily living (IADLs)
    activity intolerance and, 3
    impaired home maintenance management and, 197
Self-care assistance
    bathing/hygiene: self-care deficit in, 383
    delayed surgical recovery and, 461
    dressing/grooming deficit in, 387
    feeding deficit in, 390
    toileting deficit in, 394
Self-care deficit: bathing/hygiene (specify level), 381–384
Self-care deficit: dressing/grooming, 384–388
Self-care deficit: feeding (specify level), 388–391
Self-care deficit: toileting, 392–395
Self-esteem
    altered sexuality patterns and, 418
    body image disturbance and, 32
    chronic low, **395–398**, 396–397
    defensive coping and, 92
    self-esteem disturbance and, 402
    situational low, **398–400**, 399
Self-esteem disturbance
    body image disturbance vs., 31
    nursing diagnoses for, **400–402**
Self-esteem enhancement
    chronic low self-esteem and, 397

personal identity disturbance and, 345

powerlessness and, 357

self-esteem disturbance and, 402

Self-modification assistance, 194

ineffective therapeutic regimen management and, 271

noncompliance and, 291

Self-mutilation restraint

anxiety and, 23

post-trauma syndrome and, 351

rape-trauma syndrome and, 365

risk for impaired skin integrity and, 425

risk for self-directed violence and, 518

risk for self-mutilation and, 404

Self-mutilation, risk for, 403–407

Self-responsibility facilitation

altered growth and development and, 187

diversional activity deficit and, 128

powerlessness and, 357

relocation stress syndrome and, 375

Sensory/perceptual alterations (specify: auditory, gustatory, kinesthetic, olfactory, tactile, visual), 408–413

Sepsis, 608–609

Severe depression, 573–574

Sexual counseling, 415

See also Counseling

Sexual dysfunction, 413–417

Sexuality patterns, altered, 417–419

Shock management: cardiac, 55

altered tissue perfusion and, 483

Shock management, volume

fluid volume deficit and, 162

risk for fluid volume deficit and, 165

Sickle cell crisis, 609

Skin graft, 564

Skin integrity, impaired (specify), 419–423

Skin integrity, risk for impaired, 423–428

Skin surveillance

impaired skin integrity and, 421

risk for impaired skin integrity and, 426

risk for perioperative positioning injury and, 339

risk for trauma and, 498

Sleep

acute confusion and, 70

chronic confusion and, 74

disorganized infant behavior and, 228

hopelessness and, 200

potential for enhanced organized infant behavior and, 234

risk for disorganized infant behavior and, 232

sleep deprivation and, 430

sleep pattern disturbance and, 434, 435

Sleep deprivation, 428–431

Sleep enhancement

potential for enhanced organized infant behavior and, 235

sleep deprivation and, 430

Sleep pattern disturbance, 431–436

Social interaction, impaired, 436–439

Social interaction skills

anxiety and, 23

defensive coping and, 92

impaired social interaction and, 437

risk for loneliness and, 259

social isolation and, 442

Social involvement

diversional activity deficit and, 128

impaired social interaction and, 438

risk for loneliness and, 259

Social isolation, 440–443

Socialization enhancement

risk for loneliness and, 260

social isolation and, 442

Social support

altered health maintenance and, 190

altered parenting and, 328

risk for loneliness and, 259

social isolation and, 442

Sorrow, chronic, 443–446

Spinal surgery, 564–565

Spiritual distress, 446–449

Spiritual distress, risk for, 450–451

Spiritual support

potential for enhanced spiritual well-being and, 453

spiritual distress and, 448

Spiritual well-being

energy field disturbance and, 136

potential for enhanced and, 452

risk for spiritual distress and, 450

spiritual distress and, 447, 448

See also Well-being

Spiritual well-being, potential for enhanced, 451–453

Spontaneous ventilation, inability to sustain, 453–457

Substance abuse, 574–576

Substance addiction consequences, 458

Substance use treatment, 146

Suffocation, risk for, 457–459

Suicide, 576

Suicide self-restraint, 518

Support system enhancement
   altered health maintenance and, 191
   post-trauma syndrome and, 352
Suppression of preterm labor, 584
Surgical conditions
   abdominal surgery, 555–556
   breast surgery, 557
   chest surgery, 557–558
   craniotomy, 558–560
   ear surgery, 560
   eye surgery, 560–561
   musculoskeletal surgery, 561–562
   neck surgery, 562–564
   rectal surgery, 564
   skin graft, 564
   spinal surgery, 564–565
   urologic surgery, 565–566
   vascular surgery, 566–567
Surgical precautions, 361
Surgical recovery, delayed, 460–463
Surveillance, delayed surgical recovery and, 461
Surveillance, safety
   altered protection and, 361
   risk for poisoning and, 348
   sensory/perceptual alterations and, 411
Swallowing, impaired, 463–468
Swallowing therapy, 466
Symptom control behavior
   effective therapeutic regimen management and, 267
   ineffective airway clearance and, 16
   ineffective denial and, 112
   noncompliance and, 290

T
Teaching
   disease process, 252
   individual, 252
   infant care, 252, 319
   preoperative, 252
   prescribed activity/exercise, 252
   prescribed diet, 252
   prescribed medication, 252
   procedure/treatment, 252
   psychomotor skill, 252, 494
   safe sex, 252
   sexuality, 252
   See also Counseling
Temperature regulation: intraoperative
   hyperthermia and, 204
   hypothermia and, 207
   risk for altered body temperature and, 36
Temperature regulation
   hyperthermia and, 204
   hypothermia and, 207

   risk for altered body temperature and, 36
Therapeutic touch, 136
Thermoregulation: neonate
   disorganized infant behavior and, 228
   hyperthermia and, 203
   hypothermia and, 206
   potential for enhanced organized infant behavior and, 234
Thermoregulation
   disorganized infant behavior and, 228, 229
   hyperthermia and, 203
   hypothermia and, 206, 207
   ineffective, **468–469**
   potential for enhanced organized infant behavior and, 234
   risk for disorganized infant behavior and, 232
Thought processes, altered, 469–474
Tissue integrity: skin and mucous membranes
   altered oral mucous membrane and, 308
   impaired skin integrity and, 420, 421
   impaired tissue integrity and, 475
   peripheral altered tissue perfusion and, 490
Tissue integrity, impaired, 474–475
Tissue perfusion: peripheral
   altered tissue perfusion and, 478, 479, 490
   peripheral neurovascular dysfunction and, 341
   risk for impaired skin integrity and, 425
   risk for perioperative positioning injury and, 338
Tissue perfusion
   abdominal organs, 54
   altered (peripheral), **488–492**
   altered (specify: cardio pulmonary, cerebral, gastrointestinal, and renal), **476–488**
   cardiac, 478
Tonsillectomy, 610
Transfer ability, impaired, 492–496
Transfer performance
   impaired physical mobility and, 280
   impaired transfer ability and, 494
   impaired walking and, 522
Trauma
   chest, 538
   risk for, **496–499**
Treatment behavior: illness or injury
   altered health maintenance and, 190
   diarrhea and, 121
   impaired adjustment and, 13

ineffective airway clearance and, 16
ineffective therapeutic regimen
management and, 271
noncompliance and, 290
Tube care: umbilical line, 238

U
Ulcers, 543
Unfolding mystery, 452
Unilateral neglect, 499–502
Unilateral neglect management, 501
Urinary catheterization, intermittent,
216
Urinary continence
altered urinary elimination and, 503
functional urinary incontinence
and, 212, 213
reflex urinary incontinence and, 216
stress urinary incontinence and, 219
total urinary incontinence and, 221
urinary incontinence, urge and, 223
urinary retention and, 505
Urinary elimination
altered, **502–504**
altered tissue perfusion and, 479
altered urinary elimination and, 503
functional urinary continence and,
212
reflex urinary continence and, 216
stress urinary continence and, 219
total urinary incontinence and, 221
urinary incontinence, urge and, 223
Urinary elimination management
altered urinary elimination and, 503
delayed surgical recovery and, 461
Urinary habit training
functional urinary incontinence
and, 213
reflex urinary incontinence and, 216
urinary incontinence, urge and, 224
Urinary incontinence care
functional urinary incontinence
and, 213
stress urinary incontinence and, 219
total urinary incontinence and, 221
urinary incontinence, urge and, 224
Urinary retention, 504–506
Urinary retention care, 505
Urologic disorders, 554
Urologic surgery, 565–566

Uterine bleeding, 585

V
Vascular disease, 554–555
Vascular surgery, 566
Ventilation assistance, 455
**Ventilatory weaning response, dys-
functional (DVWR), 507–512**
**Violence: directed at others, risk for,
513–517**
**Violence: self-directed, risk for,
517–520**
Visitation facilitation, 260
Vital signs monitoring
hyperthermia and, 204
hypothermia and, 207
risk for altered body temperature
and, 36
Vital signs status
altered tissue perfusion and, 478
decreased cardiac output and, 54
DVWR and, 509
inability to sustain spontaneous
ventilation and, 454
ineffective breathing pattern and, 50

W
Walking, impaired, 520–524
Weight gain assistance, 295
Weight management
risk for more than body requirements altered nutrition and, 305
sensory/perceptual alterations and,
411
Weight reduction assistance, 301
Well-being
potential for enhanced spiritual, 452
sleep pattern disturbance and, 434
social isolation and, 442
See also Spiritual well-being
Withdrawn patient, 577
Wound care
delayed surgical recovery and, 461
impaired skin integrity and, 421
impaired tissue integrity and, 475
Wound healing: primary intention
impaired skin integrity and, 420, 421
impaired tissue integrity and, 475
Wound healing: secondary intention,
475